Quality Management for Radiographic Imaging

NOTICE

Medicine is an ever-changing science. As new research and clinical experience broaden our knowledge, changes in treatment and drug therapy are required. The authors and the publisher of this work have checked with sources believed to be reliable in their efforts to provide information that is complete and generally in accord with the standards accepted at the time of publication. However, in view of the possibility of human error or changes in medical sciences, neither the authors nor the publisher nor any other party who has been involved in the preparation or publication of this work warrants that the information contained herein is in every respect accurate or complete, and they disclaim all responsibility for any errors or omissions or for the results obtained from use of the information contained in this work. Readers are encouraged to confirm the information contained herein with other sources. For example and in particular, readers are advised to check the product information sheet included in the package of each drug they plan to administer to be certain that the information contained in this work is accurate and that changes have not been made in the recommended dose or in the contraindications for administration. This recommendation is of particular importance in connection with new or infrequently used drugs.

Quality Management for Radiographic Imaging

A Guide for Technologists

Andrea Trigg Stevens, MS, RT(R)(QM)

Quality Assurance Coordinator, Department of Radiology
Medical Center of Central Georgia
Macon, Georgia

McGraw-Hill
MEDICAL PUBLISHING DIVISION

New York   St. Louis   San Francisco   Auckland   Bogotá   Caracas   Lisbon   London
Mexico City   Milan   Montreal   New Delhi   San Juan   Singapore   Sydney   Tokyo   Toronto

McGraw-Hill

*A Division of The **McGraw·Hill** Companies*

**Quality Management for Radiographic Imaging:
A Guide for Technologists**

1 2 3 4 5 6 7 8 9 0   KGP/KGP   0 9 8 7 6 5 4 3 2 1 0

ISBN 0-8385-8249-4

This book was set in Caledonia by Rainbow Graphics, LLC.
The editors were Sally J. Barhydt and Mary E. Bele.
The interior designer was Robert Freese.
The production supervisor was Richard C. Ruzycka.
Quebecor Printing Kingsport was the printer and binder.

This book is printed on acid-free paper.

Library of Congress Cataloging-in-Publication Data

Stevens, Andrea Trigg.
    Quality management for radiographic imaging: a guide for technologists / Andrea Trigg Stevens.
       p.   cm.
    Includes bibliographical references and index.
    ISBN 0-8385-8249-4
    1. Radiography, Medical—Quality control.   I. Title.
RC78.S775 2000
616.07'572—dc21

                                                        00-055042

Dedication

This book is dedicated to:

My brother, John, who made my career possible in 1966,
My father who taught me that hard work is a worthwhile endeavor,
My husband, Frank, whose love and understanding
    made writing this book so much easier,
and David Cordova, teacher, mentor, and friend.

A special dedication to the educators of the profession:
"A teacher affects eternity: he can never tell where his influence stops."

Henry Brooks Adams

Contents

5
Fluoroscopic Systems   243

Introduction • The X-ray Tube and Image Intensifier • Fluoroscopic Quality Control Tests • Chapter Review

6
Quality Management in Mammographic Services   275

Quality Management in Mammography • Tools for Quality Management • The Darkroom • Automatic Processors • Accessory Devices • The Tube and Collimator • The Generator • Automatic Exposure Control • Half Value Layer • Compression • Chapter Review

Preface

In 1996, after several years of development, the American Registry of Radiologic Technologists announced the introduction of the advanced level certification examination for quality management. While studying for this exam, I became aware that there were few books available that comprehensively addressed the subjects of quality management, quality assurance, and quality control for medical imaging.

This book is intended to be an introductory level text geared to the needs of radiography students, radiographers, as well as people directly involved in the quality assurance process, and managers of medical imaging departments. Although the purpose of this book is to fill the void that currently exists, the book is not a "cookbook" for quality control, but a guide for those who need to know more about the quality management process.

Each chapter is devoted to some aspect of the quality management process. Chapter 1 covers the concepts of quality management, performance improvement, and image quality improvement. Chapter 2 covers the tools that are used in the quality management process. Chapters 3 through 6 are devoted to the quality control processes that pertain to the darkroom, radiographic room, fluoroscopic room, and mammography. Each chapter ends with discussion questions that may be used by an instructor to stimulate classroom activity. In addition, the chapter reviews and a practice examination at the end of the book may be used to study for the Registry's advanced level quality management examination and the advanced level mammography examination. Advanced imaging modalities like computed tomography, magnetic resonance imaging, medical sonography, digital imaging, and nuclear medicine are not covered in the text because they are not covered at the present time on the quality management examination; these topics are therefore beyond the scope of this text. The acceptance parameters for each quality control test protocol are based on the requirements of the Code of Federal Regulations and Mammography Quality Standards Act or the recommendations of the National Council on Radiation Protection and Measurements.

As you read this text you may become aware that there is redundancy in several of the quality control protocols. This is intentional; it provides the technologist with a variety of test protocols and basic information that deal with the theory and operation of the energized equipment. As discussed, each chapter is designed for easy access by the technologist, allowing for quick referral to specific protocols. For instance, if you are interested in only mammography and mammography QC protocols, you need to refer only to Chapter 6.

I sincerely hope that the reader will find this a valuable reference tool for the practice of quality management, thereby improving the quality of services provided by these critical healthcare professionals.

Andrea Trigg Stevens, MS, RT(R)(QM)

Acknowledgments

Four years ago when I started writing *Quality Management for Radiographic Imaging*, I naively thought that the book would be done in a very short time and that I would not need any assistance in seeing this text come to fruition. There have been many people along the way who have contributed to making this book possible, and I am deeply appreciative of their assistance. This assistance has come from many parts of this country.

In the last 4 years I have had two really wonderful and understanding editors—Kim Davies at Appleton & Lange and Sally Barhydt at McGraw-Hill. I am especially indebted to both editors for their support and faith in me to see the book come about.

I wish to thank all of the following individuals for their support and assistance: Charles Kircher and Michael Hayes at General Electric; Robert Meisch, Steve Proper, Dale Appleton, and Dewy Colbaugh at Marconi Medical Systems; Steve Wilson, John Fink, Stephen Pflanz, and Linda Boouchard at Eastman Kodak; A. J. Lee at Agfa; Phil Chambliss, Michael Biddy, and Thomas Ruckdeschel at Phoenix Technology in Atlanta, Georgia; William Remien at GAMMEX/RMI; and Martin Ratner at Nuclear Associates.

I want to thank Debbie Biddle, RT(R) at Portland Community College for her encouragement and support in the early stages of writing this book. A special thanks goes to Travis Ragins, RT(R) at Central Georgia Diagnostics in Macon, Georgia, Michael Mandich, RT(R) at Samaritan Medical Center in Watertown, New York, and Richard Powers, RT(R) at Massena Hospital in Massena, New York. They provided me with ideas, equipment, and resource materials for writing the book.

At the Medical Center of Central Georgia, many of my colleagues gave their time to proofread sections of the book. They also allowed me to use them as a sounding board for some of my ideas. I would like to thank Ronnie Harris, MD, Darcell Thaxton, MT(ASCP), Sandy Sumner, RT(R)(M), Melaine Kirkland-Engel, RT(R)(M), Janice Sheppard, RT(R), and Jennifer Pittard, RT(R)(M) of Focal Pointe Women.

Students have had a very special part in making this possible, and I want to thank the 1997 and 1999 graduating radiology classes at North Country Community College and at the Medical Center of Central Georgia for their assistance in Beta testing the manuscript.

I am deeply indebted and appreciative of the time and assistance that Patricia Dunaway, RT(R)(M)(QM), Carol Collings, MD, and Paula Huffmaster willingly gave to help me with completing this book.

Finally, this book would never have been possible if it had not been for my husband Frank. He gave up evenings and weekends to read my manuscript and make suggestions for improvement.

Foreword

In recent years, there has been increasing emphasis on fiscal control in medical imaging and government-mandated procedures to ensure quality outcomes. For this reason, the student and seasoned radiographer alike have a need for a concise text on quality management and quality control that permits accessibility to these increasingly important issues. This text will serve as a reference in the classroom or clinical setting.

The author has had many years of experience as a staff technologist, educator, clinical coordinator, and quality management coordinator for a large medical facility. Each of these positions has reinforced her belief that the need for quality in every form is an essential ingredient in good imaging.

Quality Management for Radiographic Imaging: A Guide for Technologists is a comprehensive guide to the current regulations that impact Radiology Quality Management Programs today. It successfully incorporates the quality assessment tests into a very readable text. It is well organized with many useful tables and charts. Furthermore, step-by-step directions have been provided for many of the quality control tests. Chapter 6, which is devoted to mammography (probably the most regulated field in radiology), provides excellent coverage of the quality control requirements mandated by the Mammography Quality Standard Act. The text is an accurate reference for all aspects of radiologic quality management.

This text is destined to become an important part of quality management teaching programs as well as a valuable addition to the thinking technologist's reference library.

Carol Collings, MD
Patricia Dunaway, RT(R)(M)(QM)

Quality Management for Radiographic Imaging

1

Introduction to Quality Management

KEY WORDS

American College of Radiology (ACR)
Bureau of Radiological Health (BRH)
Cost analysis
Customer service
Deming approach
Image quality improvement
Juran approach
Mammographic Quality Standards Act (MQSA)
Performance improvement

Quality management (QM)
Radiographic quality assurance (QA)
Radiographic quality audit
Radiographic quality control
Radiologist quality assurance (QA)
Repeat analysis
Timeliness of service
Total quality management (TQM)
Turn around time (TAT)

GOALS

1. To develop an understanding of the quality management process.
2. To learn about the benefits of a quality management program.
3. To appreciate the impact of quality management on image quality.
4. To understand the relationship that exists between quality management and image quality.
5. To develop an understanding of need for quality management in diagnostic radiology.

OBJECTIVES

1. Describe the historical development of total quality management and quality control.
2. Discuss Deming's 14 points and apply them to medical imaging.
3. State the purpose of a quality management program.
4. Identify the members of the quality management committee.
5. Differentiate between performance improvement and image quality improvement.
6. Discuss the purpose of performance improvement.
7. Identify and discuss the opportunities that exist for performance improvement.
8. Differentiate between external and internal customers.
9. Compare and contrast the three levels of customer service.
10. Discuss the ramifications of customer service as it applies to customer satisfaction.
11. Discuss the impact that timeliness of service has on medical imaging.
12. Discuss the importance of radiologist quality assurance (QA), suboptimal film tracking, and medical imaging audits.
13. State the purpose of image quality improvement.
14. Discuss the rationale for implementing an image QA program.
15. Compare and contrast radiographic QA and radiographic quality control.
16. Explain the differences between levels of equipment testing.
17. Discuss the need for a radiographic QA program.

INTRODUCTION

Medical imaging departments are complex and offer a variety of customer services that are constantly changing to meet the needs of the patients and physicians they serve. In a typical medical imaging department, the services offered include diagnostic imaging, CT, MRI, ultrasound, nuclear medicine, and vascular imaging. To determine the efficacy of the medical imaging department, it has been necessary to create a position to monitor the variety of services offered. As medical imaging departments become more attuned to the greater demands of the twenty-first century, it will be necessary to create a **quality management (QM)** program that has two specific goals: performance improvement and image quality improvement. To have an effective QM pro-gram within a medical imaging program, it is necessary to identify a dedicated individual to oversee the program. The individual selected will be responsible for overseeing both aspects of the QM program. To adequately discuss QM, performance improvement, and image quality improvement it will be essential to discuss the historical perspective for quality assurance (QA) and quality control (QC) and provide the reader with definitions of current terminology.

HISTORICAL PERSPECTIVE OF QUALITY ASSURANCE IN MEDICAL IMAGING

To understand QA and its influence on radiology it will be necessary to briefly discuss the concepts of QC and **total quality management (TQM)** from the perspective of industry, health care, and government action. A timeline (Fig. 1-1) has been provided to assist the reader in following the development of QA and QC.

Late 1930s—Introduction of the Control Chart by Bell Laboratories

Late 1940s/early 1950s—Quality management principles developed in post-war Japan

1968 Radiation Health and Safety Act

1974 Bureau of Radiological Health begins regulation of medical and dental x-ray equipment

1978 Quality assurance and quality control guidelines for radiographic equipment become available

Early 1980s—Total quality management (TQM) introduced to American industry

1981 Consumer Radiation Health and Safety Act

Late 1980s—TQM Principles incorporated by the JCAHO into the Agenda of Change

1991 Safe Medical Devices Act

1992 Mammographic Quality Standards Act

1999 Final MQSA guidelines take effect

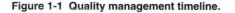

Figure 1-1 Quality management timeline.

The concept of QC originated at the Bell Laboratories in the late 1930s with the development and introduction of the control chart. The concepts of total QC and TQM were used effectively by General Douglas MacArthur in the rebuilding of the Japanese industrial base. The introduction of quality control as a management tool in the late 1940s and early 1950s came about through the efforts of Drs. W. Edwards Deming and J. M. Juran. The **Deming approach** to the use of QC as a management tool can be summarized in his 14 points in Fig. 1-2. The

1. **Create constancy of purpose toward improvement of product and service, with the aim to become competitive and to stay in business.**

2. **Adopt a new philosophy.**

3. **Cease dependence on mass inspection to achieve quality. Build quality into the product in the first place.**

4. **End the practice of awarding business on the basis of price alone. Instead, minimize total cost. Move toward a single supplier for any one item, based on a long-term relationship built on loyalty and trust.**

5. **Improve constantly and forever the system of production and service, to improve quality and productivity and thus constantly reduce costs.**

6. **Institute training on the job.**

7. **Institute leadership to help people do the job better.**

8. **Drive out fear so that everyone can work effectively for the good of the organization.**

9. **Break down barriers between departments.**

10. **Eliminate slogans, exhortations, and targets for the work force.**

11. **Eliminate work standards (quotas). Substitute leadership.**

12. **Eliminate merit rating systems.**

13. **Institute a vigorous program of education and self-improvement.**

14. **Involve everyone in the organization in the transformation to total quality improvement.**

Figure 1-2 Deming's 14 points applied to radiology. (From Adams HG, Arora S. *Total Quality in Radiology: A Guide to Implementation.* Delray Beach, FL, St. Lucie Press; 1994).

Juran approach to QC as a management tool used a trilogy of quality factors that addressed quality planning, QC, and quality improvement. The concepts developed by Deming and Juran were not introduced into the United States until the 1980s when they were successfully used by American industry. The underlying premises that TQM is based on are outlined in Fig. 1-3. In the late 1980s the Joint Commission on Accreditation of Healthcare Organizations (JCAHO) implemented the concepts of TQM into their Agenda of Change with the intent of improving quality of patient care and outcomes.

In 1968, the federal government enacted the Radiation Health and Safety Act, which mandated that the U.S. Department of Health, Education, and Welfare (which became the Department of Health and Human Services) establish and administer standards for a radiation control program. Maintaining the program became the responsibility of the **Bureau of Radiological Health** (**BRH,** which became the National Center for Devices and Radiological Health). In 1974, the BRH established regulations that were designed to reduce the amount of useless radiation being produced by medical and dental x-ray equipment. In 1978, QA and QC guidelines became available for the

---

♦ **Due to their intimate knowledge of job conditions, those workers closest to the problem are more likely to know what is wrong with a process and how to fix it.**

♦ **Every person in the organization wants to be a valuable contributor and wants to do a good job.**

♦ **Such contributions provide the employee a sense of ownership and reduce adversarial relationships between workers and management.**

♦ **Processes, not people, are the root of quality problems. The system is the cause of the problem 85% of the time; the cause is personnel 15% of the time (the 85/15 rule).**

♦ **A structured problem solving process using statistical means produces better long-term solutions than an unstructured process.**

♦ **Quality improvement is everyone's job because all processes can be improved; in healthcare, all processes are interrelated by one common factor: the patient.**

♦ **Practicing in an environment of fear is counterproductive and leads to poor performance in the long run.**

♦ **80% of the problems are the result of 20% of the causes (the 80/20 rule).**

Figure 1-3 Premises for TQM. (From Adams HG, Arora S. *Total Quality in Radiology: A Guide to Implementation.* Delray Beach, FL, St. Lucie Press; 1994).

first time. The JCAHO and most state public health agencies subsequently adopted the guidelines. The Consumer Patient Radiation Health and Safety Act of 1981 mandated the implementation of programs to reduce repeat exposures and unnecessary radiation exposure to patients, minimum standards for radiography training programs, and certification of operators of medical x-ray equipment. The Safe Medical Devices Act of 1991 simply states that all medical facilities are required to report to the Food and Drug Administration (FDA) within 10 days any medical devices that have caused serious injury or death to an employee, patient, or visitor to the medical facility. The **Mammographic Quality Standards Act (MQSA)** of 1992 requires the establishment of QA programs for all facilities performing mammographic procedures and that these facilities be approved and certified by the **American College of Radiology (ACR).** In the last quarter of 1998, MQSA underwent final revision and the final changes went into effect in April 1999.

QUALITY MANAGEMENT IN MEDICAL IMAGING

The quality management goal for the medical imaging department is to provide the highest quality of service to the customer. **Quality management** requires the dedication and commitment of management, radiologists, technical staff, and support staff. For this to occur it will take teamwork by all parties involved to reach the end result. The end result of the QM program in the medical imaging department is the reduction of radiation exposure to both the patient and staff, the reduction of costs, improvement of medical imaging services, and the improvement of diagnoses.

For this to occur it will be necessary to form a QM committee to oversee the major components of the program. The program should have two major components, one dedicated to performance improvement and the other dedicated to image quality improvement (Fig. 1-4). Both components are interrelated and equally important to the QM program of the medical imaging program. Failure of either one or both of the components will have a negative impact in the daily operations of the medical imaging department.

QUALITY MANAGEMENT COMMITTEE

The committee that oversees quality issues within the medical imaging department is often called the QA committee, the continuous quality improvement committee, performance improvement committee, or the QM committee. For the purposes of this text, "QM committee" will be used. The purpose of the QM committee is to establish criteria for performance improvement and im-

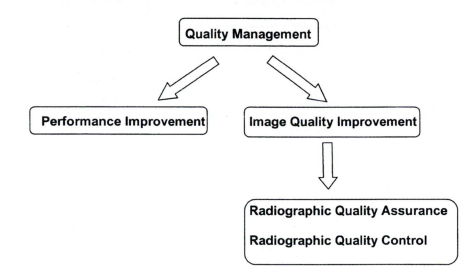

Figure 1-4 Quality management scheme.

age quality improvement. Once the criteria have been established, it is their responsibility to ensure that the criteria are met. The QM committee should include a radiologist, senior management, a representative from each of the imaging areas, and the QA coordinator for the medical imaging department.

PERFORMANCE IMPROVEMENT

Performance improvement focuses on those aspects of departmental operations that directly pertain to improving the standard of patient care and outcomes. Within the medical imaging department there are ample opportunities for obtaining data that are used in improving the overall efficiency of the department. There are a variety of activities that can be monitored for performance improvement purposes (Fig. 1-5). All of the topics discussed in this section are interrelated because they have either a direct or indirect effect on the standard of patient care. Some of these are customer satisfaction (patient and physician), employee satisfaction, timeliness of service, repeat rates, cost analysis, exam tracking, radiologist QA, suboptimal film reports, and medical imaging audits.

When discussing performance improvement, the most difficult task encountered is the retrieval of data for analysis. Data retrieval or capture may be achieved through manual or automatic acquisition. The manual acquisition of data is a labor-intensive process, and is highly inefficient. The most efficient way to obtain data for analysis is automatic acquisition by means of a radiology information system (RIS) that has data capture programs built into the system.

1. Customer Satisfaction (Patient)	26. Frequency of Film Check-out
2. Customer Satisfaction (Physician)	27. Retrieval Time for Film Jackets
3. Employee Satisfaction	28. Filing Time for Film Jackets
4. Cost Analysis	29. Delinquency Rate for Film Check-out
5. Repeat/Reject Rates	30. Duplicate Film Jackets
6. Timeliness of Service	31. Lost or Misfiled Film Jackets
7. Radiologist Quality Assurance	
8. Exam Scheduling (Availability of Examination Time)	
9. Exams Ordered but Not Performed	
10. Exams Completed but Not Interpreted	
11. Exam Demographics	
12. Crash Cart Inventory	
13. Room Inventory	
14. CPT Coding Accuracy	
15. Contrast Media Reactions	
16. I.V. Infiltration Rate	
17. Suboptimal Film Reports	
18. Report Availability	
19. Exam Repeat Rate	
20. Cost per Exam	
21. Refrigerator Temperature Checks	
22. Invasive Procedure Review	
23. Radiology/Pathology Report Correlation	
24. Radiology/Ultrasound Report Correlation	
25. Radiographic Quality Audits	

Figure 1-5 Areas for performance improvement monitoring.

Data analysis may be achieved by using commercially available statistical analysis packages or computer software that includes a database and spreadsheet (e.g., Microsoft Office).

Customers in General

A customer is an individual who uses the services of a provider. In the healthcare setting there are two distinct types of customers that are encountered—external customers and internal customers. External customers are from the outside and use the services of the hospital and medical imaging department. This particular type of customer would generally be outpatients, physicians, and other referring agencies. Internal customers are typically those individuals who are from within the facility and use the services of the medical facility. House staff, nursing staff, inpatients, personnel from the medical imaging department, and other hospital personnel would be considered internal customers.

Whether or not customers are external or internal in origin, it is important for the medical imaging department to measure the satisfaction level that those customers have with the services offered.

Levels of Customer Service

When discussing the customer, it is important to keep in mind that there are three levels of **customer service**—minimal, average, and high. When a patient receives a minimal level of service, he/she hopes to obtain the correct examination and courtesy from the staff and the ordering physician hopes to obtain a report within 7 days of the procedure. Patients receiving an average level of service are given the correct examination, it is performed in a reasonable amount of time, and the ordering physician receives a written report within 3 to 5 days. The highest level of customer service involves all personnel in the Medical Imaging Department treating the patient at all levels of the radiology visit with courtesy and respect, promptly performing the procedure, and if necessary explaining why the examination was delayed. Included in this is providing the ordering physician with a preliminary phone call upon completion of the procedure, plus a written report within 24 to 48 hours.

The highest level of customer service has three components and is best described in the customer service/expectation loop (Fig. 1-6). The first component of the service/expectation loop includes the expectations of the patient, physician, institution, and Medical Imaging Department, plus the service provided by the staff of the Medical Imaging Department. The physician, institution, department, staff, and individuals providing the specific service meet all of patient's expectations. The referring physician's expectations are met when he/she can schedule the desired procedure promptly. Institutional expectations maybe summarized as providing the highest quality of service for the lowest price. The expectation of the Medical Imaging Department is to provide the patient with prompt and expedient service with minimal expenditure

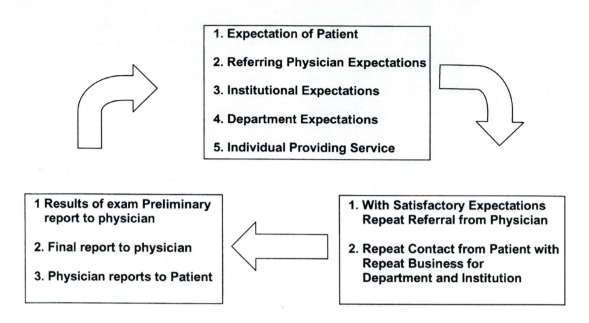

1. Expectation of Patient

2. Referring Physician Expectations

3. Institutional Expectations

4. Department Expectations

5. Individual Providing Service

1 Results of exam Preliminary report to physician

2. Final report to physician

3. Physician reports to Patient

1. With Satisfactory Expectations Repeat Referral from Physician

2. Repeat Contact from Patient with Repeat Business for Department and Institution

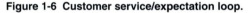

Figure 1-6 Customer service/expectation loop.

of resources. The most important component of the service/expectation loop are those individuals who are providing the service to the patient. This includes the receptionist, the radiographer, and the radiologist. The cornerstone of this component is making the patient feel that they are the most important person in the world and that there is no one else that matters.

The second component of the service/expectation loop is a result of satisfactory completion of the first component. When patient and physician expectations are satisfactorily met, there will be repeat business from the patient and the referring physician will refer additional patients to the hospital and Medical Imaging Department.

The final component of the service/expectation loop is how reports are handled when the patient's examination is completed. As part of customer service, it is important that the radiologist take the time to call the referring physician with a preliminary report. It is the responsibility of the Medical Imaging Department to ensure that the referring physician receives the final report within 24 to 48 hours of the patient's examination. Upon receiving the report, the physician has the obligation to notify the patient of the results.

Customer Satisfaction Surveys

There are essentially three types of customers that are surveyed in the Medical Imaging Department: inpatients, outpatients, and physicians. As a general rule, the majority of medical facilities conduct a survey of all patients that are dismissed from the facility. This section will discuss the customer service surveys that are directed toward outpatients and physicians. The outpatient receives the survey form upon arriving at the department or upon completion of the examination. The physician generally receives the survey through the mail. The development of a survey instrument for both outpatients and physicians is an evolutionary process that will often take several generations before a final version is achieved that measures the desired parameters. In developing a survey instrument it is very important to have questions that are well thought out and clearly stated. There are two schools of thought regarding survey development. The first school of thought maintains that the questions asked should have only two answer options which are either yes and no or agree and disagree (Figs. 1-7 and 1-8). This type of format does not provide the customer with any latitude when answering the survey questions. It locks them into one of two answers when they feel that another answer would be better. The second school of thought maintains that using a survey instrument with a multiple answer format provides the customer with a variety of options when answering questions (Figs. 1-9 and 1-10). This type of format provides better insight into the overall satisfaction of the customer.

Another important issue that needs to be considered when doing customer satisfaction surveys is the frequency of the survey, the sample size, and when the customer receives the survey. Surveys that involve outpatients should be done 1 week out of each month and should have a minimum sample size of 100. The survey instrument used for outpatients should be handed to the patient upon completion of the procedure. This will provide the best possible results. Generally when the survey is handed to a customer upon arrival in the department they will usually fill the survey out before having the examination. Physician surveys should be mailed to 20% of the physicians with privileges semiannually.

Employee Satisfaction

An important indicator of the internal health of the hospital and Medical Imaging Department is employee satisfaction. Employees should be surveyed on either a semiannual or annual basis. If the results of the employee satisfaction survey demonstrate that the employees are unhappy, then the administration of the hospital and Medical Imaging Department need to determine what the problems are and fix them. Dissatisfied employees have an enormous affect on the quality and type of service provided to the customer.

Timeliness of Service

"Time is money and money is time" is an old adage that is very true in the current atmosphere of increased demand on services and managed health care. It is very important that all personnel in the Medical Imaging Department be-

Radiology Survey

<u>Your Opinion Counts</u>

Will you take a few moments to share your thoughts with us?

Test(s) performed during your visit:

_____ X-ray   _____ Mammogram   _____ Nuclear medicine

_____ CAT scan   _____ Other

What other departments did you visit today? _____

How long did you wait to be registered at Outpatient Registration? (Circle one of the following)

No wait   Less than   Less than   Longer than   Don't know
          15 mins.   30 mins.   30 mins.

Approximate Waiting Time For Procedure (Circle one of the following):

No wait   Less than   Less than   Longer than   Don't know
          15 mins.   30 mins.   30 mins.

	YES	NO
1. Was the receptionist courteous?	____	____
2. Did the receptionist answer your questions?	____	____
3. Was the receptionist neat in appearance?	____	____
4. Was the waiting room clean?	____	____
5. Was the technologist courteous?	____	____
6. Did the technologist answer your questions?	____	____
7. Was the technologist organized?	____	____
8. Did the technologist make you feel comfortable?	____	____
9. Was your procedure(s) clearly explained?	____	____
10 Was your procedure(s) performed in a timely fashion?	____	____
11. When your procedure(s) were completed were you promptly released?	____	____
12. Was the technologist neat in appearance?	____	____
13. Was the x-ray room clean?	____	____
14. Were the rest rooms clean?	____	____

Please grade us on our services (check one): ☐ Outstanding   ☐ Good   ☐ Fair   ☐ Poor

Thank you for completing this survey.
Any suggestions may be placed on the back of the survey.

Figure 1-7 Sample outpatient customer service survey.

Department of Radiology

June 1, 1997

Dear Doctor,

The Radiology department strives to provide quality services to you and our mutual patients. As a frequent referrer to the Radiology department, your opinions regarding our level of service are very important to us.

Please take a moment to answer the following questions to help us serve you better. Any suggestions you wish to offer outside the questions asked would be appreciated. Please fax your completed survey to the Technical Director for Radiology or mail it in the enclosed envelope.

1. Are you able to schedule procedures in a timely manner?   Yes   No

    Comments:

2. Do you feel you always get the earliest appointment available?   Yes   No

    Comments:

3. Are certain procedures harder to schedule than others?   Yes   No

    Please name specific procedures.

4. Are receptionists in Radiology helpful and friendly?   Yes   No

    Comments:

5. If you view your films, do they meet your quality expectations?   Yes   No

    Comments:

6. Does report turn around time meet your expectations?   Yes   No

    If not, what is acceptable to you?

7. Do the hours the radiologist are available meet your needs?   Yes   No

    Comments:

8. What do you perceive is the greatest opportunity for improvement regarding Radiology Services at the hospital?

Figure 1-8 Sample physician customer service survey.

Radiology Survey

Directions: We are constantly striving to improve the service that we offer our customers. Please take the time to complete the following survey

1. How long did you wait in the radiology department for the start of your examination? (Circle one of the following):

   a. 1 – 10 minutes   b. 11 – 20 minutes   c. 21 – 30 minutes   d. > 30 minutes

	Poor	Fair	Good	Very Good	Excellent	NA
2. How would you rate the following qualities of the reception staff?						
a. Caring	___	___	___	___	___	___
b. Courtesy	___	___	___	___	___	___
c. Professional appearance	___	___	___	___	___	___
3. How would you rate the following qualities of the technical staff?						
a. Caring	___	___	___	___	___	___
b. Courtesy	___	___	___	___	___	___
c. Professional	___	___	___	___	___	___
4. How would you rate the following aspects of your exam?						
a. Instructions given to you by the technologist	___	___	___	___	___	___
b. Time in room until your exam began	___	___	___	___	___	___
c. Organization of the technologist	___	___	___	___	___	___
d. Procedure performed promptly	___	___	___	___	___	___
e. Prompt release following procedure	___	___	___	___	___	___
f. Courtesy of the radiologist	___	___	___	___	___	___
g. The ability of the radiologist to answer your questions	___	___	___	___	___	___
5. How would you rate the following features of the radiology department?						
a. Cleanliness of the waiting room	___	___	___	___	___	___
b. Comfort of the waiting room	___	___	___	___	___	___
c. Cleanliness of the x-ray room	___	___	___	___	___	___
d. Cleanliness of the restrooms	___	___	___	___	___	___
e. Privacy of the dressing room	___	___	___	___	___	___
6. How would you rate your visit today?	___	___	___	___	___	___
7. How would you rate us on the service provided today?	___	___	___	___	___	___
8. How would you compare today's exam with previous exams?	___	___	___	___	___	___

Thank you for completing this survey.
Any comments may be placed on the back of the survey.

Figure 1-9 Sample outpatient customer service survey with multiple option answers.

Department of Radiology

The Radiology department strives to provide quality services to you and our mutual patients. As a frequent referrer to the Radiology department, your opinions regarding our level of service are very important to us.

Please take a moment to answer the following questions to help us serve you better. Any suggestions you wish to offer outside the questikns asked would be appreciated. Please fax your completed survey to the Quality Assurance Coordinator for Radiology or mail it in the enclosed envelope.

1. How long do you wait at the customer service counter in the Radiology department to receive your films?

   a. 1 – 10 minutes   b. 11 – 20 minutes   c. 21 – 30 minutes   d. > 30 minutes

2. How long do you wait to receive your radiology reports?

   a. < 24 hours   b. 24 hours   c. 24 – 36 hours   d. 36 – 48 hours   e. > 48 hours

	Poor	Fair	Good	Very Good	Excellent	NA
3. How would you rate the following qualities of the file room staff?						
a. Caring	___	___	___	___	___	___
b. Courtesy	___	___	___	___	___	___
c. Professional appearance	___	___	___	___	___	___
4. How would you rate the following qualities of the technical staff?						
a. Caring	___	___	___	___	___	___
b. Courtesy	___	___	___	___	___	___
c. Professional	___	___	___	___	___	___
5. How would you rate the following features of radiology department?						
a. Report turn-around-time	___	___	___	___	___	___
b. Availability of appointment times	___	___	___	___	___	___
c. Customer service desk	___	___	___	___	___	___
d. Film quality	___	___	___	___	___	___
e. Availability of the radiologists	___	___	___	___	___	___
6. How would you rate the following features of the radiology department?						
a. Cleanliness of the waiting room	___	___	___	___	___	___
b. Comfort of the waiting room	___	___	___	___	___	___
c. Cleanliness of the x-ray room	___	___	___	___	___	___
d. Cleanliness of the restrooms	___	___	___	___	___	___
e. Privacy of the dressing room	___	___	___	___	___	___
7. How would you rate us on the services that we provide?	___	___	___	___	___	___

8. What do you perceive is the greatest opportunity for improvement regarding Radiology Services at the hospital?

Thank you for completing this survey.
Any comments may be placed on the back of the survey.

Figure 1-10 Sample physician customer service survey with multiple option answers.

come aware that time is a commodity that is important to both the patient and healthcare practitioner. **Timeliness of service** is an integral part of the Medical Imaging Department and studies that measure the timeliness of service can identify areas in service delivery that need to be improved. It is important that timeliness of service be measured for all imaging modalities used in the Medical Imaging Department. Timeliness of service generally covers the time of the patient's arrival in the department to the time they are released. However, a timeliness of service study should also include the time that the report is dictated and when the report goes to the referring physician. The components of timeliness of service are found in Fig. 1-11.

As part of the performance improvement program at a large medical cen-

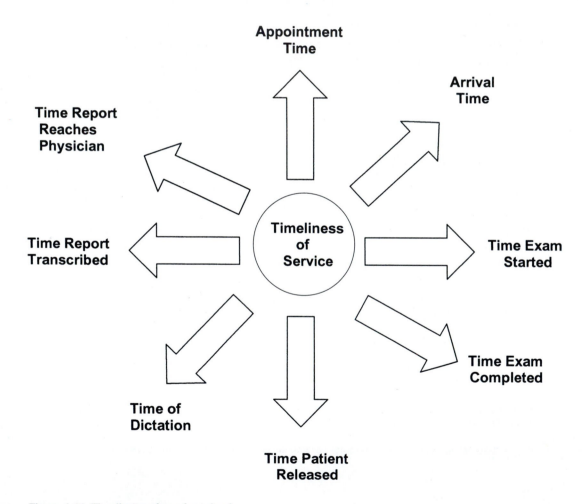

Figure 1-11 Timeliness of service wheel.

ter in the Southeastern part of the United States, they are tracking the **turn around times (TATs)** for stat portables ordered in the Neonatal Intensive Care Unit, IVPs, GI fluoroscopic examinations, and CT scans ordered from the Emergency Center. The TAT for stat portables is based on the time the examination is ordered to the time it is completed. The TAT for GI studies looks at arrival to release time, arrival to examination start time, and examination start to complete time. The TAT studies for CT scans from the Emergency Center look at verbal order time to arrival time, verbal order time to release time, and arrival time to release time. By analyzing the TATs for CT scans, management discovered that there was a serious problem with the delivery of service with respect to the time that the CT scan is ordered and the time that the patient arrives in the Medical Imaging Department. The explanation for the delay in service may be the result of several independent problems that are occurring between the two departments. The next step is to determine what is happening and develop an action plan to correct the problem.

As part of timeliness of service studies management is planning to incorporate time of dictation into their time studies. This will provide valuable data and information about how their department is functioning from a time management perspective.

Repeat Analysis

An analysis of the repeat rates is a critical component of the Medical Imaging Department's performance improvement and radiographic quality programs. The procedure for conducting a **repeat analysis** will be discussed in greater detail in Chap. 3. An increase in the repeat rate indicates that there is a major problem. The timeliness of service that the Medical Imaging Department provides is being affected and becomes a performance improvement issue. An increased repeat rate will also result in increased cost and a loss in productive manpower hours for the Medical Imaging Department.

There are two types of repeat analyses that may be performed within the imaging department. The first method involves determining the number of films repeated and the number of films rejected by anatomic area. The second method is a causal repeat rate, which determines the percentage of repeats for a specific cause. The data for this type of analysis can be obtained from the first method. Both methods provide a valuable insight into the overall operation of the Medical Imaging Department and are related to the subject of cost analysis.

Cost Analysis

Cost analysis is a budgetary means of determining the cost of services within the Medical Imaging Department. This mechanism can be used in a variety of ways to determine the financial health of the department and to pinpoint areas of waste. One such area would be the repeat rate. An increased repeat rate is an indication that film expenditure is high and timeliness of service is reduced. A reduction in timeliness of service means that the patient has to wait and there is a decrease in staff productivity. The cost per examination is another area to monitor, because it provides valuable information as to where waste is occurring.

Examination Tracking

The tracking of examinations in the Medical Imaging Department provides a unique opportunity to look at the internal operations and the type of patients that visit the department. There are several ways that examination tracking may be used to look at the internal operations of the Medical Imaging Department. One of these is TATs for all procedures or a variety of procedures, which has previously been discussed. Another is the scheduling of examinations and the availability of examination times. Examinations completed but not interpreted, examinations ordered but not performed, and examination repeat rates are other aspects of examination tracking. Each of these items provides an insight into how well the Medical Imaging Department is performing. If any or all of these items demonstrate an increase, then there is a delay in service, which translates into a reduced standard of care.

Another aspect of examination tracking is the use of examination demographics, which provide important information regarding the client base for the Medical Imaging Department. Looking at age, sex, marital status, race, socioeconomic information, and medical history affords the Imaging Department the opportunity to provide the highest level of care as the client base changes.

Radiologist Quality Assurance

Radiologist quality assurance (QA) can occur in a variety of ways, including double reading of films, correlation of radiology and ultrasound reports, correlation of radiology and pathology reports, and a monthly radiology morbidity and mortality conference. As a result of MQSA, radiologists are now required to double read mammograms. Double reading is a process by which a second radiologist reviews the same set of films previously read by another radiologist. This process was implemented to increase diagnostic sensitivity for breast cancer and studies in general have not demonstrated a significant increase in call back rate. This type of QA should be extended to include the other imaging modalities that are used in the Medical Imaging Department. The double reading of films other than mammograms should be done on a monthly basis with a different radiologist designated to read the films. The films that are to be read should be randomly pulled from the previous month (i.e., films to be read in May come from April, etc.). The number of films to be read should be approximately 5% of the total examinations performed or 30 cases, whichever is largest. The results of the double reading should be recorded on a form designed for radiologist QA (Fig. 1-12).

RADIOLOGIST QA

QA REF # _____

Radiology/Physician QA

Aspect of care: Performance improvement/peer review

Indicator: **Cross-readings**

Threshold: 100% agreement with original dictation

Radiologist: _____   Date of review: _____

Note to transcriptionist: Please send this QA form/request and typed report to the QA office.

Patient name: _____   DOB _____

Patient MR# _____

Exam/exams: _____

Pertinent HX: _____

Comparison films pulled: Yes _____   No _____

Review by QA radiologist

Were readings in agreement?   Yes _____   No _____

Peer review determination:

_____ 1. Not a variance   _____ 4. Marginal deviation from S.O.C.

_____ 2. Predictable/acceptable, within S.O.C.   _____ 5. Significant deviation from S.O.C.

_____ 3. Unpredictable, within S.O.C.

Comments:_____

_____

Signature of QA Radiologist: _____   Date: _____

Original Radiologist: _____

Figure 1-12 Radiologists QA form.

Another aspect of radiologist QA is the correlation of radiology reports between different imaging modalities, such as interventional radiology and ultrasound. As an example, the correlation of carotid arteriogram findings to Doppler ultrasound findings might be done. This type of correlation could also be carried out to include the pathology findings. The correlation of reports and pathology could be extended to several areas of the hospital. Arthrogram findings could be correlated with MRI findings and then compared to the findings of the orthopedic surgeon.

A monthly morbidity and mortality conference for the radiologists is a method to ensure the best possible care for the patient. At this type of conference films are pulled that have pathology that was missed. These conferences should have three significant outcomes. (1) They should assist the radiologists in sharpening their interpretive skills in all of the diagnostic imaging modalities. (2) They show what the most commonly missed lesions are within the Medical Imaging Department. (3) They make the radiologists aware that they are human and that they do make mistakes.

Suboptimal Film Tracking

Along with the repeat film analysis, tracking the number of suboptimal films being passed is an important component of the performance improvement program. Like the repeat film analysis, it is a mechanism for identifying and assisting radiographers who are having problems with primarily positioning and technique.

When monitoring suboptimal films, it is important to statistically track the suboptimal films by area, technologist, facility, and cause. Once this has been completed, a plan of action and a documentation process must be developed. However, the simplest way to reduce the number of suboptimal films is to station someone in the processing area to check films as they drop from the processor. If that is not possible, the action plan to reduce the number of suboptimal films being reported by the radiologist and the documentation process should be implemented. This method is not designed to instill fear into the radiographers but to enhance awareness of a problem that should be addressed. The way to address the problem is through education and a better understanding of what the problem is.

Due to the high volume of suboptimal film reports, one large Medical Center where the author worked was forced to develop an action plan (Fig. 1-13) and a documentation form (Fig. 1-14A and B). As a result of this action they are seeing a decrease in the number of suboptimal films being passed by the technologists. At this point in time, they have implemented the documentation form at the urgent care facilities that are part of their system. The image action form has provided them a method of opening a line of communications between technologists and facilities.

Medical Imaging Audits

Audits of a Medical Imaging Department provide an important insight into the overall operations of the department. Medical imaging audits should be done on a monthly basis and should include a random selection of examinations performed during the month. The QM committee should determine the number of

---

During a rotating 6 month period beginning April 1, technologists doing suboptimal work will receive an Image Quality Action form.

Technologists receiving

1. **Three Image Quality Action forms in a 6 month period will be given a verbal warning and counseling.**

2. **Four Image Quality Action forms in a 6 month period will be given a written reprimand.**

3. **Five Image Quality Action forms in a 6 month period will be given probation and/or suspension.**

4. **Six Image Quality Action forms in a 6 month period will be terminated.**

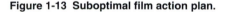

Figure 1-13 Suboptimal film action plan.

examinations to be audited, but the examinations selected for review should be randomly pulled to provide an overall impression of the department. It should be stressed that this is not a job for one person but several people. The audit team should have technical and nontechnical representation to make the audit process work. The audit should be inclusive of all imaging areas within the department. Figure 1-15 illustrates the areas that the medical imaging audit should include.

IMAGE QUALITY IMPROVEMENT

The primary purpose of image quality improvement is to maintain a standard of image quality that benefits the patient, physician, Medical Imaging Department, and the institution. **Image quality improvement** has two key components, a radiographic QA component and a radiographic QC component. Image quality improvement is a critical part of the overall QM program because of its relationship with the factors discussed in performance improvement.

Radiographic Quality Assurance

Radiographic quality assurance focuses on the improvement of image quality through a systematic program of record keeping, equipment selection and acceptance testing, imaging criteria, and continuing education. An integral part of radiographic QA is the ability to track the performance and maintenance of equipment. This can be achieved by maintaining a record on each piece of imaging equipment in the Medical Imaging Department. There are a

Diagnostic Radiology

Image Quality Action

Please return to the QA Coordinator at Box #155 within 7 days of receipt.

Technologist: _____   Number: _____

Student: _____   Number: _____

Complaint lodged by: _____

Facility: _____

Patient: _____

MR#: _____

Exam: _____

Date of procedure: _____

1. Film identification   4. Wrong exam done   _____

    a. Wrong ID stamp on film   _____   5. Wrong patient done   _____

    b. No ID stamp on film   _____   6. All views not done   _____

2. Film quality   7. No evidence of collimation   _____

    a. Overexposed   _____   8. No evidence of gonadal
                                                                    shielding   _____
    b. Underexposed   _____
                                                               9. No pertinent patient history _____
    c. Poor positioning   _____
                                                               10. Film size (too large/small) _____
    d. Motion   _____
                                                               11. Processor   _____
    e. Artifacts   _____

    f. Double exposed   _____

    g. Part excluded   _____

    h. Part obscured   _____

    i. Grid cut-off   _____

    j. Other   _____

3. Film marking

    a. No right or left marker   _____

    b. Improper marking of film   _____

    c. No technologist number   _____

    d. No date and/or time on
        portable films   _____

    e. Wrong date and/or time   _____

Figure 1-14A Obverse of the image quality action form.

QA comments:

_____

_____

_____

_____

_____

_____

_____

_____

_____

_____

Date _____ _____
Signature

Technologist comments:

_____

_____

_____

_____

_____

_____

_____

_____

_____

Date _____ _____
Signature

Supervisor comments:

_____

_____

_____

_____

_____

Date _____ _____
Signature

Figure 1-14B Reverse of the image quality action form.

- ◆ **Proper exam for clinical problem**

- ◆ **Correct number of views for exam**

- ◆ **Correct film size(s) present**

- ◆ **Films identified correctly (patient information, markers, etc.)**

- ◆ **Technical quality of films (density, contrast, image sharpness, positioning)**

- ◆ **Satisfactory image quality (free of artifacts)**

- ◆ **Gonadal shielding and collimation evident on films**

- ◆ **Satisfactory exam turn around time**

- ◆ **Satisfactory exam dictation turn around time**

- ◆ **Satisfactory report turn around time**

- ◆ **Radiology report in medical record**

- ◆ **Proper billing of exam**

- ◆ **Referring physician perspective on radiology services**

- ◆ **Patient perspective on radiology services**

Figure 1-15 Areas of the medical imaging audit.

variety of ways that this could be done. The most common way is to keep a separate logbook on each piece of equipment from installation to removal. It is advisable that the record logs be kept in a central location as opposed to having the log in the room where the equipment is installed. Centralized record keeping ensures that maintenance and repair records can be readily found and reduces the chance of them being misplaced.

Historically, individuals or groups of individuals who are not directly involved in using the equipment have made equipment selection decisions. Typically these individuals have been upper level management and radiologists. The time has come for Medical Imaging Departments to begin accepting input into equipment selection from radiographers who are directly involved in patient contact and have expertise with the equipment. Forming an equipment selection team that consists of one radiologist, one manager, one radiographer, and the person responsible for QA can solve many of the dilemmas of equipment selection. Each member of the team should have equal input into the selection of the equipment or determining equipment specifications. Failure to include radiographers' input into equipment selection can result in the purchase of equipment that has limited use and purpose. Once a piece of equipment has been selected, purchased, and installed it should undergo a formal acceptance testing process. This may be done by the company or by an independent consultant. Once the equipment has been certified as meeting the stated performance standards, it can be turned over to the facility.

Radiologists and senior management historically have dictated imaging criteria. With rapid changes occurring in the field of diagnostic medical imaging, it is time to include members of the diagnostic team in the decision loop when imaging criteria are being established. This inclusion will provide a cohesiveness and sense of purpose for the technical staff. Forming an image specifications team that consists of radiologists, management, radiographers, and the person responsible for QA can establish the desired imaging criteria for the Medical Imaging Department and the institution. The imaging criteria for a Medical Imaging Department should be reviewed annually to make appropriate changes when equipment is changed or there are significant changes in imaging related factors (i.e., film, chemistry, client base, etc.).

Continuing education has become a critical factor for all healthcare professionals. Primarily JCAHO requirements, professional certification organizations, and medical facility policies are driving the need for continuing education. Medical radiographers need to keep current with changes in the profession. The most efficient way to meet continuing education needs of the technical staff is provide an atmosphere within the Medical Imaging Department that promotes continuing education. Continuing education can be obtained in several ways. The most common are monthly in-services, participation in professional organizations, educational seminars, and directed readings. A novel way to provide continuing education is to form a journal club within the Medical Imaging Department. The journal club could meet either formally or informally. The key for success is to provide the staff with a variety of technical articles from professional journals. Once they have received the articles, have them read each article and then discuss the articles one on one or in small groups. This is a reliable technique; it is currently being used in radiology resident programs. The challenge now is for Medical Imaging Departments to implement this technique with their technical staff.

Radiographic Quality Control

Radiographic quality control focuses on the testing and monitoring of equipment in all areas of the Medical Imaging Department (Fig. 1-16). When

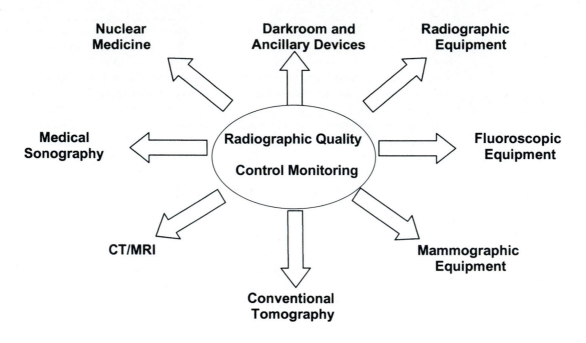

Figure 1-16 Areas for monitoring radiographic QC.

discussing equipment testing and monitoring, there are essentially two levels of testing, noninvasive and invasive. Noninvasive testing can be further divided into the areas of simple and complex testing, which can be conducted by designated technologists. Invasive testing is complex in nature and is generally done by physicists or engineers because it involves disassembly of the equipment. The routine QC tests performed in a Medical Imaging Department are listed in Figs. 1-17 and 1-18. The individual QC tests will be discussed in detail in subsequent chapters of this book.

The value of a radiographic QC program is determined by two factors—the cost of running the program and the savings that can be realized. The cost of a radiographic QC program can vary depending on the size of the institution and the institution's commitment to improving image quality. The primary cost for the QC program is in the test equipment and paying the salary of someone to run the program. The amount and type of equipment purchased will depend on the size of the Medical Imaging Department and how vigorously the department wants to pursue a monitoring and testing program. Figures 1-19, 1-20, and 1-21 demonstrate the cost for QC equipment based on the size of the Medical Imaging Department. The actual equipment costs for the QC program will vary from a few thousand dollars up to approximately $25,000. The higher the cost, the more elaborate and sophisticated the QC program will be.

Darkroom and Ancillary Areas

Automatic processors **   Film screen contact **
Safelights **   Screen blacklight **
Darkroom cleanliness **   Laser printers
Illuminator uniformity **   Repeat/reject analysis

Radiographic Equipment *

Exposure time   Exposure repeatability
SID   mAs reciprocity
Light field/beam alignment   kVp
Beam perpendicularity   mR/mAs output
Bucky/light field alignment   AEC
Bucky/beam alignment   Grids
Focal spot size

Fluoroscopic Equipment *

Fluoroscopic image size   Low contrast fluoroscopic test
Fluoroscopic beam limitation   Beam perpendicularity
Fluoroscopic exposure rate   Focal spot size
Standard fluoroscopic levels   ABC
Fluoroscopic resolution

Mammographic Equipment

Screen cleanliness   Uniformity of screen speed
Phantom images   Focal spot size
Beam quality assessment   Average glandular dose
Fixer retention analysis   Light field illumination
Compression   Radiation output
Collimation   AEC
kVp accuracy and reproducibility Breast entrance exposure
System resolution   Grids

Conventional Tomography

Slice level
Slice thickness
Resolution
Blur
Pinhole trace

* Includes both mobile radiographic and mobile fluoroscopic equipment.

** Includes mammography.

Figure 1-17 Routine QC tests for imaging equipment.

Computed Tomography

- CT number calibration
- Light field accuracy
- CT number standard deviation
- Slice width
- High contrast resolution
- Bed indexing
- Low contrast resolution
- Bed backlash
- Accuracy of distance measuring device
- CT number versus algorithm
- CT number flatness
- CT number versus slice width
- Accuracy of localization device
- Noise characteristics
- CT number versus patient position
- Radiation scatter and leakage
- CT number versus patient size
- kVp waveform

Magnetic Resonance Imaging

- Noise characteristics
- Linearity
- Uniformity
- Sensitivity profile
- Spatial resolution
- Slice contiguity
- Contrast resolution

Medical Sonography

- Sensitivity of system
- Image uniformity
- Accuracy of distance measurement
- Vertical and horizontal distance measurement
- Axial spatial resolution
- Lateral resolution

Nuclear Medicine

- Energy resolution and photopeaking
- Counting rate limits
- Field uniformity
- Spatial resolution
- Spatial linearity sensitivity
- Multiple window spatial registration

Figure 1-18 Routine QC tests for advanced imaging modalities.

Test Equipment	Average Cost
Sensitometer	$800
Densitometer	$800
Digital thermometer	$200
Screen contact wire mesh	$130
Collimator template	$150
Beam alignment tool	$200
Stepwedge penetrometer	$120
Digital light meter	$350
Total	**$2750**

Figure 1-19 Test equipment for small facilities without mammography, CT, and MRI.

Test Equipment	Average Cost
Sensitometer	$800
Densitometer	$800
Digital thermometer	$200
Screen contact wire mesh	$130
Blacklight	$200
Collimator template	$150
Beam alignment tool	$200
Digital kVp meter	$2000
Digital mAs meter	$450
Direct reading R-meter	$2000
Digital generator timer	$700
Tomography phantom	$200
2° star test pattern and stand (focal spot)	$610
Grid alignment tool	$150
Fluoroscopic beam alignment	$125
Fluoroscopic resolution	$225
Mammography phantom	$550
Mammography scales	$20
Mammography screen contact wire mesh	$140
Mammography slit camera and stand	$2500
Photometer	$1200
CT phantom	$2000
Total	**$15340**

Figure 1-20 Test equipment for medium-sized facilities with mammography and CT.

Test Equipment	Average Cost
Sensitometer	$800
Densitometer	$800
Digital thermometer	$200
Screen contact wire mesh	$130
Blacklight	$200
Comprehensive noninvasive x-ray test Device for mammography, fluoroscopy, and radiography	$6700
Remote ionization chambers	$4500
Collimator template	$150
Beam alignment tool	$200
Tomography phantom	$200
2° star test pattern and stand (focal spot)	$610
Grid alignment tool	$150
Fluoroscopic beam alignment	$125
Fluoroscopic resolution	$225
Mammography phantom	$550
Mammography slit camera and stand	$2500
Photometer	$1200
CT phantom	$2000
MRI phantom	$2000
DSA phantom	$2000
	Total $25240

Figure 1-21 Test equipment for large facilities with all imaging modalities.

The bottom line for a radiographic QC program is the savings that can be realized over the long term. The savings are both tangible and intangible. Tangible savings are primarily film and processing chemistry. Film and chemistry savings can be achieved through radiographic QC by monitoring the repeat rate and all of the automatic film processors in the Medical Imaging Department on a regular basis. Intangible savings are primarily equipment downtime, lost manpower time, and the amount of time that a patient has to wait for a particular procedure. Equipment downtime, lost manpower time due to equipment failure, and lost patient time due to the first two can be greatly reduced when all equipment in the Medical Imaging Department is routinely monitored in a radiographic quality control program.

CHAPTER REVIEW

- Historically QA began in the 1930s with the development of the control chart by Bell Laboratories. In the reconstruction of Japan after World War II, Drs. Deming and Juran introduce quality control as a management tool in the rebuilding of Japan's economy. In the 1980s, the principles developed by Deming and Juran were successfully reintroduced to American industry as TQM. In the late 1980s, the JCAHO implemented the principles of TQM as part of their Agenda for Change. Beginning in 1968 through a variety of acts enacted by Congress, the Federal government began regulating the use of ionizing radiation in health care. All of the legislation gave birth to present day radiographic quality control in medical imaging departments.
- The primary objective of QM in the Medical Imaging Department is to provide the customer the highest quality of service. Reducing costs, improving diagnosis, improvement of imaging services, and reducing radiation exposure to the patient and staff are the end results of a medical imaging quality management program.
- The QM committee is composed of representatives of management, radiologists, each imaging area, and the QA coordinator. The purpose of the QM committee is to make sure that the established criteria for performance improvement, image quality, and radiographic quality control are met.
- The purpose of performance improvement is to monitor those areas of departmental operation that directly affect the standard of patient care and patient outcomes.
- Customers to the Medical Imaging Department may be either external or internal in origin. Typical customers include patients, physicians, and hospital personnel. It is important to remember that any person who uses the services of the hospital and Medical Imaging Department is considered to be a customer.
- There are three levels of customer service. They are minimal, average, and high. A minimal level of service revolves around the concept of receiving the correct examination and the physician receiving a report within 7 days. An average level of service occurs when the correct examination is performed in a reasonable amount of time and the physician receives a report within 5 days. The highest level of customer service has components, described as a customer/service loop, where the outcome is that the customers at all levels receive the highest level of service possible.
- Customer satisfaction surveys should be designed to measure specific items or attributes that have been determined by the Medical Imaging Department. Surveys should provide the customer with a variety of answering options. Both internal and external customers should be surveyed on a regular basis. The information obtained should be used to improve service of the Medical Imaging Department.

- Employee satisfaction is a barometer for the Medical Imaging Department and is a mechanism for determining performance improvement opportunities. Monitoring the satisfaction of medical imaging personnel can provide valuable information to management about the overall health of the department. Employee satisfaction should be measured semiannually. Failure to act on employee dissatisfaction can lead to a decrease in productivity, which in turn can affect customer service.
- A critical component in the successful operation of a Medical Imaging Department is timeliness of service. An increase in the amount of time it takes to perform a procedure results in increased patient dissatisfaction and a decrease in the customer service approval rating.
- There are two ways that repeat film analysis may be done. They are the examination method and the causal method. The repeat analysis is a valuable tool for identifying areas where the technical staff are having problems.
- Cost analysis is a budgetary mechanism used to analyze the cost of services within the Medical Imaging Department. Cost analysis is an important mechanism that assists in determining the financial health of the department and pinpoints areas of waste.
- Examination tracking provides an opportunity to look at internal operations, types of examinations ordered, types of patients, TATs, cost of examinations, examination scheduling, availability of appointment times, and patient demographics. Data obtained from examination tracking can be used to improve customer service and meet customer needs.
- Quality assurance for the radiologist is a mechanism for maintaining accountability and the highest standard of patient care. The four most common methods of radiologist QA are double reading of examinations, correlation of radiology reports with the results of other imaging modalities, correlation of reports with pathology results, and monthly morbidity and mortality conferences.
- Tracking the number of suboptimal film reports is another mechanism that can provide useful information about the technical operations of the Medical Imaging Department. When tracking suboptimal film reports, it is important to have an action plan and documentation process in place to assist in data collection and education.
- The use of medical imaging audits is a way to look at the overall operations of the department and the quality of service being provided to the customer.
- The primary goal of image quality improvement is to maintain imaging standards that benefit the patient, physician, Medical Imaging Department, and institution. Imaging standards are maintained through radiographic QA and QC.
- The goal of radiographic QA is to ensure imaging standards by maintaining a systematic program of record keeping, equipment selection, imaging criteria, and continuing education.

- Radiographic QC is responsible for the testing and monitoring of all imaging equipment in the Medical Imaging Department. Depending on the size of the department test equipment will cost approximately $2,500 to $30,000. The savings realized by a QC program outweigh the investment cost.

DISCUSSION QUESTIONS

1. Discuss the historical development of total quality management.
2. How are Deming's 14 points applied in medical imaging?
3. What is quality management?
4. What is the purpose of the quality management committee?
5. What is performance improvement?
6. How are performance improvement and image quality related? How are they different?
7. What are the levels of customer service?
8. What are the differences in the levels of customer service?
9. When developing a customer service survey, what format should be used?
10. How does employee satisfaction impact performance improvement and image quality?
11. How does timeliness of service impact customer service?
12. Why are repeat analysis and cost analysis important?
13. Explain how examination tracking impacts the Medical Imaging Department.
14. Explain the importance of radiologist QA.
15. How does suboptimal film tracking impact the Medical Imaging Department?
16. What are medical imaging audits and how are they used?
17. What are the two components of image quality improvement?
18. What are the four major components of radiographic quality assurance? Why are they important?
19. How does radiographic quality assurance impact customer service?
20. What are the major components of radiographic quality control? Why are they important?
21. How does radiographic quality assurance impact customer service?

REVIEW QUESTIONS

1. Which of the following statements is correct?
   a. Quality management deals with performance improvement.
   b. Quality management deals with image quality improvement.
   c. Quality management deals with quality assurance and quality control.

d. Quality management deals with performance improvement and image quality improvement.

2. Quality control as a management tool was introduced in post-war Japan by:
    a. Dr. Deming
    b. Dr. Juran
    c. both a and b
    d. neither a nor b

3. What organization had the responsibility to establish and administer standards for a radiation control program?
    a. BRH
    b. HEW (HHS)
    c. NCRP
    d. NRC

4. Which of the following did the 1981 Consumer Patient Radiation Health and Safety Act do?
        1. Reduce repeat exposure
        2. Reduce unnecessary exposure to patients
        3. Minimum training standards for radiography programs
        4. Certification of operators
    a. 1 and 3 only
    b. 2 and 4 only
    c. 1, 2, and 3 only
    d. 1, 2, 3, and 4

5. Which of the following are components of Dr. Juran's approach to quality control as a management tool?
        1. Quality planning
        2. Quality control
        3. Quality improvement
        4. Quality systems
    a. 1 and 2 only
    b. 1 and 3 only
    c. 1, 2, and 3 only
    d. 1, 2, 3, and 4

6. The MQSA Act became final in
    a. April 1992
    b. April 1994
    c. April 1997
    d. April 1999

7. Dr. Deming's approach to quality control as management tool can be summarized in his
    a. 3 points
    b. 7 points
    c. 10 points
    d. 14 points

8. Which of the following statements would be correct about the 85/15 rule?
   a. Personnel are the cause of the problem 85% of the time and the system is the cause of the problem 15% of the time.
   b. The system is the cause of the problem 85% of the time and personnel is the cause of the problem 15% of the time.
   c. The system and personnel are the cause of the problem 85% of the time and other causes are the cause of the problem 15% of the time.
   d. Other causes are the cause of the problem 85% of the time and the system and personnel are the cause of the problem 15% of the time.
9. Which of the following statements is correct?
   a. Quality management focuses on those aspects of departmental operations that directly pertain to improving the standard of patient care and outcomes.
   b. Image quality improvement focuses on those aspects of departmental operations that directly pertain to improving the standard of patient care and outcomes.
   c. Performance improvement focuses on those aspects of departmental operations that directly pertain to improving the standard of patient care and outcomes.
   d. None of the above
10. Which of the following statements is correct?
    a. The primary purpose of QM is to maintain a standard of image quality that benefits the patient, physician, Medical Imaging Department, and institution.
    b. The primary purpose of image quality improvement is to maintain a standard of image quality that benefits the patient, physician, Medical Imaging Department, and institution.
    c. The primary purpose of performance improvement is to maintain a standard of image quality that benefits the patient, physician, Medical Imaging Department, and institution.
    d. None of the above
11. Customers that come from outside the hospital are generally referred to as
    a. external customers
    b. internal customers
    c. both a and b
    d. neither a nor b
12. Customers that come from inside the hospital are generally referred to as
    a. external customers
    b. internal customers
    c. both a and b
    d. neither a nor b
13. Which of the following are considered internal customers?
    1. Nurses
    2. House staff

    3. Inpatients

    4. Personnel from other departments

  a. 1 and 2 only

  b. 2 and 3 only

  c. 1, 2, and 3 only

  d. 1, 2, 3, and 4

14. Which of the following are considered external customers?

    1. Nurses

    2. Referring physicians

    3. Inpatients

    4. Outpatients

  a. 1 and 2 only

  b. 1 and 3 only

  c. 2 and 3 only

  d. 2 and 4 only

15. Which of the following are forms of peer review?

    1. Suboptimal film tracking

    2. Radiologist QA

    3. Medical imaging audits

  a. 1 and 2 only

  b. 1 and 3 only

  c. 2 and 3 only

  d. 1, 2, and 3

16. How many levels of customer service are there?

  a. 1

  b. 2

  c. 3

  d. 4

17. Which of the following statements are correct about the 80/20 rule?

  a. Twenty percent of the causes result in 80% of the problems.

  b. Twenty percent of the problems are the result of 80% of the causes.

  c. Both a and b

  d. Neither a nor b

18. Equipment testing and monitoring involves

  a. one level of testing and monitoring

  b. two levels of testing and monitoring

  c. three levels of testing and monitoring

  d. four levels of testing and monitoring

19. What level of customer service would a patient get if they were to receive the correct examination and the physician were to receive a report within 3 to 5 days?

  a. An average level

  b. A high level

  c. A minimal level

  d. None of the above

20. Which of the following statements is correct?
    a. Radiographic QC focuses on the improvement of image quality through a systematic program of record keeping, equipment selection, imaging criteria, and continuing education.
    b. Image quality improvement focuses on the improvement of image quality through a systematic program of record keeping, equipment selection, imaging criteria, and continuing education.
    c. Radiographic QA focuses on the improvement of image quality through a systematic program of record keeping, equipment selection, imaging criteria, and continuing education.
    d. None of the above

21. What are the levels of equipment testing and monitoring?
    a. Invasive
    b. Noninvasive
    c. Both a and b
    d. Neither a nor b

22. Which of the following statements is correct?
    a. Radiographic QC focuses on testing and monitoring of equipment in all areas of the Medical Imaging Department.
    b. Radiographic QA focuses on testing and monitoring of equipment in all areas of the Medical Imaging Department.
    c. Image quality improvement focuses on testing and monitoring of equipment in all areas of the Medical Imaging Department.
    d. None of the above

23. Which of the following is a way of looking at the overall operations of the Medical Imaging Department and the quality of service being provided to the customer?
    a. Cost analysis
    b. Examination tracking
    c. Medical imaging audits
    d. Timeliness of service

24. Invasive equipment testing is
    a. complex
    b. simple
    c. both a and b
    d. neither a nor b

25. Which of the following mechanisms provides the opportunity to look at the internal operations of the department?
    a. Cost analysis
    b. Examination tracking
    c. Medical imaging audits
    d. None of the above

2

Tools for Quality Management

GOALS

1. To learn about quality management (QM) tools.
2. To learn how to apply QM tools in the Medical Imaging Department.
3. To learn about performance improvement models and their use.
4. To learn about story books and storyboards.

OBJECTIVES

1. Identify the tools that are used in QM.
2. Apply the QM tools to given situations.
3. Discuss the importance of the computer in QM.
4. Identify and discuss the nonstatistical QM tools.
5. Identify and discuss the statistical tools that are used in QM.
6. Explain the measures of central tendency.
7. Identify and discuss three models for performance improvement.
8. Discussion story books and storyboards.

INTRODUCTION

Quality management (QM) is a process that involves the analysis of tremendous amounts of data. To make sense of the raw data, individuals involved in the QM process need to transform it into usable information. This can be achieved by utilizing tools that are specifically designed for the QM process. The tools used in the QM process are the computer, nonstatistical tools, statistical tools, and performance improvement models (Fig. 2-1). It is important that anyone involved in the QM process know how and when to use them.

THE COMPUTER AS A QUALITY MANAGEMENT TOOL

All the tools discussed in this chapter are critical to the QM process. However, the most important tool to be used is the computer. The computer is essential because it allows the individual to store and analyze a tremendous amount of data. The critical components of the computer are the storage capacity, speed, and type of software that is to be used.

The computer should have storage capacity of at least 1 gigabyte or higher. This amount of storage permits the storing of raw and computed data with ease. In addition it is important to have sufficient random access memory (RAM) to ensure that the computer runs efficiently when handling multiple programs or tasks.

Selecting and installing software that will provide the tools needed to adequately perform quality assurance (QA) and quality control (QC) duties is important. The type of software to be installed should include a word processing program, **database,** and spreadsheet.

- **Computer**

  - **Word processing**

  - **Spreadsheet**

  - **Data base**

- **Nonstatistical tools**

  - **Brainstorming**

  - **Surveys/questionnaires**

  - **Flow charts**

  - **Control charts**

  - **Matrices**

  - **Pareto charts**

  - **Cause-and-effect diagrams**

  - **Graphs in general**

- **Statistical tools**

  - **Measures of central tendency**

  - **Measures of spread (dispersion)**

  - **Frequency distributions**

  - **Sample size**

- **Process Improvement Models**

  - **FOCUS-PDCA**

  - **The Seven Step model**

Figure 2-1 Quality management tools.

NONSTATISTICAL TOOLS

The nonstatistical tools discussed in this chapter are the techniques and processes that are used in QM and the performance improvement process. The intent of this section is to provide the reader with a basic overview of the nonstatistical tools and examples of where they may be applied in the QM process. The nonstatistical tools discussed are brainstorming, surveys, flowcharts, control charts, matrices, Pareto charts, FOCUS-PDCA, cause-and-effect diagrams, and graphs in general. Each of these tools plays an important role in healthcare and medical imaging.

Brainstorming

Brainstorming is a technique that allows a team to efficiently generate a large volume of ideas on a wide range of topics or a specific topic. As a process, it is free of criticism and judgment. Brainstorming encourages free thought and gets the entire team involved. This technique provides each team member the opportunity to be creative and focused on the topic being discussed.

Brainstorming may be either structured or unstructured. When structured brainstorming is used, members give their ideas in turn. Unstructured brainstorming allows members to give their ideas as they come to mind. Figure 2-2 illustrates the brainstorming method.

Surveys

As discussed in Chap. 1, the survey plays an important role in the operation of the Medical Imaging Department. A **survey** is generally used to obtain information

---

◆ **Identify the group leader and recorder.**

◆ **Clarify the question under discussion.**

◆ **Establish the ground rules that will be followed by all participants.**

◆ **Provide a time frame (≤ 2 minutes) for participants to generate their own ideas.**

◆ **Establish a time frame for brainstorming and begin brainstorming.**

◆ **Record all responses so that all participants may see them.**

◆ **After brainstorming is complete, discuss and clarify the ideas.**

◆ **Streamline the list and establish a plan for followup.**

Figure 2-2 Brainstorming guide.

on how to improve the overall operation of the department. The success or failure of a survey is directly related to how well the instrument is designed. Figure 2-3 describes the process for creating a survey instrument. All of the items mentioned in Fig. 2-3 are important, but there are several key points that need to be stressed for the successful design of a survey instrument. When developing a survey instrument, it is important to determine what type of information is going to be obtained and who the target audience will be. Therefore, a survey instrument designed to obtain data regarding customer satisfaction and the delivery of healthcare would not be the same instrument used for physicians or employees. After the target audience has been determined, the next step is to design a survey instrument that is at the reading level of the target population. If the instrument is designed to survey the satisfaction of patients, then it would most likely need a reading level of the fourth or fifth grade. The simplest way to design a survey is to make the questions as easily understood as possible. This may be achieved by using language that is monosyllabic and not overwhelming. After the pilot survey

---

- ◆ **Determine the focus of the survey and who the respondent group will be.**

- ◆ **Provide directions at the beginning of the survey that are clear, simple, and brief.**

- ◆ **The survey instrument should not exceed 1 or 2 pages, and it must be complete enough to obtain the necessary feedback.**

- ◆ **It is important to state where the survey is to be returned.**

- ◆ **Anonymity of the respondents should be ensured.**

- ◆ **It is important to pilot test the survey with a sample of the respondent group. One should get feedback regarding:**

  - ▪ **The amount of time required to fill out the survey.**
  - ▪ **The clearness of the questions.**
  - ▪ **The suitability of the vocabulary.**
  - ▪ **General feedback regarding the survey instrument.**

- ◆ **Information obtained from the pilot test should be used to make revisions in the survey instrument.**

- ◆ **Perform a periodic review of the survey, the response rate, the method of distribution and the method of return.**

Figure 2-3 Designing a survey.

instrument has been used, it is very important that feedback be obtained from the target audience. The feedback should focus on the length of time required to answer the questions, question clarity, and readability. The information obtained from the feedback process should be used to improve the survey instrument.

Once the survey has been designed and finalized, it will be necessary to make the decision as to when the survey should be given to the target audience. The author feels that the survey should be given to the patient right after the examination has been completed. This is the most appropriate time; the experience is still fresh in the mind of the patient. Providing the survey to the patient any time prior to the examination provides the patient with the opportunity to answer the questions before the study has commenced.

Matrices

A **matrix** is a simple tool that is used to compare two or more variables. The variables are generally displayed in horizontal and vertical rows. In healthcare, the matrix has been modified to produce reference guides for employees seeking quick answers in emergency situations. A large medical center familiar to the author has developed two matrices that are used by the employees for emergency utilities shutdown and for abuse/neglect referral. The Medical Imaging Department at the same medical center developed a matrix for equipment service (Fig. 2-4). For large departments, the equipment service matrix provides all employees a means of obtaining equipment service.

Flowcharts

Flowcharts are used to picture or map a process from its beginning point to its end point. The process that is tracked can be anything from services to material and equipment to manpower. Flowcharts determine the sequence of

Equipment	Location	Vendor	Phone #	Serial #	Site ID#	Service Contract	P.O. Required
Advantx/Legacy R/F Unit	Room 1	General Electric	1-800-437-1171	34582VP4	812633MR1	No	Yes
Advantx/Legacy R/F Unit	Room 2	General Electric	1-800-437-1171	34620VP2	812633MR2	No	Yes
Tilt-C Digital Fluoroscopy Unit	Room 3	General Electric	1-800-437-1171	54366WK7	812633MR3	Warranty	Yes
Advantx/Legacy R/F Unit	Room 4	General Electric	1-800-437-1171	52877WK1	812633MR4	Warranty	Yes
SPX Tomographic/ Radiographic Unit	Room 5	General Electric	1-800-437-1171	194508WK8	812633MR5	No	Yes
MTX Radiographic Unit	Room 6	Picker	1-800-321-3346	509505803	71770	No	Yes
Panellipse II Panoramic Dental Unit	Panorex Room	General Electric	1-800-437-1171	200-101264	812633MRP	No	Yes

Figure 2-4 Typical equipment service matrix.

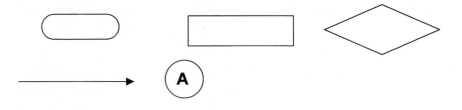

Figure 2-5 Standard flowchart symbols.

events in the process. They are able to show where there is redundancy and allow changes to be made that will simplify an existing process or procedure. When developing a flowchart or a series of flowcharts, it is important to use the universally accepted standard flowchart symbols. Essentially, there are five basic symbols that are used when developing a flowchart. The standard symbols are the oval, rectangle, diamond, arrow, and a circle with an "A" in the middle (Fig. 2-5). The oval signifies the beginning and end steps in a process. The rectangle represents a step in the process that is being described. The diamond is placed at a point in the flowchart where a decision occurs and it is generally referred to as a decision diamond or decision point. Arrows connect each symbol and represent the direction of flow. On occasion a flowchart will continue from one page to another and when that occurs it will be necessary to use circle with an "A" inside to denote continuation on the next page. It is important to remember that, when a decision point is reached, there must be "yes" and "no" alternatives given. Arrows will direct the flow in both the yes and no direction.

Developing a flowchart is a fairly easy process; however, it can be quite time consuming for those individuals who have never constructed one before. Figure 2-6 provides some guidelines for developing a flowchart. Flowcharts

---

◆ **Identify the process that will be studied.**

◆ **Determine what the beginning and end points are.**

◆ **Use the flowchart symbols in an appropriate manner with arrows to connect them.**

◆ **It is important that the flowchart demonstrate the real processes.**

◆ **The flowchart should flow from the top to the bottom of the page.**

Figure 2-6 Guidelines for developing a flowchart.

can be created by hand or computer. This author has found that computer-generated flowcharts are quite satisfactory. The flowcharts depicted later in this chapter are examples of computer-generated flowcharts. There are several flowchart software packages that are available on the market. For example, in Microsoft Office, there are flowchart symbols available in the AutoShapes portion of the drawing tools, and they work quite well for creating flowcharts.

There are two types of flowcharts that are generally used for describing a process. They are the detailed flowchart and the top-down flowchart. There are three levels of detailed flowcharts, the macro-level (Fig. 2-7), the intermediate-level (Fig. 2-8), and the micro-level (Fig. 2-9). The macro-level flowchart demonstrates the key steps in the process but does not show decision points. An intermediate-level flowchart will show all the steps in the process plus decision points. A micro-level flowchart is very detailed and will show minute items within processes.

Another way to describe a process is with a top-down flowchart. A top-down flowchart has major and minor elements. The major elements are placed in a horizontal line and the minor elements are placed under the major elements of the process. The minor elements may be subdivided into subelements of the process. Figure 2-10 describes the process for creating the top-down flowchart. The most important steps in creating a top-down flowchart are to (1) clarify the process and (2) define the beginning and ending points of the process. Failure to do this will lead to erroneous assumptions about the process. There are a variety of processes where the top-down flowchart would be useful. Essentially any process that can be described in a detailed flow can be applied to a top-down flowchart. Figure 2-11 illustrates a top-down flowchart that deals with pre-procedure wait times for outpatient myelograms.

Control Charts

Control charts are used to monitor a process over a specified time period by studying variation and its source. When used correctly, a control chart is a powerful tool that can predict how a process will behave in the future. It can also demonstrate the effect that experimental change has on the process. They may be developed from either count (i.e., repeat analysis) or measurement data (i.e., turn-around-times). Control charts have predetermined upper control limits (UCL), lower control limits (LCL), and a center line. By convention, the UCLs and LCLs are dotted lines and the center line is a solid heavy line. Control charts are used in a variety of ways throughout the hospital. An example is refrigerator temperature over time.

In medical imaging the most common type of control chart encountered is the processor control, which will be discussed in Chap. 3. The effect of turn-around-times (Fig. 2-12) and repeat rates (Fig. 2-13) in the Medical Imaging Department can also be shown using a control.

There are six basic rules used in the interpretation and analysis of control charts.

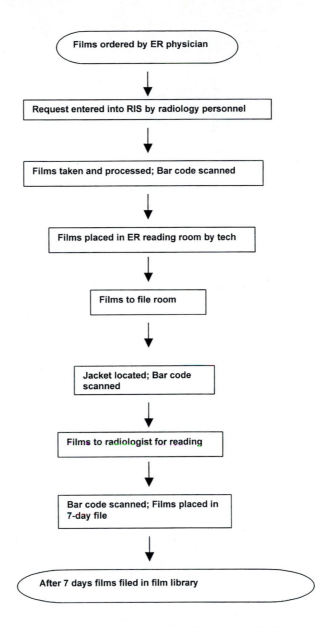

Figure 2-7 A macro-level flowchart for tracking ER films.

1. A *shift* exists when seven or more consecutive points are above or below the center line.
2. A *trend* exists when seven consecutive points all go up or all go down.
3. A single point that falls outside of the established control limits is called a *point out of control.*

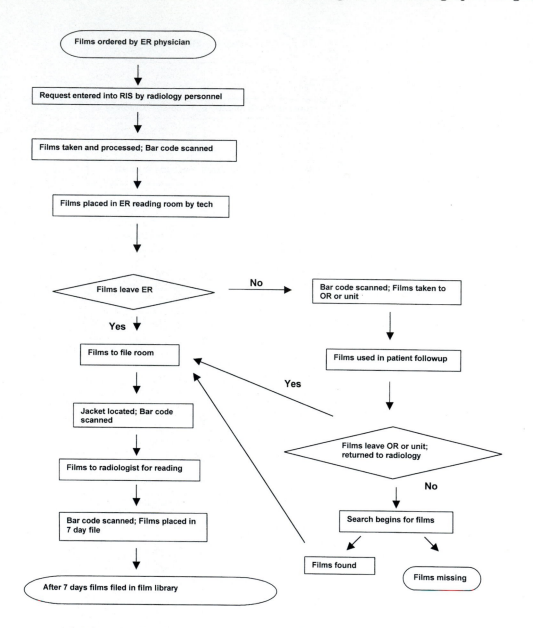

Figure 2-8 An intermediate-level flowchart for tracking ER films.

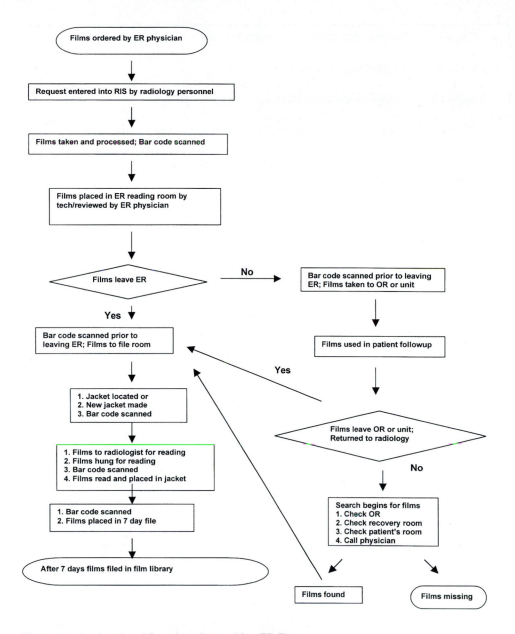

Figure 2-9 A micro-level flowchart for tracking ER films.

◆ **Clearly define the process to be considered.**

◆ **Define the beginning and ending points.**

◆ **Specify the major elements in the process.**

◆ **Across the top of the page write them in horizontal sequence.**

◆ **Below each major element, identify the minor element steps necessary to achieve it.**

Figure 2-10 Guidelines for designing a top-down flowchart.

4. The *one sigma rule* occurs when four or five consecutive points are one standard deviation on the same side of the center line.
5. The *two sigma rule* occurs when two or three consecutive points are two standard deviations on the same side of the center line.
6. *Hugging* occurs when eight or more consecutive points are within one standard deviation above or below the center line.

Run Charts (Trend Charts)

The only difference between a run chart and a control chart is the run chart does not have preset upper and lower limits. The **run chart** is used to monitor one or more processes over time to determine if there are shifts or trends. Run charts are used in a variety of ways throughout the hospital. They may be used to track patient temperature, absenteeism of employees, or other processes that need to be monitored.

In the Medical Imaging Department, run charts could be used to track the fluctuation of mAs, and mR/mAs over a specified time frame. Figure 2-14 is a run chart that illustrates the fluctuation of kVp over time.

Check Sheets

A **check sheet** is the simplest and easiest quality management tool to use. It is a quick method for documenting sample information about a process. The check sheet can be used as an ongoing monitoring tool to sample a process at random intervals for the purpose of documenting improvement or degeneration. In medical imaging a check sheet could be used in a variety of ways to measure several different processes. One process that could be measured effectively is physician satisfaction with the customer service that the film library is delivering. Another is supply availability (i.e., film). Figure 2-15 illustrates a

1. Identification of Problem → **2. Current Process** → **3. Root Causes** → **4. Solution** → **5. Evaluation**

1.1 Outpatients are waiting too long for their Myelograms.

1.2 Pre-procedure wait time approximately 2.9 hours.

2.1 Patient arrives at hospital.

2.11 Patient registers.

2.12 Patient presents at endoscopy and is prepared for myelogram.

2.13 Patient waits in endoscopy until neurosurgeon ready.

2.2 Neurosurgeon contacts Radiology when ready to perform study.

2.3 As soon as possible Radiology sends for patient and interrupts scheduled procedures in R/F rooms.

2.4 Patient transported to Radiology.

2.5 Patient is taken into room and prepped for exam by radiology staff.

2.6 Neurosurgeon is called to perform exam.

2.7 Myelogram is performed.

2.8 Patient is transported to back to endoscopy.

3.1 Neurosurgeons are performing myelograms between cases.

3.2 Radiology is performing myelograms between scheduled procedures.

4.1 Schedule myelograms.

4.11 On myelogram days, myelograms are started 30 min prior to 8 a.m.

4.12 Realign staffing schedule.

4.13 Radiology to provide staffing to operate 4 rooms on Tuesdays and Thursdays.

4.14 As a pilot study two neurosurgeons agree to participate.

4.2 Run pilot study for 6 months.

5.1 Compare pre-procedure wait times to pilot study pre-procedure wait times.

5.2 Make changes as necessary to reduce wait time.

5.3 Provide education as as needed.

Figure 2-11 Top-down flowchart for reducing pre-procedure wait time for outpatient myelograms.

51

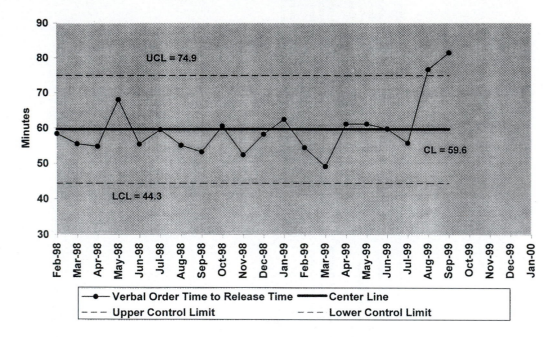

Figure 2-12 Control chart tracking the turn-around-times for ER CT scans from verbal order time to release time.

simple check sheet. Once the data have been collected, they can be pictorially displayed as either a bar chart (Fig. 2-16) or a pie chart representing the particular film size and its usage by the three shifts (Fig. 2-17).

Pareto Charts

The **Pareto chart** was developed by the nineteenth-century Italian economist Vilfredo Pareto. The Pareto chart rank orders or prioritizes some event or issue. It is a bar chart that demonstrates the event or priority being studied, ranked in descending order from left to right. In medical imaging Pareto charts may be used in a variety of ways that would help clarify an issue. Figure 2-18 illustrates the use of a Pareto chart to rank order the number of repeats by the type of radiographic examination. Figure 2-19 illustrates the use of a Pareto chart to rank order the number of waste films by cause.

Cause-and-Effect Diagrams

A **cause-and-effect diagram** is used to analyze the cause and effect of different variables on a process. In medical imaging, there are thousands of

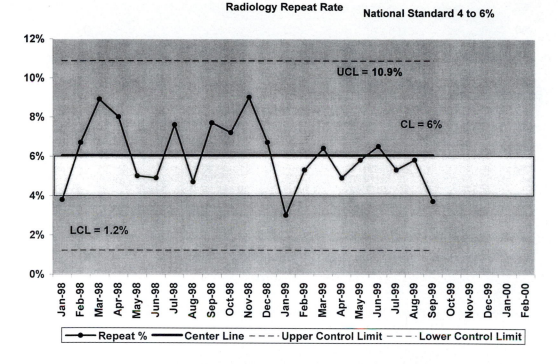

Figure 2-13 Control chart tracking the repeat rate in a Radiology Department.

processes where a cause-and-effect diagram could be used to identify areas for potential improvement. A cause-and-effect diagram could be used to discover why films are being misplaced in the film room or the reason for poor image quality (Fig. 2-20).

Scatter Plots

A **scatter plot** is an analysis tool designed to determine whether there is a relationship between two variables. It is a visual method to determine if a decrease or an increase in one variable consistently correlates with a decrease or increase in the other variable. In medical imaging, scatter plots could be used to analyze radiation intensity versus kVp or radiation intensity versus mAs (Figs. 2-21 and 2-22).

Histograms

A **histogram** is the graphic representation of a frequency distribution. It is a tool used to display data regarding the frequency of an occurrence. A histogram is an excellent tool to describe the distribution of continuous data. In the hospital and

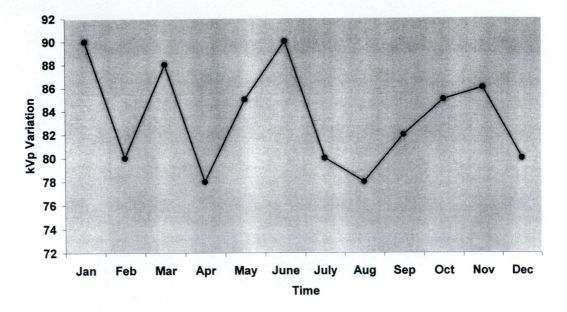

Figure 2-14 Run chart demonstrating the fluctuation of kVp over time.

Medical Imaging Department, histograms can be used to chart the frequency of absenteeism, tardiness, equipment failure, and repeats. Figure 2-23 is a histogram that demonstrates the number of repeats for a group of technologists.

Graphs in General

Graphs are a method of presenting large amounts of data in pictorial form. There are a variety of graphs that may be used to display data that have been gathered. There are bar graphs, line graphs, scatter plots, pie charts, doughnut

Film Size	7 a.m. to 3 p.m.	3 p.m. to 11 p.m.	11 p.m. to 7 a.m.
14 x 17	IIII	III	I
14 x 14	III		
11 x 14	IIII	II	I
10 x 12	IIIII	III	III
9 x 9	II		
8 x 10	IIIIII	IIII	III
7 x 17	II	I	I
5 x 12	II		

Figure 2-15 Check sheet illustrating film removed by size from film storage by shift.

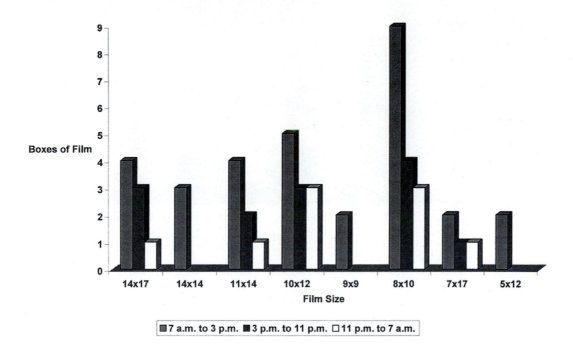

Figure 2-16 Bar chart depicting total film removed from film storage by shift.

14 x 17 Film Usage by Shift

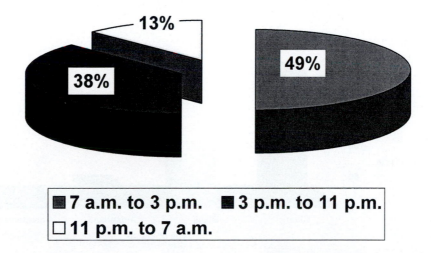

Figure 2-17 Pie chart representing 14 × 17 film usage for three shifts.

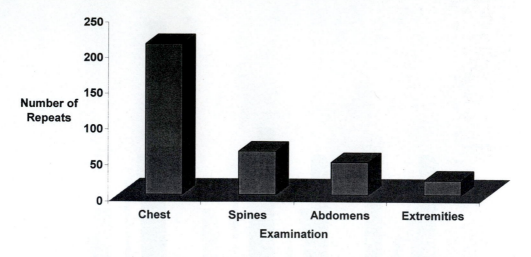

Figure 2-18 Pareto chart that demonstrates the number of repeats by the type of radiographic examination.

charts, cylinder charts, and pyramid charts. All of these graphs may be used to describe data that have been collected in the QM process. The more common graphs encountered in QM are the bar graph, pie chart, line graph, and the scatter plot. The Pareto chart and histogram are examples of bar graphs that are used in medical imaging. The line graph is an excellent tool to display turn-around-times. The pie chart fits quite well in displaying the data obtained from analyzing casual repeat rates. Graphs are an essential element of the QM process and should be used as often as possible to display the data obtained.

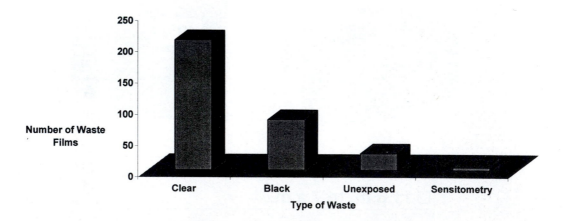
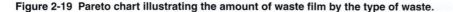

Figure 2-19 Pareto chart illustrating the amount of waste film by the type of waste.

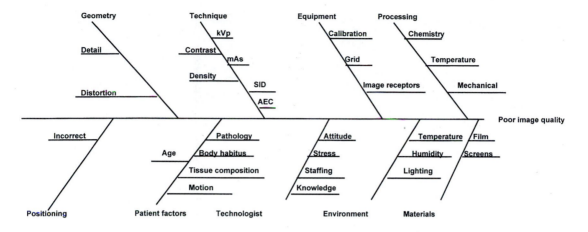

Figure 2-20 Cause-and-effect diagram demonstrating the potential causes for poor image quality.

STATISTICAL TOOLS

The statistical analysis tools that are discussed in this chapter are referred to as *descriptive statistics* because they are used to describe an event. The intent of this section is to provide the reader with a basic overview of descriptive statistics and examples of where they may be applied in the QM process. The descriptive statistics discussed here can be calculated by using a personal com-

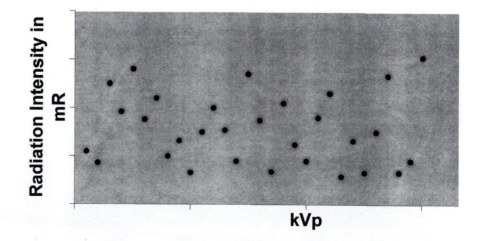

Figure 2-21 Scatter plot representing the non-linear relationship between kVp and radiation intensity.

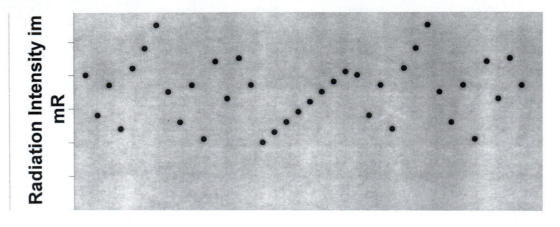

Figure 2-22 Scatter plot representing the correlation between mAs and radiation intensity in mR.

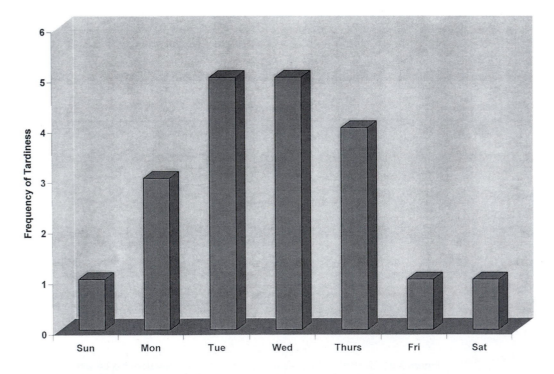

Figure 2-23 Histogram illustrating the frequency of tardiness in a 7-day period.

puter that has a commercially available statistical package or **spreadsheet,** which is the most efficient way to calculate any of the descriptive statistics discussed in this chapter. Descriptive statistics that are used in QM include measures of central tendency, percentile, standard deviation, frequency distributions (histograms), and scatter plots.

Measures of Central Tendency

A number that is used to describe or characterize a distribution of numbers is called a **measure of central tendency.** The mean, median, and mode are measures of central tendency.

- **Mean** The **mean** is the average of a group of numbers. It is the most commonly used measure of central tendency because of its stability. The mean is determined by adding the values and dividing by the number of values (Fig. 2-24). From a medical imaging perspective, the mean may be used when describing the average turn-around-times for procedures done in the Medical Imaging Department, the average number of films repeated per technologist for a group of technologists, the average cost of a procedure, or the average number of films per examination.

- **Median** When the values of a group of numbers are very large or very small, the mean may not be representative of that group and the median should be used. Before determining the median, it is important to arrange the values either from the highest to lowest or the lowest to the highest value. The **median** is the midpoint of the values after they been arranged. Figure 2-25 illustrates how the median is determined. In QM and medical imaging the median is rarely used because of it's instability.

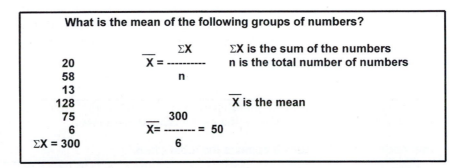

Figure 2-24 Determining the mean of a group of numbers.

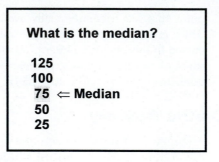

Figure 2-25 Determining the median.

- **Mode**   The mode is the most frequently observed number in a set of numbers. The mode does not require any calculation. From the medical imaging perspective, the mode has little or no application in the handling of raw data. Figure 2-26 demonstrates the determination of mode.

Measures of Spread (Dispersion)

Numbers that describe the spread around the mean are called **measures of spread** or dispersion. Typically these are range, percentile, standard deviation, and coefficient of variation.

- **Range**   The **range** is the lowest and highest number in a group of numbers. The easiest way to determine the range of a set of number is to rank order them from lowest to highest or vice versa (Fig. 2-27). Range has very little real application in medical imaging.

- **Percentile**   The **percentile** is a number or score that falls at or below a given percentage. The percentile scale is used to describe percentiles. The most commonly used percentiles are the 25th, 50th, and 75th percentiles. Percentiles are frequently used in health care to compare some specific procedure or operation of the institution with the same procedure or operation at other institutions in the same area or nationally. Percentiles can be readily used in medical imaging to compare

---

The repeat/reject rate for a 12 month period is 10%, 5.5%, 15%, 10%, 4.5%, 6%, 7%, 5%, 10%, 9%, 6.5%, and 11%. What is the modal repeat/reject rate?

The mode is 10% because it appears the most often.

Figure 2-26 Determining the mode.

What is the range of the following 4.5, 10, 8, 23, 6, and 15?

23⇐ Highest number
15
20   The range is 4.5 and 23.
 8
 6
4.5⇐ Lowest Number

Figure 2-27 Determining the range of a group of numbers.

turn-around-times of various procedures (e.g., CTs, stat portables, etc.), repeat/reject rates, radiologist QA, and potentially many other items that are done as performance improvement opportunities. The most efficient way to calculate percentile is to use the statistical analysis package that comes with the majority of spreadsheet programs that are on the market today.

- **Standard Deviation**   The range of variation around the mean is called the **standard deviation.** This is the most commonly used dispersion measure in health care. In medical imaging it is used to calculate mA repeatability, which is discussed in Chap. 4. Standard deviation is typically shown as SD or the small Greek letter sigma (σ). Standard deviation is calculated by using the following formula:

$$SD\ (\sigma) = \sqrt{\frac{\Sigma\ (X - \overline{X})^2}{N}}$$

Where X = the raw score or number, $\overline{X}$ = the mean, and N is the number of scores. Figure 2-28 illustrates how the standard deviation is calculated.

- **Coefficient of Variation**   There are times that it will be necessary to compare two or more measures of dispersion. When that time comes, a direct comparison may lead to a false conclusion. The best way to avoid this is to use the coefficient of variation. The coefficient of variation is a useful statistic because it is a relative measure of dispersion. The **coefficient of variation** (CV) is the standard deviation (σ) divided by the mean (X). The number that expresses CV is always stated as a fraction (i.e., 0.01). The coefficient of variation is expressed as the following formula:

$$CV = \frac{\sigma}{\overline{X}}$$

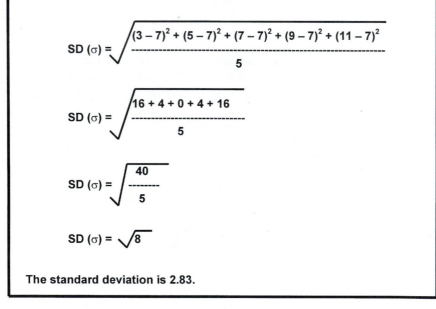

What is the standard deviation of the following group of numbers?

    3, 5, 7, 9, and 11

Step 1: Determine the mean ($\bar{X}$)

    The mean is 7.

Step 2: Calculate the standard deviation

$$SD\ (\sigma) = \sqrt{\frac{(3-7)^2 + (5-7)^2 + (7-7)^2 + (9-7)^2 + (11-7)^2}{5}}$$

$$SD\ (\sigma) = \sqrt{\frac{16 + 4 + 0 + 4 + 16}{5}}$$

$$SD\ (\sigma) = \sqrt{\frac{40}{5}}$$

$$SD\ (\sigma) = \sqrt{8}$$

The standard deviation is 2.83.

Figure 2-28 Calculating the standard deviation.

In medical imaging the coefficient of variation is used in conjunction with the mean and standard deviation when measuring reproducibility of x-ray generators. Figure 2-29 illustrates the application of the formula in medical imaging.

Frequency Distributions

A **frequency distribution** is used to describe data by how often an event or a situation occurs. The simplest way to use a frequency distribution is to group the data into categories. Frequency distributions could be used in medical imaging to determine how often a particular situation or event is oc-

What is the coefficient of variation for four exposures using a technique of 200 mA 0.5 sec and 80 kVp? The four exposures yielded mR readings of 425, 420, 423, 426.

$$CV = \frac{\sigma}{\bar{X}}$$

Step 1: Determine the mean and standard deviation.

$$\bar{X} = 423.5 \qquad SD\ (\sigma) = 2.29$$

Step 2: Calculate the coefficient of variation.

$$CV = \frac{2.29}{423.5}$$

$$CV = 0.005$$

The estimated coefficient of variation of radiation exposures shall be no greater than 0.05. The CV for this exposure is within the accepted limits.

Figure 2-29 Calculating the coefficient of variation.

curring. For instance, frequency distributions are ideally used in suboptimal film tracking, repeat analysis, causal repeat rates, duplicate film folders, and lost or misplaced film folders. Figure 2-30 shows how a frequency distribution might be used in medical imaging.

Sample Size

Sample size is determined by what is being studied. It should be adequate to obtain the required data for the problem. When the sample size is too small, the tabulated results will not be accurate. When the sample size is too large, the volume of data will be too cumbersome to calculate. It is important to select a sample size that will meet the current need. In medical imaging there are no clear-cut guidelines for selecting the size of the sample. To obtain data that are reliable it is critical that the sample be selected in a random fashion (i.e., one out of five, etc.). Randomization reduces the possibility of skewing. The ideal sample size should be be no less than 30 and no greater than 100. This range provides an adequate sampling base for almost any study that would occur in the medical imaging department.

Tech	# of Repeats/Week	Tech	# of Repeats/Week
A	0	K	5
B	2	L	2
C	1	M	3
D	2	N	4
E	4	O	1
F	3	P	1
G	2	Q	3
H	2	R	2
I	3	S	3
J	4	T	4

Figure 2-30 Frequency distribution showing the number of repeat films per week for a selected group of technologists.

PROCESS IMPROVEMENT MODELS

As a result of their Agenda of Change, the Joint Commission on Accreditation of Healthcare Organization (JCAHO) developed and implemented a 10-step monitoring and evaluation process (Fig. 2-31). This 10-step process is still in use today but the emphasis has changed from QA to **process improvement.** Current models of process improvement have evolved from the 10-step process. There are a variety of process improvement models available for use, but the author has found that the FOCUS-PDCA model and the Seven-Step model are easily adapted to any process improvement action that is needed in the Medical Imaging Department. It is important to recognize that processes are complex and any attempt to shortcut them can have major and lasting effects on the institution. It is critical that, when process improvement is undertaken, the model selected is followed without deviation.

FOCUS-PDCA Model

This model is the most commonly used process improvement model in healthcare today. It is a straight forward model with precise steps that follow a logical sequence (Fig. 2-32). There are three critical components of the **FOCUS-PDCA model.** These components are the

- team given the task to initiate the process improvement.
- selection of the problem.
- tools that are used to bring about the improvement.

- **Step 1: Assign responsibility.**

- **Step 2: Delineate the scope of care and service.**

- **Step 3: Identify important aspects of care and service.**

- **Step 4: Identify indicators.**

- **Step 5: Establish a means to trigger evaluation.**

- **Step 6: Collect and organize data.**

- **Step 7: Initiate evaluation.**

- **Step 8: Take actions to improve care and service.**

- **Step 9: Assess effectiveness of actions and maintain improvements.**

- **Step 10: Communicate results to affected individuals and groups.**

Figure 2-31 The JCAHO 10-step model.

Failure to select the right mix of personnel will impact the success of the improvement project. It is critical to select and use the correct QM tools throughout the process of improvement. Figure 2-33 identifies the QM tools that are appropriate for use with the FOCUS-PDCA model.

The Seven-Step Model

The Seven-Step model is an alternative to the FOCUS-PDCA model. It uses the same principles and tools as the other model. Figure 2-34 illustrates the major components of the Seven-Step model. Like the FOCUS-PDCA model, team selection, problem identification, and use of appropriate tools are essential for the success of the process.

Storyboards and Storybooks

Storyboards and storybooks are methods of presenting the information that is obtained from a performance improvement project. The storyboard can be various shapes and sizes. A storybook is a storyboard in book form.

Find a problem to solve or a process to improve.

- Prioritize the problem.
- Review the plan of operation.
- Identify the important process characteristics.

Organize a team that knows the process.

- Select the team.
- Identify individuals who have process experience.
- Create a plan.

Clarify current knowledge of the process.

- Familiarize team with current process.

Understand causes of process variation.

- Measure the important process characteristics.
- Identify the process variables.
- Measure potential process variables.
- Determine if there is a relationship between the process. characteristics and process variables.

Select the process improvement.

- Analyze improvement alternatives for their effectiveness and feasibility.
- Select the improvement.

Plan the implementation and continue data collection.

- Plan the implementation of the improvement.
- Plan continued data collection.

Do the improvements.

- Make the change.
- Measure the impact of the change.

Check the results.

- Analyze the data to find out whether the change has led to the anticipated improvement.

Act to hold gains and continue improvement.
- Develop and implement a strategy for maintaining the Improvements.

Figure 2-32 The FOCUS-PDCA model.

> ◆ **Brainstorming**
>
> ◆ **Data collection**
>
> ◆ **Pareto charts**
>
> ◆ **Flowcharts**
>
> ◆ **Cause-and-effect diagrams**
>
> ◆ **Histograms**
>
> ◆ **Control charts**
>
> ◆ **Run charts**
>
> ◆ **General graphs and charts**

Figure 2-33 Quality management tools that are frequently used with the FOCUS-PDCA model.

> ◆ **Step 1: Select the problem or process**
>
> ◆ **Step 2: Describe the current process**
>
> ◆ **Step 3: Identify the root causes**
>
> ◆ **Step 4: Develop a solution and action plan**
>
> ◆ **Step 5: Implement the solution or process change**
>
> ◆ **Step 6: Evaluate the result of change**
>
> ◆ **Step 7: Apply experience**

Figure 2-34 The Seven-Step model for process improvement.

CHAPTER REVIEW

- There are four categories of tools that are used in QM—the computer, nonstatistical tools, statistical tools, and performance improvement models.
- The computer is the most powerful tool that can be used in QM because of its ability to store and manipulate tremendous amounts of data. The ability of the computer to perform the necessary tasks is directly related to its processing speed and storage capabilities.
- Nonstatistical tools include brainstorming, surveys, flowcharts, control charts, run charts, check sheets, Pareto charts, cause-and-effect diagrams, scatter plots, histograms, and graphs in general.
- Statistical tools include measures of central tendency, measures of spread, frequency distributions, and sample size.
- There are a variety of process improvement models available for use in QM. The process improvement models include the 10-step JCAHO model, the FOCUS-PCDA model, and the Seven-Step model.
- Brainstorming is a method that is used to generate large volume of ideas on a wide range of topics. It may be either structured or unstructured.
- Surveys are used to collect data and improve customer service.
- Matrices are used to compare two variables. The variables are displayed in horizontal and vertical rows. Matrices used in healthcare have been modified to be quick reference guides for employees.
- Flowcharts map a process from beginning to end and use five basic symbols. There are two types of flowcharts that may be used to describe a process, the detailed flowchart and the top-down flowchart. The detailed flowchart is the most complex because it consists of three levels. The top-down flowchart places the major elements in horizontal row with minor elements under them.
- Control charts are used to monitor a process over a specified period of time. They are derived from either count or measurement data. A control chart has predetermined upper, middle, and lower limits. The two most common control charts used in a Medical Imaging Department are the refrigerator temperature chart and the processor control chart. Control charts may also be used to track and identify the effect of turn-around-times on customer service in the Medical Imaging Department.
- Run charts measure a process over a specified period of time, but they do not have predetermined upper and lower limits. In the Medical Imaging Department, run charts could be used to document the fluctuations in kVp, mA, mAs, and mR/mAs over a period of time.
- The check sheet is the easiest QM tool to use. It is a simple and fast method for documenting information about a process. In medical imaging, it could be used to obtain information regarding supply use within the imaging department.
- The Pareto chart rank orders or prioritizes events and issues. It is a bar graph that describes the event being monitored in descending order from left to right. In the Medical Imaging Department, it might be used to

illustrate the number of repeat films by the type of examination or the number of waste films to the type of waste.

- Cause-and-effect diagrams are used to analyze the cause and effect of different variables on a process.
- Scatter plots are used to determine whether or not a relationship exists between two variables.
- Histograms are the graphic representation of a frequency distribution. They are bar graphs that display the frequency of an occurrence.
- Graphs are used to describe or represent the data that have been obtained through other methods. The most common graphs used to describe data are bar graphs, pie charts, and line charts.
- Measures of central tendency include the mean, median, and mode. The most commonly used measure of central tendency is the mean. The mean is the average of a group of numbers. The mean is very stable. The median and mode are not used as frequently because they are unstable measures.
- Measures of spread (dispersion) are the range, percentile, standard deviation, and coefficient of variation. The range is the highest and lowest number in a group of numbers. The most commonly used percentiles are the 25th, 50th, and 75th. Standard deviation is the range of variation around the mean. Coefficient of variation is a relative measure of dispersion and is used to compare two or more measures of dispersion.
- Frequency distributions are used to describe data by how often an event or a situation occurs.
- Sample size is dictated by what is being studied. The ideal sample size should be no less than 30 and no greater than 100.
- Process improvement models evolved from the JCAHO 10-step monitoring and evaluation process. The most commonly used process improvement model is the FOCUS-PDCA model. Another model that is gaining acceptance is the Seven-Step process improvement model.
- Storybooks and storyboards are pictorial methods of describing a performance improvement process.

DISCUSSION QUESTIONS

1. What are the four types of QM tools?
2. Why is the computer an important QM tool?
3. What are the nonstatistical QM tools? Give an example of each.
4. What are the measures of central tendency? Give an example of their use.
5. Discuss percentile and frequency distributions.
6. Discuss standard deviation and its use.
7. Explain the importance of sample size.
8. Discuss process improvement models and their application.
9. Discuss how storybooks and storyboards are used.

REVIEW QUESTIONS

1. What is the mean of 2, 4, 6, 8, 10, and 12?
   a. 5
   b. 7
   c. 8
   d. 9
2. What is the standard deviation of 2, 4, 6, 8, 10, and 12?
   a. 11.66
   b. 6.66
   c. 3.42
   d. 2.83
3. Based on the answer obtained in question 2, what is the coefficient of variation?
   a. 0.95
   b. 0.48
   c. 0.41
   d. 0.17
4. What is the range of 33, 25, 55, 44, 66, 18, and 22?
   a. 18 and 66
   b. 25 and 66
   c. 33 and 55
   d. 25 and 44
5. What is the mode of the following data 5%, 15%, 20%, 10%, 5%, 8%, 9%, 25%, 5%, 15%, and 10%?
   a. 25%
   b. 15%
   c. 10%
   d. 5%
6. Which of the following are considered measures of central tendency?
   1. Mean
   2. Mode
   3. Median
   4. Standard deviation
   a. 1, 2, and 4 only
   b. 1, 2, and 3 only
   c. 2, 3, and 4 only
   d. 1, 2, 3, and 4
7. Which of the following are considered measures of dispersion?
   1. Coefficient of variation
   2. Percentile
   3. Range
   4. Standard deviation
   a. 1, 2, and 4 only
   b. 1, 2, and 3 only

    c. 2, 3, and 4 only

    d. 1, 2, 3, and 4

8. Which of the following allows a team to generate a large volume of ideas?

    a. Brainstorming

    b. FOCUS-PDCA

    c. Flowcharts

    d. Surveys

9. Which of the following statements is correct?

    a. The ideal sample size should be no less than 5 and no greater than 10.

    b. The ideal sample size should be no less than 25 and no greater than 50.

    c. The ideal sample size should be no less than 30 and no greater than 100.

    d. Sample size is of no importance.

10. Which of the following is pictorial representation of a frequency distribution?

    a. Histogram

    b. Pareto chart

    c. Pie chart

    d. Scatter plot

11. Which of the following statements correctly describes a control chart?

    a. Control charts measure a process over a specified period of time.

    b. Control charts do not have predetermined upper and lower limits.

    c. Controls charts have predetermined upper and lower limits.

    d. Control charts have predetermined upper, middle, and lower limits.

12. Which of the following statements is correct?

    a. Pareto charts describe the event being monitored in ascending order from right to left.

    b. Pareto charts describe the event being monitored in descending order from right to left.

    c. Pareto charts describe the event being monitored in a random fashion.

    d. None of the above.

13. Which of the following statements correctly describes a run chart?

    a. Run charts do not have predetermined upper and lower limits.

    b. Run charts have predetermined upper and lower limits.

    c. Run charts have predetermined upper, middle, and lower limits.

    d. None of the above.

14. Which of the following detailed flowcharts is the most complex?

    a. Intermediate-level

    b. Macro-level

    c. Micro-level

    d. None of the above

15. Which of the following tools is used to compare two or more variables?

    a. Check sheet

    b. Control chart

    c. Flowchart

    d. Matrices

16. Which of the following is the simplest QM tool to use?

    a. Check sheet

    b. Control chart

    c. Flowchart

    d. Run chart

17. What statistical tool is used to describe how often an event or situation occurs?

    a. Check sheet

    b. Frequency distribution

    c. Mode

    d. Range

18. Process improvement models evolved from the

    a. FOCUS-PDCA Model

    b. JCAHO 10-Step Model

    c. The Seven-Step Model

    d. None of the above

19. What type of chart is used to analyze the cause and effect of different variables on a process?

    a. A detailed flowchart

    b. A histogram

    c. A fishbone diagram

    d. A top-down flowchart

20. Which of the following statements is true?

    a. Pareto charts sorts events and issues.

    b. Pareto charts ranks events and issues.

    c. Pareto charts rank order events and issues.

    d. None of the above.

21. The number or score that falls at or below a certain percentage is called the

    a. mean

    b. median

    c. percentile

    d. range

22. Which of the following are methods of presenting the information obtained from a performance improvement project?

    a. Storyboards

    b. Storybooks

    c. Both a and b

    d. Neither a nor b

23. Numbers that describe the spread around the mean are called

    a. measures of central tendency

      b. measures of dispersion

      c. both a and b

      d. neither a nor b

24. The range of variation around the mean is called

      a. range

      b. standard deviation

      c. percentile

      d. coefficient of variation

25. Which of the following quality management tools would be used with the FOCUS-PDCA model?

      1. Brainstorming

      2. Flowcharts

      3. Cause-and-effect diagrams

      4. Pareto charts

      a. 1 and 3 only

      b. 2 and 3 only

      c. 1, 2, and 3 only

      d. 1, 2, 3, and 4

3

The Darkroom
and Accessory Devices

KEY WORDS

Causal repeat rate	Image receptor
Crossover procedures	Immersion time
Cycling	Lead protective devices
Densitometer	Processor monitoring
Environmental factors	Repeat/reject analysis
Film artifacts	Run
Film transport time	Sensitometer
Illuminators	Trend

GOALS

1. To learn about processor quality control.
2. To learn about safelight and darkroom cleanliness checks.
3. To learn about repeat/reject analysis procedures.
4. To understand the importance of repeat/reject analysis procedures.
5. To learn about illuminator uniformity checks.
6. To learn about film-screen contact procedures.
7. To learn about proper film storage.
8. To learn about processor and film handling artifacts.

OBJECTIVES

1. Identify the quality control procedures associated with the darkroom and accessory devices.
2. Discuss the rationale for doing each quality control test.
3. State the testing frequency for each test.
4. Identify the required equipment for each test.
5. Explain the procedure for performing each quality control test.
6. Discuss the acceptance parameters for each test.
7. Explain the importance of record keeping.
8. Identify and discuss potential problems that might arise while performing each test.
9. Calculate the speed and contrast indices.
10. Discuss the crossover procedure.
11. Define trend, run, and point out of control.
12. Given a processor monitoring chart, evaluate the chart for abnormal trends.
13. Explain the rationale for doing repeat analysis.
14. Identify the key components of a repeat analysis program.
15. Discuss the procedure for doing repeat analysis.
16. State the accepted range of values for repeat analysis.
17. Explain why a repeat analysis of less than 3% is not an accurate reflection of a department's repeat rate.
18. Discuss the commonly occurring film artifacts.
19. Analyze several films for artifacts.
20. Discuss the impact of elevated processor control parameters on image quality.

INTRODUCTION

This chapter is divided into two major sections, the film processing area and accessory devices. The film processing area includes the automatic processor, darkroom, safelight, repeat analysis, and analysis of film artifacts. Illuminators, film-screen contact, and lead protective devices are included in the category of accessory devices.

When discussing the concept of radiographic quality assurance, it is important to remember that each component of the master quality management plan plays an integral and critical role. However, the film processing area is the most critical link in the overall scheme. If the film processing systems are not functioning within specified parameters, the remainder of the medical imaging facility cannot function properly. Imaging costs, patient dose, and patient diagnosis are drastically affected when the film processing systems are compromised.

It is important that a regular quality control schedule be implemented in order to achieve optimum results. Table 3-1 provides the reader with the commonly performed quality control tests, how often each test should be performed, and the minimum acceptance parameter for the test. Tests that are performed on a quarterly, semiannual, or annual basis may be staggered throughout the year so that the imaging department and patients are not inconvenienced.

The length of time required to perform each test described in this chapter will vary according to the size of the Medical Imaging Department, the number of processors, the number of darkrooms, and the workload. Each quality control test will take approximately 30 minutes for small departments to perform. For medium-sized departments, this will increase to about 1 hour. Approximately 2 hours or more will be needed for larger departments.

Table 3-1
Film Processing Area and Ancillary Devices/Areas: Testing Frequency and Acceptance Parameters

Quality Control Test	Frequency of Test	Acceptance Parameters
Processor: crossover racks	Daily	0
Processor: developer temp	Daily	$\pm 0.5°F$
Processor: base plus fog	Daily	$+ 0.03$ of total b + f
Processor: speed index	Daily	± 0.15
Processor: contrast index	Daily	± 0.15
Ultraviolet light: darkroom	Weekly	0%
Processor PMs	Monthly	0
Repeat analysis	Monthly/quarterly	4–6%
Film transport time	Quarterly	Should not exceed 2% of the recommended manufacturer's processing time
Illuminator uniformity: group	Semiannually	Should not exceed 20%
Illuminator uniformity: single	Semiannually	Should not exceed 10%
Lead protective devices	Annually	0%
Safelight	Annually	For 2-min exposure: density should not exceed 0.05 density
		For 1-min exposure: density must not exceed 0.05 density
Screen contact	Annually	0%
Ultraviolet light: screen	Annually	0%
Developer immersion time	Annually	Manufacturer's specifications

THE DARKROOM

There are no strict guidelines on the size of a darkroom. Over the span of my career, I have seen darkrooms from the size of two offices to the size of small closets. Darkrooms should have ample room to allow unimpeded movement and adequate storage space. All darkrooms should share some commonalties, such as ventilation, lighting (ambient and safe), temperature control, humidity control, storage, loading benches, and easy access.

One problem being encountered in darkrooms today is the control of dust and dirt when a dropped ceiling is used. There are several ways to control this problem. The least expensive method involves covering the ceiling tiles with shrink wrap plastic. This will prevent dust and dirt from falling onto work surfaces and into cassettes.

The temperature and relative humidity of the darkroom room and film storage area should be checked on a daily or weekly basis, whichever is deemed appropriate by the administration of the Medical Imaging Department. Air circulation of the darkroom must be checked by plant operations of the institution on a semiannually or annually. The people who are actually doing the checks will determine the frequency of air circulation checks (Fig. 3-1).

Film Storage

Proper storage of x-ray film in the Medical Imaging Department is a crucial part of any radiographic quality assurance (QA) program. Failure to properly store film will result in film artifacts, loss of image quality, repeat films, missed diagnoses, and increased cost to the department and consumer.

Film should be stored in an area free of temperature and humidity extremes and any potential exposure to x-radiation. The storage room should be environmentally controlled with the relative humidity between **30%** and **50%** and the room temperature maintained between **10°** and **21°C** (**50°** and **70°F**). These environmental conditions also apply to the darkroom.

Film should be stored vertically either on end or on the side. Boxes of film should never be stored flat or stacked on top of each other. Always rotate stock and use the oldest stock first. The easiest way to do this is to store the film by

---

- ◆ **Air Circulation: 10 complete air exchanges per hour**

- ◆ **Temperature: 50° to 70° F**

- ◆ **Relative Humidity: 30 to 50 percent**

Figure 3-1 Darkroom and film storage environment guide.

expiration date. X-ray film will start aging (base plus fog [b + f] increases) approximately 6 months after the expiration date. Base plus fog is the inherent density in a sheet of x-ray film prior to exposure to x-rays. Some departments use a color-coding system for rotating film stock. Poor or improper film storage can result in poor image quality and film artifacts such as static.

Film Artifacts

Film artifacts originate from the automatic processor or are due to improper film handling by department personnel in the darkroom. Common automatic processor artifacts are described in Tables 3-2 through 3-18. Common film handling artifacts are described in Tables 3-19 and 3-20.

Artifacts that originate in the automatic processor may be reduced or even eliminated by instituting a careful preventative maintenance program. Whenever the processor chemistry is changed and the processor is cleaned, deep racks and crossover assemblies should be checked for rollers that are bad (worn, pitted, etc.), gears that are worn or have missing teeth, and chains that are loose. A quick visual inspection should be performed on a daily basis when the crossover rollers and the exposed rollers of the deep racks are wiped off. Any damage or anomaly should be reported to the appropriate person.

Film handling artifacts will never be eliminated in a Medical Imaging Department. This type of artifact can be reduced with proper inservice training

Table 3-2
Common Parallel Processing Artifacts: Guide Shoe Marks

Artifact Appearance	Cause
Lines that are parallel to the direction of film travel	Guide shoe set too close to the adjacent roller
Plus-density, minus-density, or minus-density with surface damage	Crossover guide shoes on single-emulsion film processed emulsion side up
Evenly spaced intervals (1 inch, 1/8 inch)	Turnaround guide shoes on single emulsion film processed emulsion side down
Continuous or short length	Appear as plus-density when pressure is exerted on the emulsion side of the film, usually from guide shoes in the developer section of the processor
Usually found on the leading edge and/or the trailing edge of the film, but can be found anywhere	Appear as minus-density without surface damage when pressure is exerted on the emulsion side of the film, usually from guide shoes in the fixer-to-wash crossover
	Appear as minus-density with surface damage when emulsion is gouged off the film base anywhere in the film path

Courtesy of Eastman Kodak.

Table 3-3
Common Parallel Processing Artifacts: Delay Streaks

Artifact Appearance	Cause
Randomly spaced narrow bands of varying widths	Buildup of oxidized developer on the developer-to-fixer crossover assembly (buildup prevents uniform development of the film(s) leading edge)
Parallel to the direction of film travel	Low solution levels can cause delay streaks when rollers are not kept wet
Usually plus-density	
Usually seen starting at the leading edge of the first film fed into the processor after it has been unused for an extended period of time	

Courtesy of Eastman Kodak.

Table 3-4
Common Parallel Processing Artifacts: Entrance Roller Marks

Artifact Appearance	Cause
Plus-density bands 1/8-inch wide	Excessive pressure on the emulsion of the film from the entrance rollers
Parallel to the direction of film travel	Moisture on the entrance rollers

Courtesy of Eastman Kodak.

Table 3-5
Common Perpendicular Processing Artifacts: Film Hesitation Marks and Stub Lines

Artifact Appearance	Cause
Plus-density located 1⅝-inches from the leading edge of the film	Improper guide shoe positioning in the developer turnaround assembly
Perpendicular to the direction of film travel	Nonuniform film speed resulting from malfunctioning rack or drive component (warped or rough rollers, rack drive chain too loose or too tight, malfunctioning gears)
	Poor quality, exhausted, or contaminated chemicals
	Buildup of chemicals on the rollers
	Processor or film emulsion design

Courtesy of Eastman Kodak.

Table 3-6
Common Perpendicular Processing Artifacts: Chatter

Artifact Appearance	Cause
Plus-density lines consistently spaced	Too loose or too tight developer rack drive chain, gears, or developer-to-fixer crossover assembly drive mechanism
Perpendicular to the direction of film travel	

Courtesy of Eastman Kodak.

Table 3-7
Common Perpendicular Artifacts: Slap Lines

Artifact Appearance	Cause
Broad, plus-density line located 2⅛–2¼ inches in from the trailing edge of the film	Occurs when the trailing edge of a film releases abruptly from the developer-to-fixer crossover and slaps the top center roller of the fix rack
Perpendicular to the direction of film travel	

Courtesy of Eastman Kodak.

Table 3-8
Common Perpendicular Processing Artifacts: Pi Lines

Artifact Appearance	Cause
Plus-density line just short of film edge with stub lines that go almost to the film edge 3.14 inches from leading edge	Emulsion on the roller
	A problem with the air/solution interface rollers
	Dirty rollers
	Newly-cleaned rollers

Courtesy of Eastman Kodak.

Table 3-9
Common Random Processing Artifacts: Drying Patterns/Water Spots

Artifact Appearance	Cause
Narrow wavering bands or spots with a mottled, wash-out, or shiny appearance	Depleted photochemicals
Readily seen by reflected light	Under-replenished photochemicals
Can be seen by transmitted light when severe	Poor squeegee action at wash rack exit
Occur at random intervals parallel or perpendicular to the direction of film travel	Air tube missing or clogged
	Dirty or inoperative dryer rollers
	Excessive dryer temperature

Courtesy of Eastman Kodak.

Table 3-10
Common Random Processing Artifacts: Wet Pressure

Artifact Appearance	Cause
Random plus-density fluctuations that may look like noise or quantum mottle on film	Rough, blistered, or warped rollers in the developer rack or developer-to-fix crossover, exerting excessive pressure on the film emulsion Exhausted developer

Courtesy of Eastman Kodak.

Table 3-11
Common Random Processing Artifacts: Surface Scratches

Artifact Appearance	Cause
Random, plus-density marks indicating pressure on the film emulsion	Processor components, especially dryer rollers and airtubes, improperly maintained or out of position after maintenance
Random, minus-density marks indicating the emulsion was scraped off the film base	

Courtesy of Eastman Kodak.

Table 3-12
Common Random Processing Artifacts: Flame Patterns

Artifact Appearance	Cause
Variations in film density resembling a flame	Low recirculation rates Less likely to occur with seasoned chemicals

Courtesy of Eastman Kodak.

Table 3-13
Common Random Processing Artifacts: Run Back

Artifact Appearance	Cause
Random, plus-density "dribble" or "scallop" on the trailing edge of the film	Developer solution runs back down the trailing edge of the film as the film enters the fixer causing increased and uncontrolled development

Courtesy of Eastman Kodak.

Table 3-14
Common Random Processing Artifacts: Bent Corners

Artifact Appearance	Cause
A corner of the film is bent	Excessive recirculation of changes in the path of the film as it is transported through the processor

Courtesy of Eastman Kodak.

Table 3-15
Common Random Processing Artifacts: Pick-Off

Artifact Appearance	Cause
Random, small minus-density spots	Rough and dirty rollers in poorly maintained processors
Readily detectable on single-emulsion film	Non-uniform or inconsistent transport speed
Emulsion has been removed down to the film base	Poor quality chemicals

Courtesy of Eastman Kodak.

Table 3-16
Common Random Processing Artifacts: Dye Stain

Artifact Appearance	Cause
A pink color seen in the clear area of the film	Incomplete removal of sensitizing dye during processing due to incomplete or inadequate fixing or washing

Courtesy of Eastman Kodak.

Table 3-17
Common Random Processing Artifacts: Brown Films

Artifact Appearance	Cause
Processed film has turned brown	Inadequate washing or fixing of the film

Courtesy of Eastman Kodak.

Table 3-18
Common Random Processing Artifacts: Skivings

Artifact Appearance	Cause
Emulsion appears 3.14 inches distance from the leading edge of the film	Non-uniform film transport speed, poor processor film path design, film slitting, cutting, or finishing
	Film emulsion formulation or inadequate or hardener-depleted developer solution

Courtesy of Eastman Kodak.

of all personnel. It is important that environmental conditions and film storage practices be monitored to help in reducing film artifacts.

Repeat Analysis

As discussed in Chap. 1, the repeat analysis program is a critical element of both the performance improvement and radiographic quality programs of the Medical Imaging Department. The **repeat analysis** process is a well-defined method that determines if problems exist, and the causes of these problems. An analysis of repeats looks at the number of repeat films, the number of rejected films, and the number of waste films. Repeat films are those films that are repeated for a reason (i.e., positioning, technique, motion, etc,). Waste films are films that are thrown away because they are black, green (unexposed), clear, sensitometric, or laser. Rejected films are a reflection of the total number of films that are used in the Medical Imaging Department. Adding the total number of repeat films and the total number of wasted films gives the number of rejected films.

There are two types of repeat analysis tools that may be used be used by the imaging department. They are repeat analysis by examination and causal repeat analysis for specific cause. The actual repeat analysis must be performed prior to doing a causal repeat analysis.

Currently there is a great deal of debate going on concerning the frequency of repeat analysis performance. Some advocate a 2-week analysis every

Table 3-19
Common Random Processing Artifacts: Static

Artifact Appearance	Cause
Random, plus-density marks that resemble tree branches, smudges, or dots and dashes	Static infrequently occurs as a result of processing; it is usually caused by low relative humidity in the darkroom, synthetic clothing worn by operators, etc.

Courtesy of Eastman Kodak.

Table 3-20
Film Handling Artifacts

Artifact Appearance	Cause
Shadow images (minus density)	Dirt and dust in darkroom and image receptors
	Screens and image receptors must be thoroughly cleaned to eliminate shadow images
	The darkroom must be as clean as possible
	Use UV light device to help detect areas where dust and dirt accumulate
Scratches (minus and plus density)	More likely to occur from handling, not processing
	Carelessly placing film in the film bin
	Routinely slamming the film bin
	Carelessly removing film from the film and loading image receptor
	Sliding film across dirty film feed tray
Static (plus density)	Usually caused by handling film in a darkroom with low relative humidity
	Use a humidifier to raise relative humidity to 30–50%
	Personnel should wear natural fibers and use anti-static laundry products
Fingerprints (minus and plus density)	Minus-density fingerprints result from moisture on the film prior to exposure
	Plus-density fingerprints result from moisture on the film after exposure and prior to processing
	Keep hands clean and dry
Pressure marks (plus density)	Stacked cases of film
	Exposed film carelessly loaded
Stress marks	Holding film incorrectly
Kink marks (minus and plus density)	Pressure from fingernails
Film feeding errors	May cause many different types of artifacts

Courtesy of Eastman Kodak.

6 months. Others advocate a 2-week analysis every quarter. The drawback to both of these opinions is that insufficient data is generated to provide a comprehensive insight into how the Medical Imaging Department is doing overall with respect to repeat, reject, and waste films. The most logical way to perform a repeat analysis is to collect and count the films in the reject box on a weekly basis, then tabulate the results monthly. This method is more accurate because more data have been generated.

Over the last 15 to 20 years, there has been a great deal of discussion regarding the acceptable standards for repeat rates. The currently accepted standard is between 4% and 6%. As a rule the repeat rate for a Medical Imaging

Department realistically should not be less than 3% or greater than 10% in any given month. Based on human nature and equipment failures, a repeat rate of less than 3% is not a realistic value for an imaging department. If the repeat rate were less than 3%, the most likely explanation would be a failure to account for all repeated or wasted films. If either the repeat rate or reject rate were to exceed 10% in any given month, the reasons would have to be identified and corrective action taken (i.e., education, equipment malfunction, etc.) This discussion has focused on the Medical Imaging Department as a whole and does preclude the possibility that an individual's overall repeat rate could be less than 3%. If this is the case, the individual should be recognized in some fashion.

Repeat Analysis Procedure

Rationale
The repeat analysis is designed to provide the Medical Imaging Department with a means for analyzing causes of repeat and reject films.

Testing Frequency
The reject analysis should be performed on a weekly basis and tabulated monthly.

Equipment
- Pencil
- Calculator
- Repeat analysis form
- Illuminator
- Reject films

Procedure
A. At the end of the repeat analysis phase, calculate the total number of films used during the time being analyzed. This number may be obtained by using the inventory method or the film estimation method. The film inventory method is more accurate and takes a little more time than the estimation method.
B. Methods for calculating total films used.
   - Film inventory method
      At the beginning of the repeat analysis phase take an initial inventory (II) of all film in the department and record this number on the film inventory log (Fig. 3-2).
      At the end of repeat analysis phase, take a final film inventory (FFI) of all film in the department and record this number on the film inventory log.
      At this time, determine if any new film shipments (NFS) have been received, and record this number on the film inventory log.

Area	8 x 10	9 x 9	10 x 12	11 x 14	14 x 14	14 x17	7 x 17	Other	Total
ACC	200		200	200	200				800
EC	400		300	200		200	300		1400
Surgery	200		200			400	100		900
NNICU	200		400	200					800
Main	300	400	100	100	100	200	100	100	1400
Storage	900	500	1000	900	200	1900	400	300	6100
Cassettes	27	23	37	18	4	67	14	2	192
Total	2227	923	2237	1618	504	2767	914	402	11592

IFI =	12492
NFS =	16100
FFI =	11592
TFU =	17000

IFI = Initial Film Inventory   **NFS = New Film Shipments**

FFI = Final Film Inventory   **TFU = Total Films Used**

Figure 3-2 Film inventory log sheet for April 1998.

Determine the total films used (TFU) with the formula:

$$TFU = (II + NFS) - FF$$

- Film estimation method
  Total films used = 3.5 × the number of examinations performed.
    3.5 is a constant that reflects the average number of films used per examination.
    The number of examinations performed reflects the number of examinations done during the analysis period.
C. Obtain repeat and waste films from designated areas.
D. Determine the cause of each repeat and waste film; record the films in the appropriate area of the repeat analysis form (Fig. 3-3).
E. Perform the following tasks.
  - Calculate the number of repeat films, reject films, and waste films.
  - Calculate the repeat percentage:

$$\text{Repeat } \% = \frac{\text{\# Repeat Films}}{\text{TFU}} \times 100\%$$

Repeat Analysis Record Form

Department Area: <u>Entire Department</u>   Quarter: 2nd   Month: <u>April</u>   Year: <u>1998</u>

	Cause	Chest	Abd	Extremity	Shoulder Girdle	Cranium	C. Spine	T. Spine	L. Spine	Sacrum Coccyx	Pelvic Girdle	Bony Thorax	UGI	BE	GU	Total
1	Positioning	238	49	32	10	68	96	28	39	1	21	4	8	4	3	601
2	Motion	15	4	2		1	2	1	1			1			1	28
3	Overexposed	65	25	28	4	5	18	18	3		8	3		1	1	179
4	Underexposed	61	27	18	8	12	10	21	7	1	10	11			2	188
5	Artifact	61	17	7	3	6	20	6	6		3		3		1	133
6	Fogged	163														163
7	Processor	46														46
8	Misc (?)	143														143
9	Total	792	122	87	25	92	146	74	56	2	42	19	11	5	8	1481

10	Black	283
11	Green	149
12	Clear	160
13	Sensitometry	39
14	Copy Film	33
15	Laser Film	473
	Total	1137

Total Waste = 1137   Total Rejects = 2618   Total Repeats = 1481

Total Films Used = (12492 + 16100) – 11592 = 17000   or   Total Films Used = 3.5 x Number of Exams

$$\text{Repeat Rate (\%)} = \frac{1481}{17000} \times 100 = 8.7\%$$

$$\text{Reject Rate (\%)} = \frac{2618}{17000} \times 100 = 15.4\%$$

$$\text{Waste Rate (\%)} = \frac{1137}{17000} \times 100 = 6.7\%$$

Figure 3-3 Completed repeat analysis utilizing actual data.

- Calculate the reject percentage:

$$\text{Reject \%} = \frac{\text{\# Repeat Films plus Waste Films}}{\text{TFU}} \times 100\%$$

- Calculate the waste percentage:

$$\text{Waste \%} = \frac{\text{\# Waste Films}}{\text{TFU}} \times 100\%$$

F. Record the data in the appropriate log book.

Acceptance Parameters
- The overall repeat rate should be less than 10%.
- The ideal repeat rate should be 4% to 6%.
- If the overall repeat rate is less than 3%, it is likely that there has been an error in counting.

Record Keeping
A record should be kept that documents the date of the test, who performed the test, the results of the test, and the corrective action taken.

Potential Problems
- The most often encountered problem is the failure to account for all repeat films. This will result in an inaccurate repeat rate.
- Another frequently encountered problem is the failure to account for all films that are wasted. This will result in an inaccurate reject rate.

IMPORTANT REMINDER
- Staff radiographers should be reminded that the repeat analysis is a routine undertaking and should not be viewed as a mechanism for punishing the personnel of the department.
- Copy and laser film should be counted in the repeat analysis because they represent a cost to the Medical Imaging Department.
- Copy and laser film should be included in the waste and reject calculations.

CAUSAL REPEAT ANALYSIS

The implementation of a casual repeat analysis as part of a quality management (QM) program is strongly recommended. Causal repeat analysis is an additional tool that will enhance the overall repeat analysis program of the Medical Imaging Department. The causal repeat analysis can determine what portion of the overall repeat rate is the result of a specific cause (i.e., positioning), and it can determine the causal repeat rate by radiographic examination.

All that is necessary to calculate the causal repeat rate is the repeat analysis form (Fig. 3-3), a calculator, and the following formula:

$$\text{Causal Repeat Rate } (\%) = \frac{\text{\# of Repeats for a Specific Cause}}{\text{\# of Total Repeats}} \times 100$$

EXAMPLE 1

What is the causal repeat rate for positioning?
The total number of repeats for the month of April was 1481.
The total number of films repeated for positioning during the month of April was 601.

$$\text{Causal Repeat Rate } (\%) = \frac{601}{1481} \times 100 = 40.6\%$$

Thus, 40.6% of the Medical Imaging Department's repeat rate was due to positioning.

EXAMPLE 2

What is the causal repeat rate for technique (overexposure/underexposure)?
The total number of repeats for April was 1481.
The total number of repeats that resulted from overexposure and underexposure was 367.

$$\text{Causal Repeat Rate } (\%) = \frac{367}{1481} \times 100 = 24.9\%$$

Therefore, 24.9% of the Medical Imaging Department's repeat rate was due to improper technique selection.

EXAMPLE 3

What is the causal repeat rate for chest positioning?
The total number of repeats for the month of April was 1481.
The total number of films repeated for positioning during the month of April was 238.

$$\text{Causal Repeat Rate } (\%) = \frac{238}{1481} \times 100 = 16.1\%$$

Therefore, 16.1% of the Medical Imaging Department's repeat rate was due to improper chest positioning.

Analysis of the **causal repeat rate** in the three examples raises questions that should be addressed by the senior management of the Medical Imaging Department. There are a variety of questions that could be asked, such as

- Are the positioning problems related to an individual or a group of individuals?
- Are the technique problems related to equipment malfunction?
- Are the technique problems related to the positioning and automatic exposure control?

It is imperative that the cause of the problems be found and remedied as soon as possible.

From a quality control (QC) perspective there are only two darkroom quality control tests that should be performed on a regular basis. They are the ultraviolet (UV) light test for darkroom cleanliness and the safelight test.

Ultraviolet Light Test for Darkroom Cleanliness

Rationale

This test is designed to confirm that the darkroom is free of dirt, dust, and any foreign material.

Testing Frequency

This test should be performed on a weekly basis, preferably at the beginning of the workweek.

Equipment

- Ultraviolet light (5 to 10 V) (Fig. 3-4)

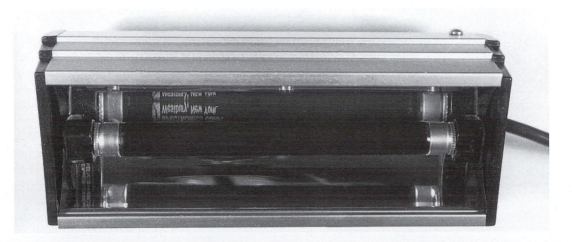

Figure 3-4 Ultraviolet light used for checking darkroom cleanliness.

Procedure

A. Plug in the UV light at a convenient outlet in the darkroom.
B. If applicable, close all doors leading into the darkroom.
C. Turn on the UV light.
D. Turn off all safelights and overhead lights.
E. Carefully examine all work surfaces with the UV light. Dirt, dust, and particulate matter will glow under the UV light.
F. Carefully examine all walls, corners, ceilings, and other areas where dirt and dust might accumulate with the UV light.
G. Record the results.

Acceptance Parameters

Acceptance parameters are determined by the American College of Radiology (ACR) and are based on the Mammography Quality Standards Act (MQSA). MQSA requires that the darkroom be totally free of dust and dirt.

Record Keeping

A record should be kept that documents the date of the test, who performed the test, the results of the test, and the corrective action taken.

Potential Problems

Suspended or dropped ceilings pose a problem because they trap dust and dirt. Every time the darkroom door is slammed, this type of ceiling generally vibrates and dust, dirt, and particulate matter come free, contaminating the work surfaces of the darkroom and image receptors.

Safelights

There are a variety ways to perform the safelight test; the safelight test described in this chapter is a modified version of the safelight test developed by Eastman Kodak. If doing the safelight test for the first time, contact your film representative for assistance.

There are essentially two types of safelights found in a medical imaging darkroom, the safelight used with calcium tungstate films and the safelight used with rare earth films. The safelight used with calcium tungstate films has a Wratten 6-B filter and the safelight for rare earth films has a GBX-2 filter. The most commonly used safelight is the GBX-2.

When installing or servicing a safelight, it is important that a visual check be done to ensure that the filter is intact and that there are no apparent light leaks in the filter housing. It is just as important to check the wattage of the light bulb being used and the distance the safelight is from the loading bench. The light bulb used for a safelight should be 7½ watts. The safelight should be mounted no less than 36 inches from the loading bench. Mounting a safelight less than 36 inches away will result in fogging of the film. A 15-watt bulb may be used with the GBX-2 safelight filter if it is 4 feet or higher from the loading bench or it is pointed toward the ceiling.

Modified Safelight Test

Rationale

This test is designed to confirm that the safelights and other unsafe light will not fog the film(s) being handled in the darkroom.

Testing Frequency

Safelights should be tested annually or when films exiting the processor are fogged.

Equipment

- An 8 × 10 image receptor (cassettes and screens as per Thompson et al., 1994; MQSA, 1999) and film
- Fastest film in the department
- Lead mat
- Timer or a clock with a secondhand or a stopwatch
- Densitometer
- One piece of 8- × 10-inch cardboard or opaque paper
- Two pieces of 2- × 10-inch cardboard or opaque paper
- Four paperclips

Procedure

A. Mark the two pieces of 2- × 10-inch cardboard or opaque paper in 2-inch increments.

B. Turn off the safelights in the darkroom and load the 8 × 10 image receptor with the fastest film in the department. The fastest film is the film most sensitive to the light from the intensifying screens.

C. Place the image receptor on the tabletop and cover the lengthwise left half of the image receptor with the lead mat.

D. The tube should be set at a 40-inch SID.

E. On the generator, set a technique that would produce an optical density of 0.6 to 1.0 on the exposed half of the film. The technique selected will depend on generator phase and the speed of the image receptor being used.

F. With the safelights off, unload the film from the image receptor.

G. Place the film on the loading bench under the safelight to be tested.

H. Cover the left one-fourth of the lengthwise portion of the film with one piece of 2- × 10-inch cardboard or opaque paper. Fasten the cardboard or paper to the film with two paper clips.

I. Cover the right one-fourth of the lengthwise portion of the film with the second piece of 2- × 10-inch cardboard or opaque paper. Fasten the cardboard or paper to the film with two paper clips.

J. Place the third piece of cardboard or opaque paper approximately lengthwise on the film 2 inches from the top of the film.

K. Turn on the safelight to be tested.

L. Every 30 seconds, move the crosswise piece of cardboard or opaque paper down approximately 2 inches until the film has been completely exposed to the safelight.

M. Immediately turn off the safelight and process the film.

N. The final film will contain 4 columns and 10 rows.

O. Starting at the left side of the film the columns are labeled A through D.
- Column A is an area of no exposure; it is used to measure base plus fog.
- Column B is exposed to safelight only.
- Column C is exposed to safelight and x-radiation.
- Column D is used to assure that the x-ray exposure range is between an optical density of 0.6 and 1.0.

P. If desired, the rows may be labeled from the top down as row 1 through 4.
- Row 1 is equal to an exposure of 120 seconds (2 minutes).
- Row 2 is equal to an exposure of 90 seconds (1½ minutes).
- Row 3 is equal to an exposure of 60 seconds (1 minute).
- Row 4 is equal to an exposure of 30 seconds.

Q. Using the densitometer, read the densities for all of the rows (Figs. 3-5A and B).

R. Record the density for rows 1 and 3 in the QC log.

Acceptance Parameters

- For the 2-minute exposure area, the density difference between the exposed and unexposed areas should not exceed an optical density of 0.05.
- For the 1-minute exposure area, the density difference between the exposed and unexposed area must not exceed an optical density of 0.05.

Record Keeping

A record should be kept that documents the date of the test, who performed the test, the results of the test, and the corrective action taken.

Potential Problems

- Light leaks in the darkroom will cause erroneous results.
- Leaving the safelight on while loading the image receptor may result in error.
- Exposing sections of film for longer than 30 seconds may result in increased density readings.
- Having the wrong wattage of bulb in the safelight may result in increased density readings.
- Using the wrong type of film will result in inaccurate density readings.
- Having safelights at less than the prescribed distance will result in increased fog and increased density readings.

IMPORTANT REMINDER

- This test is performed on every safelight in the Medical Imaging Department.
- Safelights should be at 36 inches above the loading bench and feed tray of the processor.
- All safelights should be checked to see if they have the proper light bulb installed.

Figure 3-5 *A.* Normal safelight test film.

Modified Safelight Test: Stepwedge Method

Rationale

This test is designed to confirm that the safelights and other unsafe light will not fog the film(s) being handled in the darkroom.

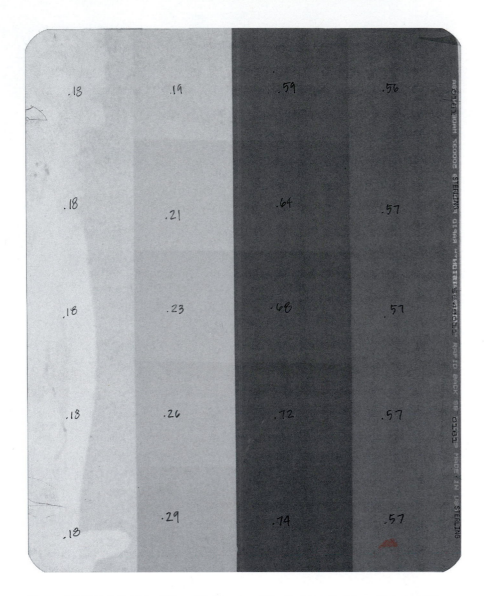

Figure 3-5 *B*. Safelight test film with increased fog that resulted from the use of the wrong wattage of light bulb.

Testing Frequency
Safelights should be tested annually or when films exit the processor fogged.

Equipment
- 8 × 10 image receptor
- Lead mats

- Timer or a clock with a secondhand or a stopwatch
- Densitometer
- Stepwedge
- Darkroom fog template

Procedure

A. Perform the following tasks prior to performing the safelight test.
   - Turn off the safelights in the darkroom and load the 8 × 10 image receptor with the most commonly used film in the department.
   - Place the image receptor on the table.
   - Place the stepwedge on the image receptor, perpendicular to the long axis of the image receptor.
   - Center the stepwedge on the image receptor.
   - Place lead mats on each side of the stepwedge and collimate the beam to the stepwedge.
   - Expose the film using the following factors:
     40″ SID
     2.5 mAs at 60 kVp
     > The exposure factors selected will be determined by the speed of the imaging system and the generator phase.
B. With the safelights off, unload the film from the image receptor.
C. Insert the film in the darkroom fog template and place them under the safelight to be tested.
D. Turn on the safelight to be tested.
E. Expose the uncovered half of the film for 2 minutes.
F. Immediately turn off the safelight and process the film.
G. Using the densitometer, measure the density difference between the exposed and unexposed sections of the film (Figs. 3-5C and D).
H. Record the density readings in the QC log.

Acceptance Parameters

For the 2-minute exposure area, the density difference between the exposed and unexposed areas should not exceed an optical density of 0.05.

Record Keeping

A record should be kept that documents the date of the test, who performed the test, the results of the test, and the corrective action taken.

Potential Problems

- Light leaks in the darkroom will cause erroneous results.
- Leaving the safelight on while loading the image receptor may result in error.
- Exposing sections of film for longer than 30 seconds may result in increased density readings.
- Having the wrong wattage of bulb in the safelight may result in increased density readings.

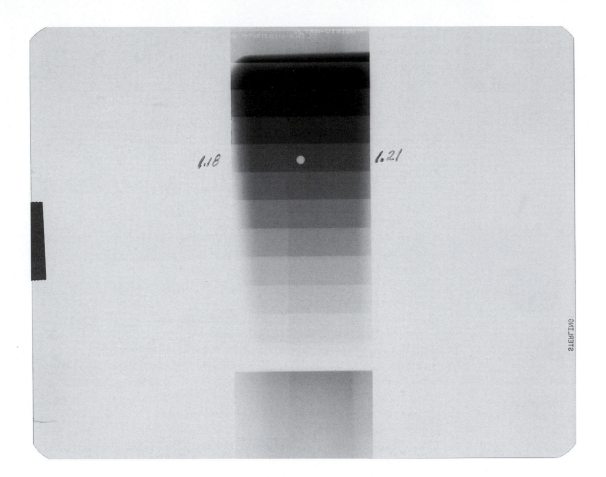

Figure 3-5 *C*. Normal safelight test film (stepwedge method).

- Using the wrong type of film will result in inaccurate density readings.
- Having safelights at less than the prescribed distance will result in increased fog and density readings.

AUTOMATIC PROCESSORS

Automatic processors may be purchased with a variety of processing times. The available processing times range from 45 seconds to 3½ minutes. Processors that have a 45-second processing time are called *rapid action processors*, and processors that have a processing time greater than 90 seconds are referred to as *extended time processors*. The standard processor in most Medical

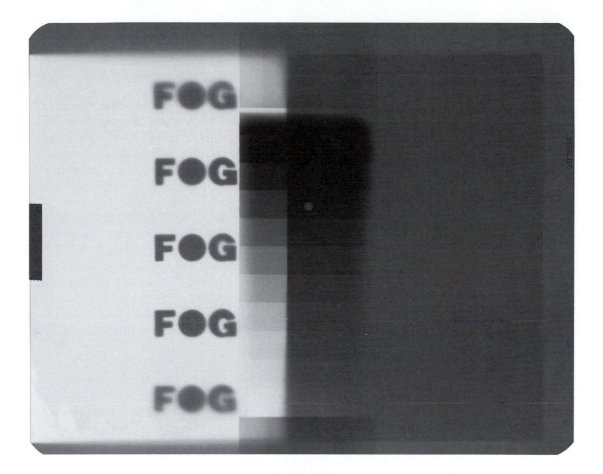

Figure 3-5 *D.* Safelight test film (stepwedge method) with increased fog.

Imaging Departments is the 90-second processor, which serves a variety of imaging demands. There are three QC tests that should be performed on automatic processors on a routine basis. They are sensitometry or processing monitoring, **immersion time,** and film transport time. Of these tests, processor monitoring and immersion are the most critical tests to perform. **Film transport time** is an excellent test to perform when a film transport problem is suspected, and should be followed up with the time in solution test as a method to confirm a film transport problem.

Establishing and Maintaining a Processor Monitoring Program

Processor monitoring is a fairly routine task that is done daily at approximately the same time and on all processors in the Medical Imaging Department. The standard for processor monitoring has been established by the MQSA guidelines and should be used for both mammography film processors and diagnostic film processors. All that is needed to perform processor monitoring is the film, processor control chart, sensitometer, densitometer, and thermometer.

The type of film used for processor monitoring will be either mammography film or the most commonly used film in the Medical Imaging Department. If a processor is serving double duty, running both mammography films and diagnostic films, then mammography film should be used for processor monitoring. If a processor is being used for strictly mammography, then mammography film should be used for processor monitoring. Processors that have only a diagnostic workload should use the most commonly run film as the monitoring film.

The processor control chart is the permanent record of the processor's performance over a specific period of time. Processor performance is tracked on a daily basis and recorded on the control chart, which has room for 31 days of data. A new control chart should be started at the beginning of each month. Processor control charts should be kept on file for at least 24 months to provide a performance history of the processor. The processor control chart is divided into six specific sections for the recording of information. The upper section is for documenting the processor, type of film, emulsion number, year, date crossover performed, and crossover emulsion number. The next section is the area for the month, date, and initials of who performed the test. The third, fourth, fifth, and sixth sections of the control chart are for recording the medium density (speed index), density difference (contrast index), base plus fog, and developer temperature. On the reverse side of the control chart is an area for making comments about processor performance (Figs. 3-6A and B). The medium density and density difference portions of the processor control chart have upper and lower limits established. These limits are ±0.15 of the midpoint of the graph. If either speed or contrast exceed or fall below this number, it is important to stop running films and find the cause of the problem. If processor values should either exceed or fall below ±0.10 of the midpoint, potential problems with the processor chemistry should be suspected. When this occurs, it will be necessary to run several filmstrips to monitor the performance of the processor and make the determination if the service engineer should be called. Table 3-21 is a trouble shooting guide for processor control charts. Once the data have been plotted on the control chart, it will be necessary to connect each point on the individual charts. It is critical to plot the points accurately and evaluate the chart for runs, trends, and points out of control. A **run** is a series of seven points that fall above or below the midpoint or target aim of the graph. A **trend** is a series of five consecutive points that present either as an upward or downward pattern on the graph. A point out of control is a data point that is outside of the established control limits. **Cycling** is a series of points alternating above or below the mean. Usually, seven points are needed to make a decision. Figure 3-7 illustrates a run, a trend, a **point out of control,** and cycling.

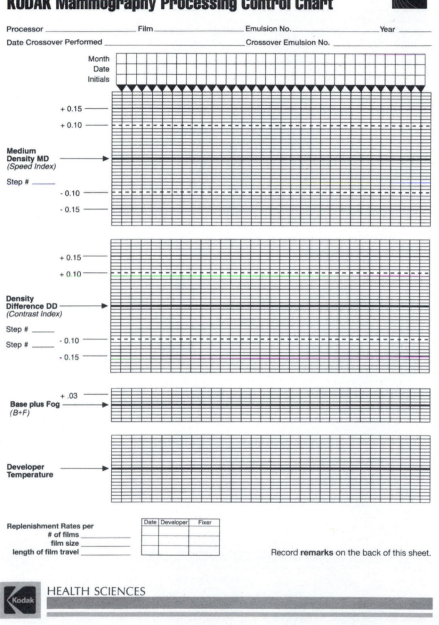

Figure 3-6 *A.* Obverse side of the Kodak Processor Control Chart. *(Eastman Kodak Company, used with permission.)*

Remarks

Date	Action

Remarks

Date	Action

More than quality imaging

Kodak

M7-173   Printed in U.S.A.   © Eastman Kodak Company, 1995   Kodak is a trademark.

Figure 3-6 *B.* **Reverse side of the Kodak Processor Control Chart.** *(Eastman Kodak Company, used with permission.)*

Table 3-21
Troubleshooting Guide for Processor Control Charts

Control Parameter	Film Appearance	Probable Causes	Corrective Action
↑ Speed index	Film density too high	Developer temperature too high	Check developer thermostat setting; check incoming water temperature
↑ Contrast index		Developer replenisher improperly mixed	Drain and remix developer
↑ Base + fog		Developer contaminated with fixer	Drain and rinse tanks and mix fresh chemistry
			Use splash guard when removing fixer rack to avoid contamination
↓ Speed index	Film density too low	Developer temperature too low	Adjust developer thermostat to correct setting
↓ Contrast index		Developer exhausted	Check replenishment rates and/or mix fresh chemistry
↓ Base + fog			Change chemistry; follow mixing instructions included with chemistry
		Developer improperly mixed	Check processor overflow drain
		Developer diluted	Check tanks for possible leaks
↑ Fog level		Developer contaminated with fixer	Drain and rinse tanks, mix fresh chemistry, and replace filter
↓ In overall film density		Fixer replenishment rate inadequate	Drain tank and reset fixer replenishment rate to correct level
↑ Speed index	↑ Fog level	Fixer contaminated with developer	Drain and rinse tanks and mix fresh chemistry
↑ Contrast index	↓ In overall film density	Developer improperly mixed	Change chemistry; follow mixing instructions included with chemistry
↓ Base + fog		Developer starter inadequate	Drain and rinse tanks and mix fresh chemistry; add correct amount of starter
		Excessive developer replenishment	Drain developer tank and refill with fresh developer and add correct amount of starter
		Developer completely oxidized	Adjust developer replenishment rates
			Check replenishment rates and/or mix fresh chemistry
↑ Speed index	Loss of image contrast	Developer improperly mixed, overdiluted, or oxidized	Remix fresh chemistry
↓ Contrast index			Consider making a limited amount of chemistry
↓ Base + fog		Developer replenishment rate inadequate	Drain developer tank and refill with fresh developer; add correct amount of starter

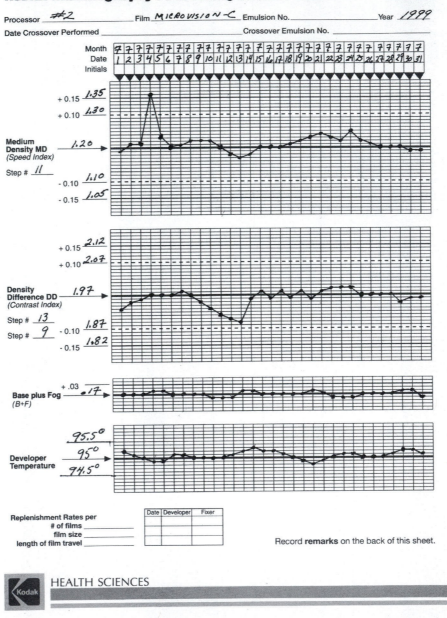

Figure 3-7 Control chart illustrating a point out of control and a run in the speed index, and a trend and cycling in the contrast index.

A device called a sensitometer (Fig. 3-8) produces the filmstrip that is used for processor monitoring. The **sensitometer** is a battery-operated electro-mechanical device that imprints a 21-step wedge on a piece of film (Fig. 3-9).

Sensitometers used in medical imaging have two exposure settings identified as blue and green. The exposure switch is located on the front corner of the sensitometer. The purpose of this switch is to allow for the use of film that is sensitive to either blue or green light. It is important to check that the proper switch position is used for the type of film used. When exposing a film with the sensitometer, a sound is emitted to denote that the film has been exposed. The quality of the sound and the duration of the exposure are different for the blue and the green settings. The blue exposure setting emits a lower and quicker sound than the green exposure setting. When exposing a film with the sensitometer, it is important to wait approximately 15 to 20 seconds between exposures. This should be done to allow the sensitometer to stabilize. The sensitometer should be sent back to the manufacturer for calibration every 12 to 18 months. The ACR requires that sensitometers be recalibrated every 18 months.

It is important that all sources of potential error be controlled as much as possible. One potential source of error that can occur with the sensitometer is how frequently the battery is changed. The battery in the sensitometer should be changed either quarterly or semiannually. When the decision is made to replace the battery, it is also very important to run film strips pre- and post-battery change. This is the only method that will confirm that speed and con-

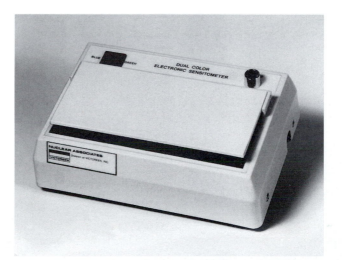

Figure 3-8 Handheld dual color sensitometer. *(Courtesy of Nuclear Associates, used with permission.)*

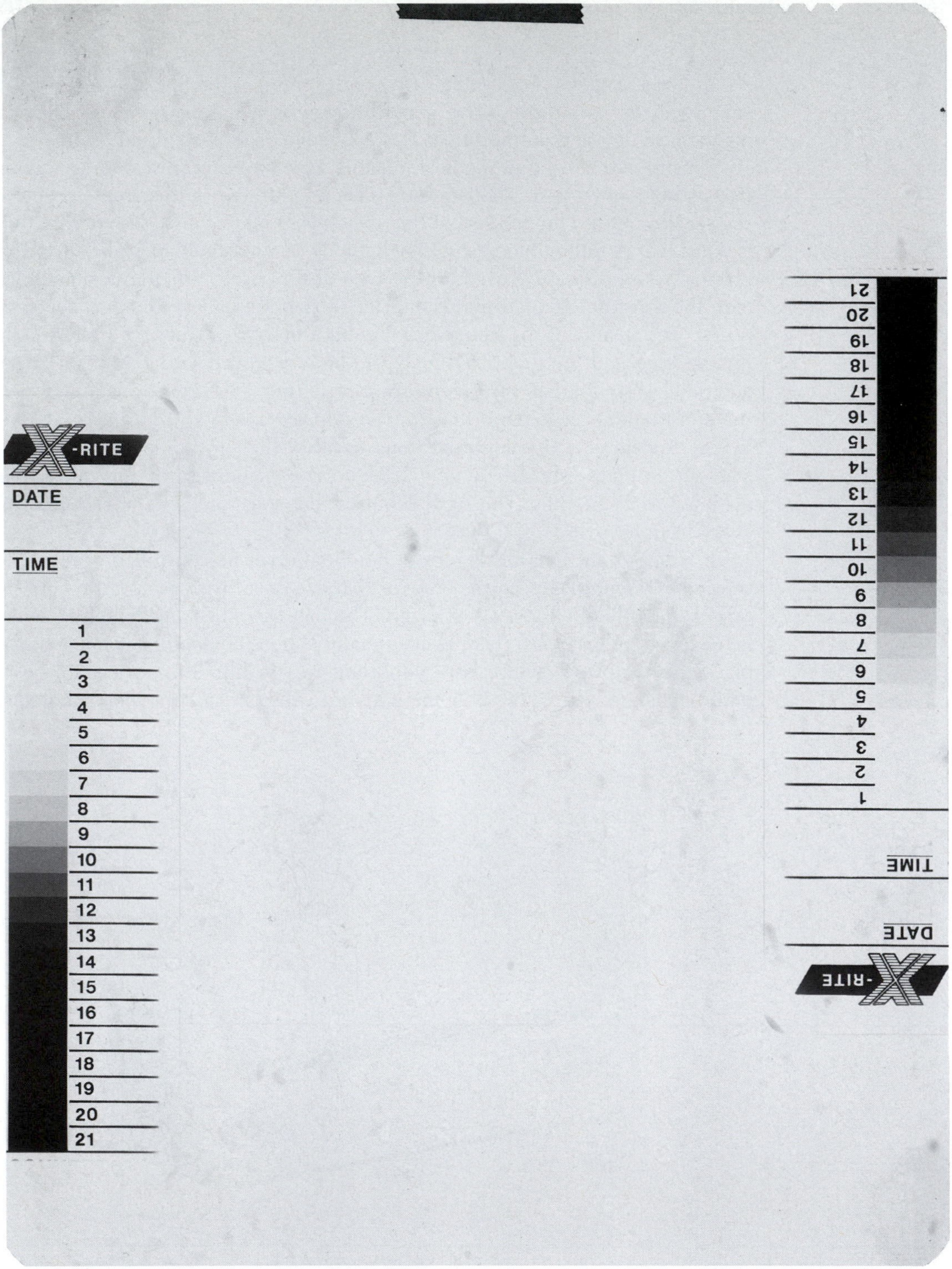

Figure 3-9 Sensitometry filmstrip.

106

trast values have not changed between battery changes. Failure to change the battery of the sensitometer either quarterly or semiannually may result in erroneous data being plotted on the processor control chart. Figure 3-10 is an example of a processor control chart that demonstrated a downward trend in the contrast index over a period of several days. Processor service was called in and the specific gravity of the developer and fixer were checked and found to be within normal limits. The serviceman changed the developer and ran a filmstrip to check the values, which were the same as the previous filmstrip. The serviceman and person in charge of processor monitoring were baffled by the problem. After some discussion and problem solving they decided to change the battery of the sensitometer. Figures 3-11 and 3-12 demonstrate the importance of changing the battery on a regular basis.

The **densitometer** (Figs. 3-13A, B, and C) is an electromechanical device used to read the optical density of a film or the pre-selected density steps from a film that has been exposed. When a densitometer is purchased, there is a pre-exposed calibration strip (Fig. 3-14) that may be used to periodically check the calibration of the unit. It is important to remember that the calibration strip has an expiration date and should be replaced every 18 to 24 months because it is an organic material and degrades when exposed to any light source. When using the densitometer, it is important to turn the unit on and let it warm up. Once it has warmed up, it will be necessary to zero the unit prior to use. Each time a density reading is taken, the unit should be zeroed again to ensure that the next reading is accurate. Like the sensitometer, the densitometer has to be periodically recalibrated. It should be sent back to the manufacturer for calibration every 12 to 18 months. The ACR requires that densitometers be recalibrated every 18 months.

The temperature of the developer should be checked on a daily basis and recorded on the processor control chart. The temperature should be measured with either a digital thermometer (Fig. 3-15) or a nonmercury analog thermometer. Do not use a mercury-filled glass thermometer to measure the temperature of the developer because there is always the possibility of the thermometer breaking and contaminating the developer. The temperature for the developer should be within ± 0.5 degrees of the aim temperature, generally 35°C (95°F).

When starting a processor monitoring program from scratch, the processor or processors to be monitored should be thoroughly cleaned, new chemistry mixed, solution temperatures checked, and the replenishment rates checked and adjusted if necessary. Once this has been accomplished, aim values should be established for the processors being monitored. The simplest way to do this is with a 5-day average of the b + f, the mid-density step (speed index), and the density difference between high and low density steps (contrast index). The new aim values are the average b + f, speed index, and contrast index. The steps and values associated with these terms are described in the automatic processor monitoring protocol.

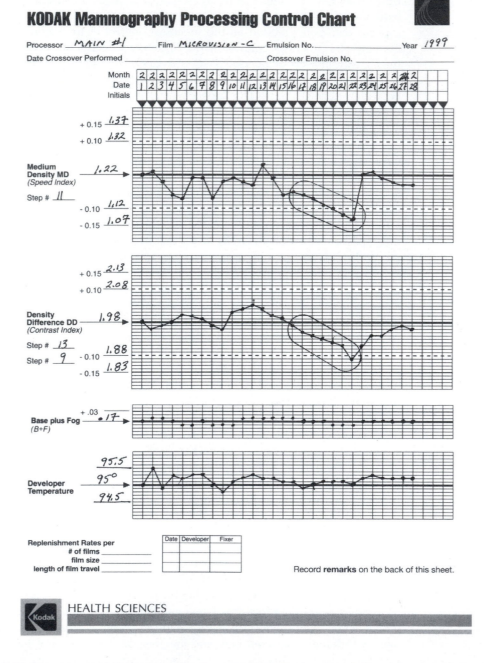

Figure 3-10 Processor control chart showing downward trend in the speed index and contrast index that is the result of battery failure.

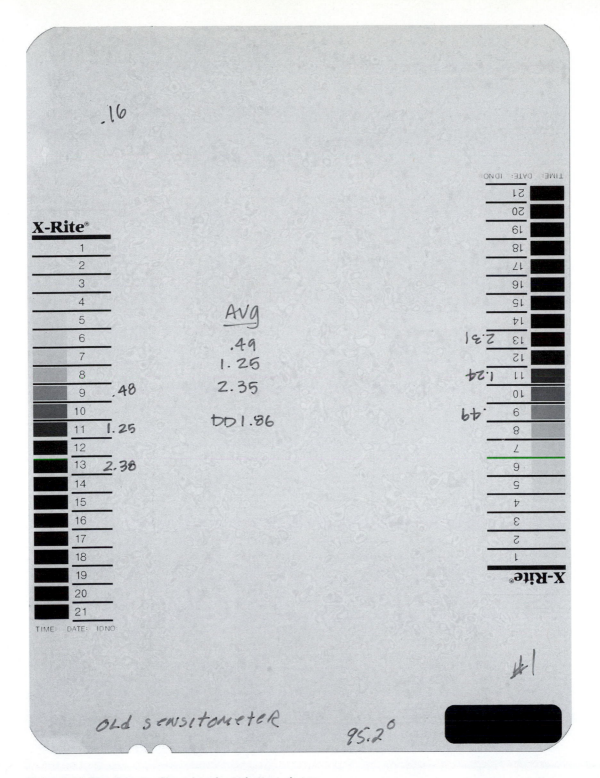

Figure 3-11 Sensitometry filmstrip prior to battery change.

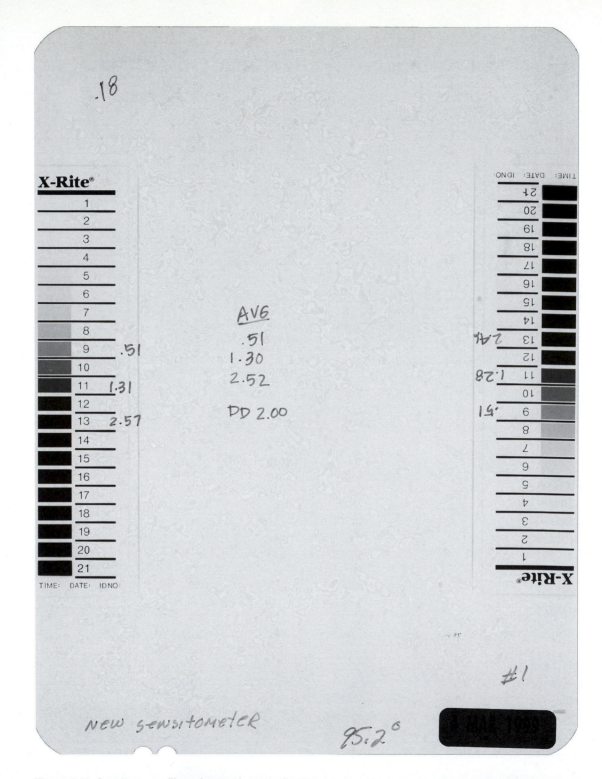

Figure 3-12 Sensitometry filmstrip post-battery change.

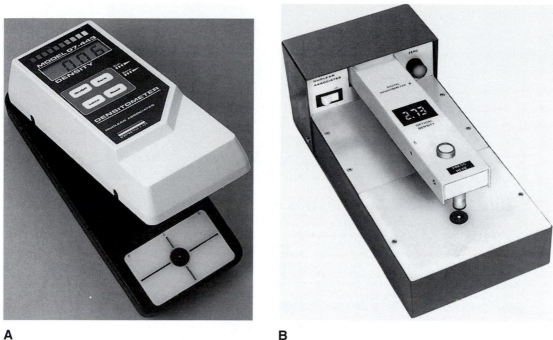

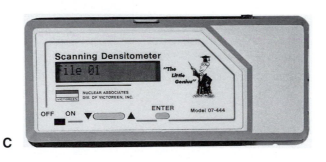

Figure 3-13 *A.* Deluxe "clamshell" digital densitometer. *(Courtesy of Nuclear Associates, used with permission.) B.* Digital tabletop densitometer with RS-232. *(Courtesy of Nuclear Associates, used with permission.) C.* Little Genius Scanning Densitometer. *(Courtesy of Nuclear Associates, used with permission.)*

Processor Preventive Maintenance

Processor preventive maintenance is a critical and integral component of the processor monitoring program. Failure to have a preventive maintenance schedule can lead to needless downtime and loss of revenue. Preventive maintenance is an ongoing task that has daily and monthly components (Table 3-22). A qualified processor service engineer should perform the monthly component of the preventive maintenance program. It is important that, when the

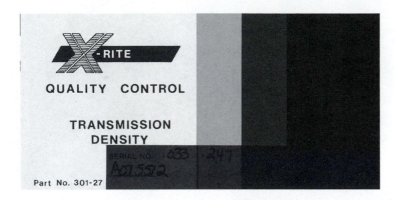

X-Rite®   CERTIFICATION OF CALIBRATION

The densities of this transmission reference are traceable to the National Institute of Standards and Technology (NIST) Standard Reference Material No. 1008 by measurements from an X-Rite, Incorporated Standard Densitometer that conforms to conditions specified in American National Standards Diffuse Transmission Density - ANSI PH2.19-1986 and ISO 5/2-1985. The measurements were made with a 3mm aperture at the center of each step and are valid in this area only.

The densities listed on the reference are the averages of several measurements taken in such a way that the maximum error is +/- 0.02D or 1%, whichever is greater. The revision letter "A" prefix on the serial number of the reference indicates the densities conform to ANSI PH2.19-1986 and ISO 5/2-1985. These densities may be changed so that they conform to ANSI PH2.19-1976 by adding the density value in the table below to the density of the corresponding step number on the reference. This reference expires 18 months from the date below or when physical abuse is noted.

	STEP NUMBER	Visual
	1	0.00D
	2	0.00D
	3	0.03D
CAL. HI	4	0.06D
	5	0.08D

Part No.: **301-27**   Serial No.: **A075512**   Date: **6/21/94**

Calibration Measurements By: _____   Title: Quality Assurance

SD43-301-27 REV. A-12/02/92

Figure 3-14 Densitometer calibration strip.

monthly preventive maintenance is done, all worn or damaged parts are replaced.

Automatic Processor Monitoring Protocol

Rationale

- This test is designed to confirm that there is consistency in density from radiograph to radiograph.
- This test is designed to confirm that uniformity exists between processors when more than one processor is found in the Medical Imaging Department and adjacent areas.

Testing Frequency

Monitoring of the processor is done on a daily basis.

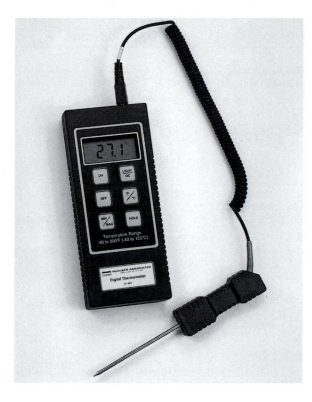

Figure 3-15 Digital thermometer used to monitor processor temperatures. *(Courtesy of Nuclear Associates, used with permission.)*

Equipment
- Sensitometer
- Densitometer
- 8 × 10 film (most critical or frequently used)
- Thermometer (nonmercury)—may be either digital or analog
- Processor control chart
- Felt tip marker
- Pencil

Procedure
A. Warm up the processor for a minimum of 30 minutes.
B. Check the developer temperature.
C. Record the developer temperature on the processor control chart.
D. Expose the emulsion side of the film with the sensitometer. The film is generally exposed on the right and left sides.
E. Process the film by feeding the long axis of the film emulsion side up into the processor.

Table 3-22
Preventive Maintenance Chart

Daily	Monthly
Wash evaporation covers with warm water.	Check replenishment rates.
Clean crossover racks with warm water; rotate and clean rollers.	Check feed tray alignment.
Check for deposits above solution level and clean if necessary.	Clean and check deep racks for any needed repairs.
Check dryer area for deposits and clean if necessary.	Clean and check crossover racks for any needed repairs.
Keep top of processor open overnight to vent trapped fumes and reduce chemical buildup.	Drain and clean processor tanks.
Run and check clearing films.	Follow manufacturer's recommendation for lubrication of gears.
	Check all tubing and connections for leaks.
	Check entrance roller detector switches for proper engaging and disengaging.

    F. Use the densitometer to measure b + f, which may be any clear area on the film or the first step of the stepwedge. Base plus fog is generally around 0.18.

    G. Use the densitometer to measure the following data points on each side of the film strip.
- The speed index, which is a midrange density (usually Step 11). The midrange density should be near but not less than 1.2 (1.0 above b + f).
- The high-density step (usually Step 13), which should have a density near 2.2 (2.0 above b + f).
- The low-density step (usually Step 9), which should have a density near but not less then 0.45 (0.25 above b + f).
- Average the data points for the low-, mid-, and high-density steps.

    H. Calculate the contrast index, which is determined by subtracting the high minus low densities.

    I. Record the b + f, the speed index, and contrast index on the processor control chart.

    J. Developer temperature, b + f, speed, and contrast are recorded on a daily basis. It is important for the technologist to observe any trends that occur and report them.

    K. If the numbers obtained for speed and contrast exceed the upper dotted line of the graph or go below the lower dotted line of the graph it will be necessary to run another strip to verify the accuracy of the original reading.

Acceptance Parameters

- The b + f should be within ±0.03 of the total b + f.
- The speed index should be within ±0.15.
- The contrast index should be within ±0.15.
- The developer temperature should be within ± 0.7°C (± 0.5°F).

Record Keeping

A record should be kept that documents the date of the test, who performed the test, the results of the test, and the corrective action taken.

IMPORTANT REMINDER

- Processor control strips should be kept for at least 1 year.
- The temperature, density values, date, and time should recorded daily on the processor strips with a felt tip marker.

Potential Problems

- Over- or under-replenishment of the chemistry will have an impact on the speed and contrast indices.
- Increased or decreased developer temperature will impact the speed and contrast indices and b + f.

IMPORTANT REMINDER

- Separate processor monitoring strips should be maintained for processors that develop radiographic films and mammographic films in the extended time.
- Processor monitoring needs to be done at the same time everyday.
- A trend is a series of points in either a downward or upward pattern on the processor control chart. If the points fall out of established limits, corrective action needs to be taken.

Film Transport Time

Rationale

This test is designed to confirm that the amount of time required to process a film, from dry film to dry film, is within the manufacturer's recommended processing time.

Testing Frequency

Film transport time should be checked on a quarterly basis, when the processor is serviced, or when a motor or chain has been replaced.

Equipment

- A stopwatch
- 14 × 17 unexposed scrap film

Procedure

A. Place the film crosswise on the feed tray of the automatic processor.
B. Begin feeding the film into the processor and start the stopwatch when the leading edge of the film enters the entrance roller.
C. Stop the stopwatch when the trailing edge of the film exits the dryer.
D. Steps A through C should be repeated 5 to 10 times.
E. The film transport time is the average of the times.
F. Record the results.

Acceptance Parameters

Film transport time should not exceed 2% of the manufacturer's recommended processing time.

Processing Time	Variance
45 seconds	± 0.9 seconds
90 seconds	± 1.8 seconds
150 seconds	± 3.0 seconds

Record Keeping

A record should be kept that documents the date of the test, who performed the test, the results of the test, and the corrective action taken.

Potential Problems

Failure to start and stop the timing device at the appropriate times will lead to erroneous test results.

Immersion Time: Time-in-Solution Test

Rationale

This test is performed to confirm that the immersion time of a film is within the manufacturer's specifications.

Testing Frequency

This test should be performed annually or when there is a suspected problem with development time.

Equipment

- TIS tool (Fig. 3-16)
- Stopwatch
- Magnet
- Calculator

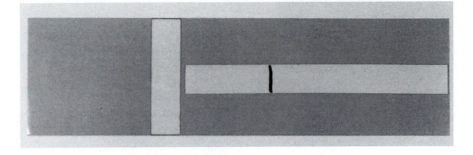

Figure 3-16 Time-in-solution (TIS) test tool.

Procedure

A. Remove the lid of the processor.
  • For newer processors, once the lid has been removed, a magnet should be placed near the microswitch to keep the processor running. This not necessary for older processors.
B. Locate the following mechanisms in the processor:
  • The 1/4-inch gap between the entrance roller assembly and the guide shoe.
  • The gap between the developer to fixer crossover and the guide shoe.
C. Place the test tool against the feed tray guide on the right side and feed the leading edge of the test tool into the processor.
  • The leading edge of the test tool will be the T.
D. Prepare to begin timing when the black line on the test tool crosses the gap in the entrance roller assembly. The stopwatch should be your hand.
E. Start timing when the top of the T reaches the gap of the entrance roller.
F. Stop timing when the top of the T reaches the gap in the developer to fixer crossover rack.
G. The timing sequences should be done a minimum of five times, and then take an average to determine the developer time.

Acceptance Parameters

Check with the manufacturer to see what the acceptance parameters for immersion time should be.

Record Keeping

A record should be kept that documents the date of the test, who performed the test, the results of the test, and the corrective action taken.

Potential Problems

Failure to start the stopwatch at the correct time will lead to misinterpretation of test results.

Crossover Procedures

Crossover procedures are done to ensure that there is consistency between the film emulsions that are being used for processor sensitometry. A crossover procedure should be performed about every 45 to 60 days or sooner, depending on the number of processors being monitored. It is important that crossover procedures be done for all processors. For example, if you have a processor in the emergency room, a processor in neonatal intensive care, the main department, and mammography, you should do a crossover for each of these processors. The mammography processor crossover would use a mammography film emulsion and the remaining processor crossovers would require the most commonly used film emulsion. When monitoring multiple processors using the same emulsion, it will become necessary to perform a crossover procedure on a more frequent basis. When doing crossover procedures, it is important to remember that the crossover should be done when the processor chemistry is stable and not immediately after a preventive maintenance task has been done.

Crossover Procedure for Processor Monitoring Film

Rationale
This procedure is designed to reference the speed index, contrast index, and b + f of a new box of film to the old box of film currently used for processor monitoring.

Equipment
- Crossover film (old and new emulsions)
- Sensitometer
- Densitometer
- Calculator
- Pencil
- Processor control chart
- Felt tip marker
- Red pen
- Crossover worksheet (Fig. 3-17)

Procedure
A. When a new box of film is used for processor monitoring, a cardboard should be placed in front of the last 5 or 10 sheets of film in the box.
B. The crossover procedure should be performed when there are five sheets of film left in the old box of film.
C. The crossover procedure should be performed in total darkness to eliminate any possibility of unwanted fog from the safelight.
D. When the cardboard is reached, expose the emulsion sides of last five sheets of film with the sensitometer.
E. Take the first five of the new box of film and repeat Step D.

Processor: <u>Main #2</u>   **Date: <u>12-15-98</u>**

Old Emulsion # <u>597 8062 0046 01</u>

Strip #	B + F	MD (Step 11)	HD (Step 13)	LD (Step 9)	DD (13-9)
1	0.16	1.25	2.50	0.46	2.04
2	0.17	1.27	2.46	0.46	2.00
3	0.18	1.27	2.50	0.46	2.04
4	0.17	1.26	2.49	0.46	2.03
5	0.16	1.30	2.53	0.47	2.06
Average	0.17	1.27	2.50	0.46	2.03

New Emulsion # <u>597 8072 0039 05</u>

Strip #	B + F	MD (Step 11)	HD (Step 13)	LD (Step 9)	DD (13-9)
1	0.17	1.24	2.43	0.46	1.97
2	0.17	1.23	2.41	0.45	1.96
3	0.17	1.23	2.43	0.46	1.97
4	0.17	1.23	2.44	0.45	1.99
5	0.17	1.25	2.46	0.47	1.99
Average	0.17	1.24	2.43	0.46	1.98

Calculate the change in film by subtracting the old average from the new average for each aim value.

	B + F	MD	DD
New Average	0.17	1.24	1.98
(-) Old Average	0.17	1.27	2.03
Change	0	-0.03	-0.05

New Aim Values: Add the change in film by subtracting the old average from the new average for each film.

	B + F	MD	DD
Present Aim	0.17	1.26	2.05
Change	0	-0.03	-0.05
New Aim	0.17	1.23	2

To obtain the new aim add the change to the present aim.

If the new B+F aim greater than 0.02 of the present aim investigate the cause or contact the service engineer and/or the film manufacturer.

Figure 3-17 Sample crossover procedure.

F. Distinguish the new film from the old film by marking the emulsion side of the film with a lead pencil. Some sources recommend that this be done in the area of the film notches.

G. In total darkness alternately process the old and new films. Feed lengthwise into the processor.

H. With a densitometer read the densities normally used for determining b + f, low density, mid density, and high density.

I. Calculate the contrast index for each film.

J. For the five old and new films, determine the average b + f, speed index, and contrast index. Record these values on the crossover calculation form (Fig. 3-17).

K. Subtract the old film values from the new film values.
- New b + f − Old b + f = Difference (+ or − or no change)
- New Speed Index − Old Speed Index = Difference (+ or − or no change)
- New Contrast Index − Old Contrast Index = Difference (+ or − or no change)

L. If there is a negative difference between the new and old values, the original processor control parameters should be reduced and a new processor control chart started.

M. If there is a positive difference between the new and old values, the original processor control parameters should be increased and a new processor control chart started.
- Instead of starting a new control chart, it is acceptable to take a red pen and draw a line on the old chart between the previous day and the day of the crossover.
- The new aim values for the processor should be written in red in the right hand margin of the control chart and identified as "New Aim Values." On the back of the control chart there should be a notation that the crossover was performed.

N. If there is no difference, the processor control parameters will stay the same.

O. The new processor control parameters will need to be put in statement form and included in the processor quality control log.

Record Keeping
- If all values are identical, the date of the crossover procedure must be indicated on the processor control chart.
- If there is a positive or negative difference between old and new values, new processor control charts must be started.
- All control strips should be kept in a notebook or file.
- The temperature, density values, date, and time should be recorded daily on the processor strips with a felt tip marker.
- The crossover procedure worksheet should be kept as a reference in the processor QC notebook.

Potential Problems
- Failure to do the crossover procedure in total darkness may lead to inaccurate results.
- Failure to follow the described procedure may cause erroneous results.

IMPORTANT REMINDER

- If for some reason the box of film that is set aside for processor monitoring is used up before a crossover procedure can be done, an average of the previous 30 days will need to be done to establish new aims for the b + f, speed index, and contrast index.

ACCESSORY DEVICES

Accessory devices include image receptors, illuminators, and lead protective devices. Although grids are considered an accessory device, they will be discussed in Chap. 4.

Image Receptors

The **image receptor** in the context of this book deals with the total film-screen imaging system used in medical imaging (Thompson et al., 1994; MQSA, 1999). The intensifying screens of the image receptor are constructed in such a way that they are durable and can last for many years. However, the longevity of intensifying screens is in direct proportion to the care that is provided by the user. Failure to take proper care of intensifying screens will lead to decreased imaging capabilities and a loss of imaging quality. Both radiographic and mammographic intensifying screens should be cleaned on a regular basis. The MQSA requires that mammographic screens be cleaned weekly. Ideally, this should also apply to screens used for general radiography. However, this is not practical because of the number of image receptors found in the typical Medical Imaging Department. Therefore it has become necessary to clean all intensifying screens on a rotating quarterly basis (Fig. 3-18).

Quarter	Image Receptor Size
First Quarter	14 x 17's
Second Quarter	10 x 12's
Third Quarter	8 x 10's
Fourth Quarter	9 x 9's and 7 x 17's

Figure 3-18 Suggested image receptor cleaning, screen contact test, and blacklight test schedule.

With everyday use, intensifying screens receive scratches, nicks, and stains to the phosphor layer, which can result in the appearance of artifacts on the radiographic image. It is critical that care be exercised when unloading the image receptors. At the time of cleaning, it is also important to carefully inspect the screens for any type of defect. It is possible that there are stains and scratches that are not readily visible to the naked eye. To ensure that there are no invisible defects, a blacklight (Fig. 3-19) should be used to examine the image receptor for defects. Figure 3-20 demonstrates an artifact that was not detected on visual inspection but was seen by the radiologist on a radiograph. The use of a blacklight demonstrated a large invisible stain in the intensifying screen.

Another aspect of intensifying screen care is the routine checks that should be performed to assure that there is proper film-screen contact in all of the image receptors of the Medical Imaging Department. Again, because of the sheer number of image receptors in the department, it is recommended that a rotating schedule be established for this task. The easiest way to achieve this is to perform the screen contact test and the blacklight test at the same time that the intensifying screens are cleaned.

Film/Screen Contact Test

Rationale

This test is designed to confirm that all image receptors in the Medical Imaging Department have perfect film-screen contact.

Testing Frequency

Image receptor film-screen contact should be checked annually or when there is a suspicion or indication that imaging resolution is being lost due to poor film-screen contact.

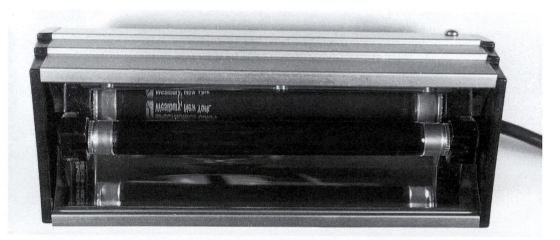

Figure 3-19 Ultraviolet light used for checking image receptor screens.

Figure 3-20 Radiograph of an intensifying screen defect that was detected with the ultraviolet light.

Equipment
- Radiographic room
- Wire mesh test tool (Fig. 3-21)
- All image receptors in the department
- Densitometer

Procedure
A. Place the image receptor on the table top and place the wire mesh test tool on top of the image receptor.
B. Collimate to the size of the image receptor.
C. Place the tube at a 40-inch SID.
D. Set an approximate technique of 2 mAs at 70 kVp.
E. Expose the image receptor.
F. Process the film.
G. Use the densitometer to measure the density of the film. The exposed film should have an optical density of between 1.5 and 2.0.
H. Repeat steps A through G for all remaining image receptors.
I. All radiographs of the image receptors should be viewed at a distance of 6 feet on a single illuminator in a dimly lit room (Figs. 3-22A, B, and C).

Acceptance Parameters
Poor film-screen contact results in a degraded image because the image resolution has been lost. Currently there are no established acceptance parameters for this test. It is the opinion of the author there should be a zero percent tolerance for this test. If an image receptor is found have poor film-screen contact it should be removed from service.

IMPORTANT REMINDER
- Areas of poor contact will appear darker than areas of good contact.
- Areas of poor contact will demonstrate loss of detail or blurring of the wire mesh.

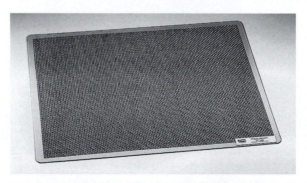

Figure 3-21 Screen contact tool. *(Courtesy of Nuclear Associates, used with permission.)*

Figure 3-22 *A*. Radiograph demonstrating satisfactory film-screen contact.

Record Keeping

A record should be kept that documents the date of the test, who performed the test, the results of the test, and the corrective action taken.

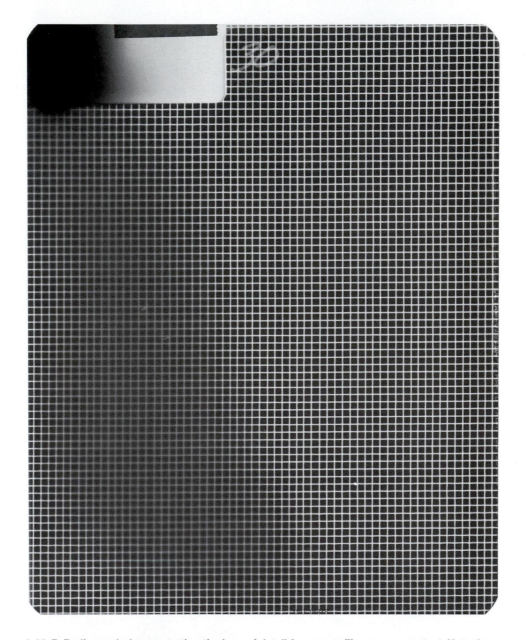

Figure 3-22 *B.* Radiograph demonstrating the loss of detail from poor film-screen contact. Note the increased density on the left half of the radiograph.

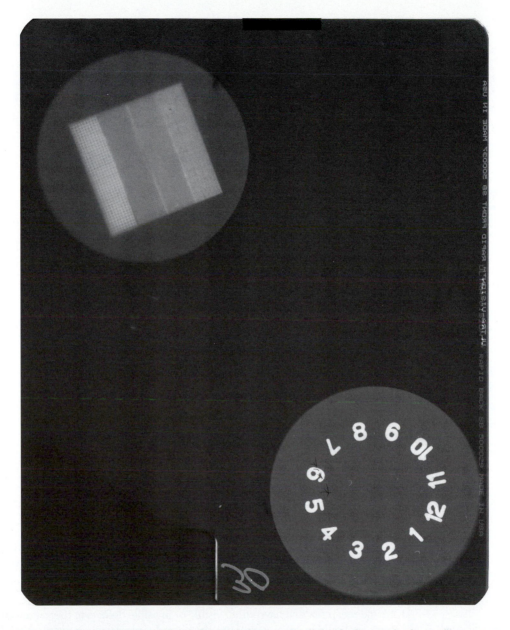

Figure 3-22 *C.* Radiograph demonstrating the loss of image detail that is the result of poor film-screen contact.

Potential Problems

Films that are overexposed or underexposed cannot be easily analyzed for film-screen contact.

IMPORTANT REMINDER

- Because Medical Imaging Departments have numerous image receptors, it would be more convenient to establish a quarterly schedule based on image receptor size for checking film-screen contact.

Ultraviolet Light Test

Rationale

This test is designed to confirm that the image receptors in the Medical Imaging Department are free of dirt, dust, foreign material, and invisible flaws or impurities in the intensifying screens.

Testing Frequency

This test should be performed annually, when image quality appears to be degraded, when an image receptor appears to be damaged, or when the screens of the image receptor are cleaned.

Equipment

- Ultraviolet light/blacklight (5 to 10 V)
- All image receptors in the department

Procedure

A. After the screens of the image receptor have been cleaned, take them into the darkroom and place them open on the loading bench.
B. Plug in the UV light at a convenient outlet in the darkroom.
C. If applicable, close all doors leading into the darkroom.
D. Turn on the UV light.
E. Turn off all safelights and overhead lights.
F. Carefully examine the open image receptors with the UV light. Dirt, dust, and invisible and visible defects in the screens will glow under the UV light.
G. If there is dust or dirt still on the image receptors, they should be cleaned again.
H. Image receptors that have either visible or invisible defects in their intensifying screens should be taken out of circulation and replaced when possible.

Acceptance Parameters

Currently there are no stated parameters for image receptors.

Record Keeping

A record should be kept that documents the date of the test, who performed the test, the results of the test, and the corrective action taken.

Potential Problems

- Suspended or dropped ceilings pose a problem because they trap dust and dirt. Every time the darkroom door is slammed, this type of ceiling generally vibrates and dust, dirt, and particulate matter come free, contaminating the work surfaces of the darkroom and image receptors.
- The NCRP states that freshly loaded image receptors may exhibit poor film-screen contact because of entrapped air. Waiting approximately 15 minutes between loading and exposing of the image receptor may reduce this problem.

IMPORTANT REMINDER

- Because Medical Imaging Departments have numerous image receptors, it would be more convenient to establish a quarterly schedule based on image receptor size for cleaning and examination of the intensifying screens.

ILLUMINATORS

Film illuminators (viewboxes) are commercially available in a variety of formats. They may be purchased as a single unit or in multiple units. Over the last 25 years, film **illuminators** have evolved into sophisticated motorized devices with the capability of displaying films on as many as 50 different patients. Illuminators whether or not they are motorized or nonmotorized have a variety of commonalities, but the two most important are they must have a light and power source for the physician to view radiographs. There are film illuminators used for viewing diagnostic radiographic images and illuminators for viewing mammographic images. The film illuminators used for reading mammographic images are governed by MQSA regulations. Currently there are no regulations governing film illuminators used for reading routine diagnostic images.

The ability of the radiologist to accurately read radiographs depends on the viewing conditions that are present in the reading room environment. The primary nontechnical factors are the brightness of the illuminator and the ambient light levels in the viewing room. It is important that the light bulbs of the illuminator be spectrally matched and have the same intensity. Therefore, it will be necessary to replace all light bulbs in the illuminator when one goes out. This will provide a uniform viewing environment. It is critical that the ambient lighting of the viewing room be kept at a standard level to help assure the accuracy of film reading.

When discussing film illuminators, two characteristics that should be mentioned are illuminance and luminance. The basic unit for illuminance is the lux; 1 lux is equal to 1 lumen per square meter. *Illuminance* is generally defined as the quantity of light that falls on a surface. The typical radiographic film illuminator should have a minimum illuminance level of 5382 lux (500 footcandles). Illuminance can be measured using a photographic light meter (Fig. 3-23). When measuring illuminance using a light meter, the light meter should be set for an ASA of 100. When the light meter is placed against the surface of the illuminator, the illuminance level of between 13 EV (500 footcandles) and 14 EV (1000 footcandles). It should be understood that illuminance levels would not be accepted by MQSA standards.

The basic unit for luminance is the nit; 1 nit is equal to 1 candela per square meter (cd/m^2). *Luminance* is the amount of light being emitted from the surface of the light source. It is the brightness of the illuminator. In medical imaging, luminance is the standard that is used when monitoring the brightness level of film illuminators. Film illuminators used to view radiographs should have a brightness level of 1500 nit. The maximum density that can be visualized at 1500 nit is an optical density of 2.80. Very bright film illuminators will have a luminance level of 3000 nit. The maximum density that can be visualized at 3000 nit is an optical density of 3.10. Determining the

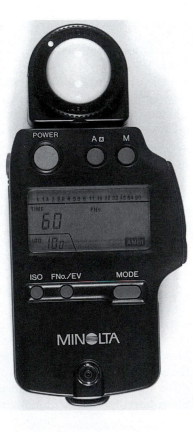

Figure 3-23 Photographic light meter used to measure the illuminance level of a film illuminator.

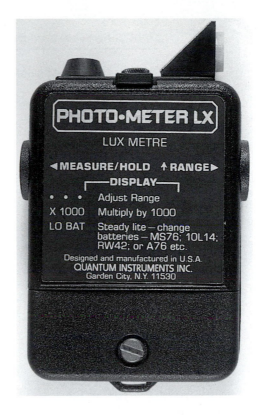

Figure 3-24 Photometer used to measure the luminance level of a film illuminator. *(Courtesy of Nuclear Associates, used with permission.)*

brightness output of an illuminator can be achieved by using a photometer (Fig. 3-24). The photometer is the more accurate than the light meter. Table 3-23 is a simple conversion table for light units. Table 3-24 is a table of light units commonly used in medical imaging.

Table 3-23
Conversion Table for Luminance

To Convert From	To	Multiply By
Lux	Footcandles	10.8
Footcandles	Lux	0.093
Nit (candela/m² [cd/m²])	Footlamberts	3.43
Footlamberts	Nit	0.292

Table 3-24
Light Units Used in Medical Imaging

Unit	Equivalent Unit
1 nit	1 cd/m^2
1 footlambert	3.426 nits
1 lux	1 lumen/m^2
1 footcandle	10.764 lux

Illuminator Uniformity: Illuminance

Rationale

This test is designed to confirm that all illuminators in the Medical Imaging Department and adjacent areas are of the same illumination intensity.

Testing Frequency

All illuminators within the Medical Imaging Department and adjacent areas should be checked semiannually or when light bulbs are replaced.

Equipment

- Photographic light meter with an EV scale
- Illuminators
- Mask with five holes cut in it

Procedure

A. Make the mask.
   - Take a 14 × 17 film from the film bin and expose it to white light.
   - Process the film.
   - In the center of the black film cut a hole approximately a half-inch square.
   - Then cut a half-inch square hole in the center of each of the four quadrants of the film.
B. Reduce the ambient light to normal viewing levels.
C. Place the mask on the illuminator.
D. Set the photographic light meter at an ASA of 100.
E. Place the light meter over the hole in the upper left quadrant of the mask and take a reading on the EV scale. EV is a measure of total exposure.
F. Place the light meter over the hole in the upper right quadrant of the mask and take a reading on the EV scale.
G. Place the light meter over the hole in the lower right quadrant of the mask and take a reading on the EV scale.
H. Place the light meter over the hole in the lower left quadrant of the mask and take a reading on the EV scale.

I. Place the light meter over the hole in the center of the mask and take a reading on the EV scale.
J. Average the five readings to obtain the illumination level of the illuminator in footcandles.
K. Record the results.
L. Repeat steps B through K for the remaining illuminators in the Medical Imaging Department.

Acceptance Parameters

- Illumination intensity should not be less than 500 footcandles or more than 1000 footcandles.
- An EV of 13 at an ASA of 100 is equal to 500 footcandles.
- An EV of 14 at an ASA of 100 is equal to 1000 footcandles.
- In a given illuminator, illumination variations should not exceed 10%.
- In a group of illuminators, illumination variations should not exceed 20%.

Record Keeping

A record should be kept that documents the date of the test, who performed the test, the results of the test, and the corrective action taken.

Potential Problems

Illuminators that have different bulb wattages and colors will lead to reading errors.

IMPORTANT REMINDER

- It is critical that all illuminator readings be conducted in the same lighting conditions that a radiologist would read films. Ambient light should be strictly controlled.
- Illumination intensity for illuminators should be between 500 and 1000 footcandles (EV 13 to 14).
- The viewing surface of the illuminator should be cleaned on a regular basis.
- When one light bulb in an illuminator is replaced, the other light bulbs in the bank of illuminators should be replaced to ensure that uniformity is maintained.

Analysis of the data in Fig. 3-25 demonstrates that the film illuminators do not have the required or necessary illumination levels to adequately view radiographs. The minimum illumination level for film illuminators is 500 footcandles or 13 EV. These particular illuminators have an average illumination level of 9 EV or approximately 31.25 footcandles.

Illuminator Uniformity: Luminance Test

Rationale

This test is designed to confirm that all illuminators in the Medical Imaging Department and adjacent areas are of the same illumination intensity.

Date: 5-18-98				Units of Measurement (Check the appropriate box)		
Location: Radiologist's Office #9				Illuminance: [x] EV □ foot-candles Luminance: □ nits □ cd/m²		
Lower Panel (Left to Right)	**LUQ**	**LLQ**	**Middle**	**RUQ**	**RLQ**	**Average**
Panel #1	8.8	9.0	9.0	9.0	9.1	9.0
Panel #2	9.0	9.2	9.1	9.1	9.2	9.1
Panel #3	8.3	8.9	8.7	8.7	8.5	8.6
Panel #4	8.7	8.9	8.5	8.6	8.4	8.7
Panel #5	8.3	8.6	8.7	8.4	8.5	8.5
Panel #6	8.5	9.0	8.6	8.7	8.9	8.7
Panel #7						
Panel #8						
Upper Panel (Left to Right)						
Panel #1	8.7	9.0	8.8	8.8	8.8	8.8
Panel #2	8.6	9.0	9.0	9.2	9.0	9.0
Panel #3	8.7	9.1	9.0	8.9	8.8	8.9
Panel #4	8.7	9.1	8.4	8.7	8.8	8.7
Panel #5	8.5	8.8	8.3	8.8	8	8.5
Panel #6	8.5	9.1	8.4	8.3	8.9	8.6
Panel #7						
Panel #8						

Figure 3-25 Actual illuminance data from an illuminator permanent record.

Testing Frequency

All illuminators within the Medical Imaging Department and adjacent areas should be checked semiannually or when light bulbs are replaced.

Equipment

- Photometer
- Illuminators
- Calculator
- Record Form

Procedure

A. Reduce the ambient light to normal viewing levels.
B. Set the photometer to read nit (cd/m²). Follow the manufacturer's guidelines.
C. Place the photometer 18 to 24 inches from the illuminator. It is important that the exact distance be duplicated for each illuminator.

D. With the photometer in hand, take readings from different areas of the illuminator. The author suggests that readings be taken from the center, right and left upper quadrants, and the right and left lower quadrants of the illuminator.

E. Once the readings have been obtained they should be averaged and the final value recorded.

F. Repeat steps A through E for all remaining illuminators in the imaging department and ancillary areas.

Acceptance Parameters

- Luminance for general radiographic illuminators should be between 1500 and 3000 nit.
- In a given illuminator, illumination variations should not exceed 10%.
- In a group of illuminators, illumination variations should not exceed 20%.

Record Keeping

A record should be kept that documents the date of the test, who performed the test, the results of the test, and the corrective action taken.

Potential Problems

Illuminators that have different bulb wattages and colors will lead to reading errors.

IMPORTANT REMINDER

- It is critical that all illuminator readings be conducted in the same lighting conditions that a radiologist would read films. Ambient light should be strictly controlled.
- Luminance levels for general radiographic illuminators should be between 1500 and 3000 nits.
- The viewing surface of the illuminator should be cleaned on a regular basis.
- When one light bulb in illuminator is replaced the other light bulbs in the bank of illuminators should be replaced to ensure that uniformity is maintained.

Analysis of the data in Fig. 3-26 demonstrates that these film illuminators meet or exceed the luminance levels that are needed to adequately view radiographs. The recommended luminance level for radiographic film illuminators is 1500 nit. These particular illuminators have an average luminance level of between 2700 and 3400 nit.

LEAD PROTECTIVE DEVICES

There are a variety of **lead protective devices** found in the majority of all Medical Imaging Departments. They include aprons, gloves, thyroid shields, and gonad shields. The lead protective devices used in general diagnostic

Date: February 26, 1999			Units of Measurement (Check the appropriate box)		
Location: Radiologist Office #9			Illuminance: ☐ EV ☐ foot-candles		
			Luminance: ☒ nits ☐ cd/m²		
Lower Panel (Left to Right)	LUQ	LLQ	Middle	RUQ	RLQ	Average
Panel #1	2500	2700	2900	2800	2900	2760
Panel #2	2800	2700	2900	2800	2900	2820
Panel #3	2800	2800	3000	2800	2800	2840
Panel #4	2800	3000	3000	2900	3000	2900
Panel #5	2600	2500	3100	2900	3000	2820
Panel #6	2700	3200	3200	3100	3000	3040
Panel #7						
Panel #8						
Upper Panel (Left to Right)						
Panel #1	2900	3100	3600	3100	3400	3220
Panel #2	2400	3400	3400	2800	3400	3080
Panel #3	2600	3000	3100	2400	3100	2840
Panel #4	2400	3600	3500	2900	3000	3080
Panel #5	2800	3000	3000	2800	3300	2980
Panel #6	2700	3600	4000	2900	3700	3380
Panel #7						
Panel #8						

Figure 3-26 Actual luminance data illuminator permanent record.

imaging are constructed from lead-impregnated vinyl-like materials and have a thickness of between 0.25 and 1.0 mm. Typically the standard is 0.5 mm. Lead protective devices may be evaluated either radiographically or fluoroscopically. The most expedient and cost-effective method is to use fluoroscopy for the evaluation. Although there is no Federal law mandating the frequency that lead protective devices are to be checked for cracks and tears, it should be done regularly. Lead protective devices should be surveyed on receipt and at least annually (Lin et al., May 1988). Depending on the number of lead protective devices in the Medical Imaging Department, it may be necessary to establish a quarterly evaluation system (i.e., for 120 aprons, do the first 40 during the first quarter, etc.). It is important to have a permanent record (Fig. 3-27) of the survey conducted on all protective lead devices in the Medical Imaging Department. The survey should include all areas within the hospital

Lead Protective Devices Survey

Date of Survey: March 8 & 10, 1999   Date of Survey: _____   Date of Survey: _____

Date of Survey: _____   Date of Survey: _____

Location of Device	Inventory Number	Description of Lead Protective Device	Inspection Results					Inspector	Comments
			99	00	01	02	03		
Surgery	10	Light Blue Double Wrap	4					A. Stevens	
Surgery		Green Apron	4					A. Stevens	
Surgery		Green Apron	2					A. Stevens	
Surgery		Dark Blue	1					A. Stevens	
Surgery	66	Light Blue Double Wrap	2					A. Stevens	
Surgery	2	Light Blue Double Wrap	4					A. Stevens	
Surgery	79	Light Blue Wrap Around	1					A. Stevens	
Surgery	Ortho Pod B	Black Multi Color Wrap Around	3					A. Stevens	Re-survey in six months
Surgery	Ortho	Dark Blue with Pocket; Wrap	1					A. Stevens	
Surgery	Ortho	Dark Blue with Pocket; Wrap	1					A. Stevens	
Surgery	Neuro	Dark Blue Wrap	4					A. Stevens	
Surgery	General	Dark Blue Wrap	3					A. Stevens	Re-survey in six months
Surgery	Picker	Royal Blue Wrap	4					A. Stevens	
Surgery	O.R. 17	Medium Blue Wrap	3					A. Stevens	Re-survey in six months
Surgery			4					A. Stevens	
Surgery		Green with Pocket	1					A. Stevens	
Surgery	O.R. Pod D	Medium Blue Wrap	1					A. Stevens	

1 = No defects   2 = Small pinholes; left in service   3 = Small holes\Small Multiple defects; left in service   4 = Large holes\Multiple defects; Remove from service

Figure 3-27 Lead protective devices survey.

137

using ionizing radiation. The permanent record can also serve as an inventory for the department.

Lead Protective Devices Test

Rationale

This test is designed to confirm that all lead protective devices are free of cracks and other defects.

Testing Frequency

All lead protective devices should be checked annually.

Equipment

- All lead protective devices
- Fluoroscopic room

Procedure

A. Set the generator for fluoroscopic mode.
B. Place the lead protective devices individually on the tabletop.
C. Carefully examine each protective device under fluoroscopy for any flaws or defects.
D. When a protective device is found to be flawed, it should be removed from circulation and identified in some fashion (Figs. 3-28A, B, and C).

Acceptance Parameters

There is a zero percent tolerance for lead protective devices.

Record Keeping

A record should be kept that documents the date of the test, who performed the test, the results of the test, and the corrective action taken.

Potential Problems

There are no potential problems that are encountered with this test.

IMPORTANT REMINDER

- Lead aprons, gloves, and mats used for shielding *should never* be folded. Lead aprons and half aprons should be hung correctly on the apron racks. Lead gloves should be placed on the glove stand on the apron rack. Lead mats should be placed in their designated areas. Lead protective devices should be properly cared for.

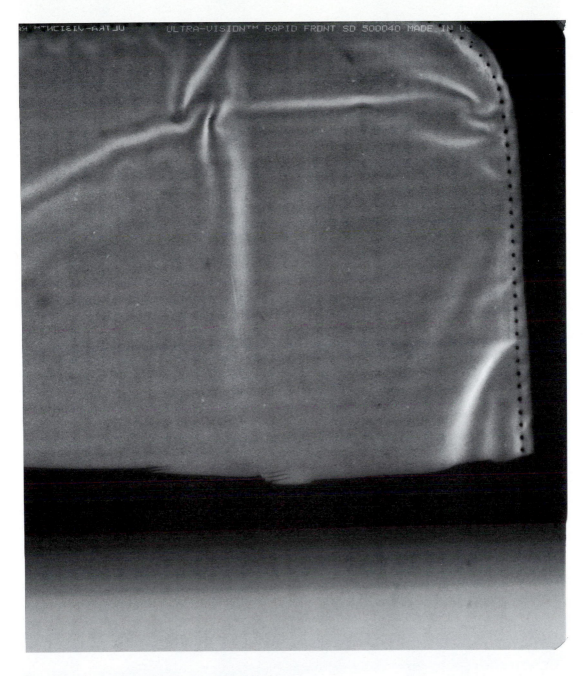

Figure 3-28 *A*. Radiograph of an undamaged lead apron.

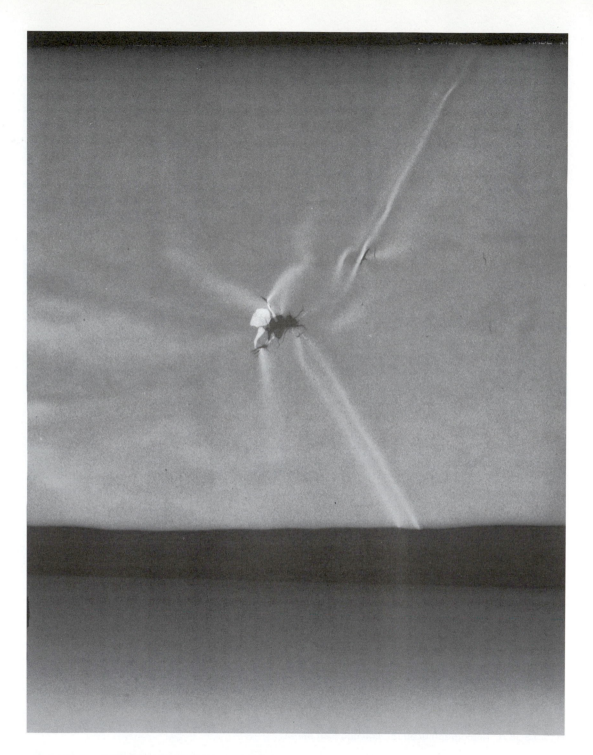

Figure 3-28 *B*. Radiograph of lead apron with a hole.

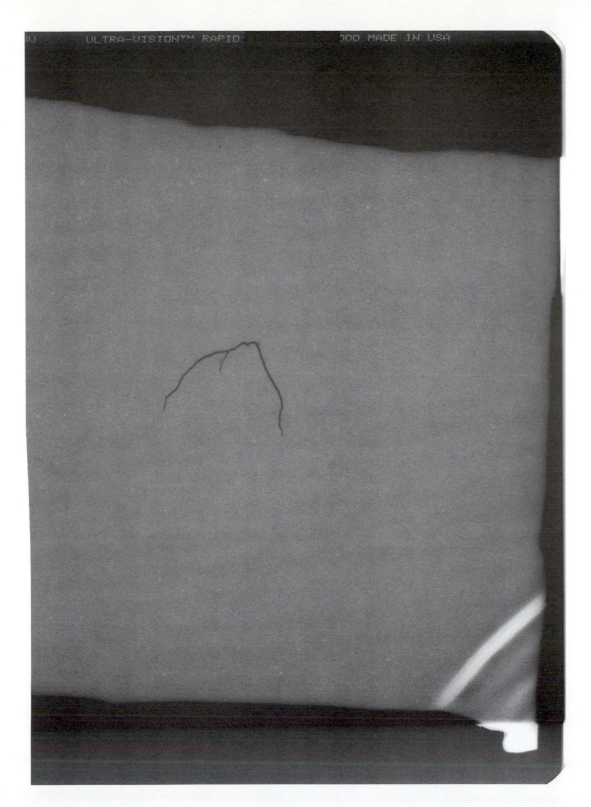

Figure 3-28 *C.* Radiograph of lead apron with a crack.

CHAPTER REVIEW

- The most important QC area in the overall QA program is the darkroom area. The automatic processors of a Medical Imaging Department will have the greatest impact on image quality if they are not operating within established parameters.
- The amount of time required to perform each individual test will be determined by the size of the Medical Imaging Department and the workload volume.
- X-ray film should be stored in an area that is environmentally controlled area where the relative humidity is between 30% and 50% and the temperature is between 10° and 21°C (50° and 70°F).
- Boxes of x-ray film should be stored vertically either on end or on the side.
- Artifacts that appear on a finished radiograph are caused either by the processor or inappropriate handling of the film before or after exposure and prior to processing. Processor artifacts can be eliminated through processor maintenance. Film-handling artifacts can be reduced through proper education of the darkroom personnel and department staff. Artifacts will never be eliminated.
- Repeat analysis within the Medical Imaging Department is used to identify areas where there are problems or potential problems. This type of analysis should never be used as a method for punishing departmental personnel. Repeat rates should be between 4% and 6%, and should never be less than 3% or more than 10%.
- Causal repeat analysis is used to determine what portion of the overall repeat rate is the result of a specific cause.
- The UV light is used to determine how clean and dust free the darkroom is. The acceptance parameters for this test are established by the ACR and MQSA standards.
- The safelight test is used determine if fog on the film is being caused by a crack in the filter or the wrong wattage of bulb in the safelight. The density readings from the 1- and 2-minute rows are used determine if the safelight is functioning properly.
- The tools that are required for processor monitoring are the thermometer, sensitometer, densitometer, the box of QC film, and processor control chart. All processors in the Medical Imaging Department should be included in the processor monitoring program.
- The ACR requires that both the sensitometer and densitometer be recalibrated every 18 months.
- It is important to analyze the processor control charts for runs and trends. A run is a series of seven or more points that fall above or below the midpoint or target aim on any section of the processor control chart. A trend is a series of five consecutive points that present as an upward or downward

pattern on any section of the processor control chart.

- Monitoring of the automatic processor is done on a daily basis and it is important for the person responsible to analyze the processor control charts for any trends that develop. Failure to do this will have an impact on image quality. Sensitometric films are run through each processor at the same time every day. Processor control charts reflect the b + f density, speed index, contrast index, and developer temperature. The midrange density of the control strip reflects the speed index. The density difference between the high and low densities reflects the contrast index.
- Processor control strips should be kept as part of the permanent record for at least 12 months to ensure continuity should a problem with the processors arise. They will serve as a reference point for trouble shooting problems that might arise.
- Film transport time should not exceed 2% of the manufacturer's recommended processing time. If the processing time is in excess of the recommended time, the films will be too dark and of questionable diagnostic value.
- The time-in-solution test is a critical test that should be done annually to ensure that the film is in the developer for the proper amount of time. The manufacturer of the specific processor being tested sets the acceptance parameters for this test.
- The crossover procedure has been developed to assure that established processing parameters are maintained from one film lot to another.
- The loss of image receptor film-screen contact will result in a loss of detail and resolution within the image. The loss of image detail results in increased exposure to the patient and increased departmental costs. Image receptors that cause a loss of detail should be removed from circulation.
- All image receptors should be checked with a UV light after they have been cleaned. The UV light will demonstrate visible and invisible defects in the intensifying screens. The use of the UV light will confirm that the image receptor is free of dirt, dust, and particulate matter.
- All radiographs should be viewed in reduced ambient light. All illuminators in the Medical Imaging Department and ancillary areas should provide the same amount of illumination. When light bulbs are replaced in illuminators, the amount of illumination should not exceed 10% of the illumination provided by a single illuminator or 20% of the illumination provided by a group of illuminators.
- Illuminance is the amount of light that falls on a surface. The unit for illuminance is the lux; 1 lux is equal to 1 lumen/m^2. Illumination intensity for illuminators should be between 500 footcandles and 1000 footcandles.
- Luminance is the brightness of the illuminator. The unit for luminance is the nit; 1 nit is equal 1 cd/m^2. Film illuminators that are used to view radiographs should have a brightness level of 1500 nit. The maximum optical density that can be visualized at 1500 nit is 2.80.
- Lead protective devices need to be checked on a regular basis by either

radiographic or fluoroscopic means. When a defect is demonstrated, that particular protective device must be removed from use. A defect allows radiation through, exposing the person wearing the device.

DISCUSSION QUESTIONS

1. Why is trend analysis important in processor monitoring?
2. Why is darkroom cleanliness important?
3. How is image quality affected when processor control parameters are increased or decreased?
4. Why is the crossover procedure important?
5. What viewing conditions are necessary for viewing finished radiographs?
6. How is image quality affected by poor film-screen contact?
7. What is the rationale for performing repeat analysis?
8. How should x-ray film be stored?
9. What environmental conditions need to be established for x-ray film storage and usage?
10. How do film artifacts affect film quality?
11. What is the procedure for caring for lead protective devices?
12. What should be done if a lead protective device is found to have a defect?
13. What are acceptance parameters for the quality control tests described in this chapter?
14. Why are the darkroom UV test and the image receptor test necessary?
15. Who is responsible for doing the repeat/reject analysis?
16. What unit is used to express illumination intensity?

REVIEW QUESTIONS

1. How often should lead protective devices be checked for defects?
   a. Weekly
   b. Monthly
   c. Quarterly
   d. Annually
2. Which of the following devices would be used to detect poor screen contact?
   a. Penetrometer
   b. Resolution test tool
   c. Ultraviolet light
   d. Wire mesh tool
3. Which of the following statements is correct?
   a. The amount of light either scattered or emitted by a surface is called illuminance.
   b. The amount of light falling on a surface is called illuminance.

    c. The amount of light being reflected is called illuminance.

    d. The amount of light falling, being scattered, or emitted by a surface is called illuminance.

4. The acceptable variations of illumination quadrants in a given illuminator should not exceed

    a. 5%

    b. 10%

    c. 15%

    d. 20%

5. What are the acceptable base plus fog parameters in processor monitoring?

    a. ±0.01 of the total base plus fog

    b. ±0.03 of the total base plus fog

    c. ±0.05 of the total base plus fog

    d. ±0.1 of the total base plus fog

6. What are the acceptable temperature parameters in processor monitoring?

    a. ±0.5°F

    b. ±1°F

    c. ±1.5°F

    d. ±2°F

7. When performing processor quality control, what is the acceptable contrast index parameters?

    a. ±0.20

    b. ±0.15

    c. ±0.10

    d. ±0.05

8. What are the acceptable speed index parameters for processor monitoring?

    a. ±0.05

    b. ±0.10

    c. ±0.15

    d. ±0.20

9. Which of the following statements is correct regarding optimum viewing conditions for radiographic images?

    a. Background or ambient lighting should be as bright as possible.

    b. The color of light produced by illuminators is not important.

    c. Individual light bulbs should be replaced as they burn out.

    d. All illuminators in the department should produce the same light level.

10. Group-to-group illuminator variations within the department should not exceed

    a. 5%

    b. 10%

    c. 15%

    d. 20%

11. The overall repeat rate of a department should not fall below
    a. 3%
    b. 5%
    c. 7%
    d. 10%

12. The primary purpose of including repeat analysis as part of a QA program in radiology is to determine
    a. how much film to purchase
    b. which quality control tests to perform
    c. the most common source of error
    d. the need for changes in staffing

13. Which of the following statements is correct?
    a. The amount of light either scattered or emitted by a surface is called luminance.
    b. The amount of light falling on a surface is called luminance.
    c. The amount of light being reflected is called luminance.
    d. The amount of light falling, being scattered, or emitted by a surface is called luminance.

14. Which of the following devices is used to imprint a 21-step stepwedge on a film?
    a. Densitometer
    b. Sensitometer
    c. Ultraviolet light
    d. Wire mesh tool

15. If the total processing time from dry film to dry film exceeds 2% of the manufacturer's recommended processing time, what will the finished radiograph look like?
    a. The finished film will not be affected.
    b. The finished film will be light.
    c. The finished film will be dark.
    d. There is not enough information given.

16. Film illuminators for general radiography should have a luminance level of
    a. 1500 cd/m²
    b. 2000 cd/m²
    c. 2500 cd/m²
    d. 3500 cd/m²

17. What is the recommended storage conditions for radiographic film?
    1. 30% to 50% relative humidity
    2. 50% to 70% relative humidity
    3. Between 50° and 70°F
    4. Between 70° and 90°F
    a. 1 only
    b. 3 only

    c. 1 and 3 only
    d. 2 and 4 only
18. Base plus fog is measured on
    a. any clear area of the film
    b. a high-density step
    c. a medium-density step
    d. a low-density step
19. Which of the following statements is correct?
    a. The contrast index is determined by the density difference between the high density and midrange density of the processor control strip.
    b. The contrast index is determined by the density difference between the high density and low density of the processor control strip.
    c. The contrast index is determined by the density difference between the midrange density and low density of the processor control strip.
    d. The contrast index is determined by the density difference between the high density and base plus fog density of the processor control strip.
20. Which of the following statements is correct?
    a. The base plus fog density of the processor control determines the speed index strip.
    b. The high density of the processor control strip determines the speed index.
    c. The low fog density of the processor control strip determines the speed index.
    d. The midrange density of the processor control strip determines the speed index.
21. The luminance level of a group of viewboxes used in general radiography was tested and found to have a luminance of 2500 nit. What conclusion could be made regarding these particular viewboxes?
    a. The luminance level of the viewboxes is within the acceptance parameters.
    b. The luminance level of the viewboxes is not within the acceptance parameters.
    c. The luminance level of the viewboxes exceeds the acceptance parameters.
22. Densitometers and sensitometers should be recalibrated every
    a. 6 to 12 months
    b. 12 to 18 months
    c. 18 to 24 months
    d. 24 to 36 months
23. The battery of the sensitometer should be changed at least every
    a. month
    b. 6 months
    c. 9 months
    d. 12 months

24. The density difference between the exposed and unexposed portion a safelight test film should not exceed a density of
    a. 0.01
    b. 0.03
    c. 0.05
    d. 0.06
25. A point on the graph that exceeds the control limits is called
    a. cycling
    b. a point out of control
    c. a run
    d. a trend

4

Radiographic Systems

GOALS

1. To learn the required and optional quality control tests for radiographic equipment.
2. To understand the findings from radiographic quality control tests.
3. To understand the required procedures for performing radiographic quality control tests.
4. To learn the required quality control tests for mobile radiographic equipment.

OBJECTIVES

1. Identify the routine quality control tests performed on a radiographic suite.
2. State the rationale for performing each quality control test.
3. Explain the rationale behind testing frequency.
4. Identify and discuss how often each test is performed.
5. Identify and describe the equipment used for all quality control tests.
6. Describe and discuss the procedure for doing each test.
7. State the acceptance parameters for each test.
8. Identify and discuss potential problems that might arise during or after each test.
9. Discuss problems that might result in erroneous findings for each test.
10. Discuss and explain the importance of record keeping.
11. Analyze and interpret test results.
12. Identify and discuss the tests performed on mobile radiographic equipment.

INTRODUCTION

As stated, a quality assurance (QA) program has many components and regular quality control (QC) is a critical part that is intended to minimize cost, improve diagnosis, and minimize radiation exposure to the patient and technical staff. There are a variety of QC tests performed on fixed radiographic systems, and many of them also carry over to mobile radiographic systems (Table 4-1). The radiographic QC tests presented in this chapter are noninvasive tests. The tests are both simple and complex. QC testing of both fixed and mobile radiographic systems should be carried out on a routine schedule by the person assigned. There is nothing written that says the technical staff assigned to rotate through a particular radiographic room cannot assist in the testing program. In fact, it is an excellent idea because the technical staff can provide valuable information to the quality control technologist. This chapter is divided into four sections—the x-ray tube, the collimator, the generator, and grids.

THE TUBE AND COLLIMATOR

When discussing the x-ray tube and collimator, it is necessary to briefly discuss how x-rays are produced, the formation of the focal spot, and the basic construction of the collimator. The production of x-rays requires a source of elec-

Table 4-1
Radiographic Equipment: Testing Frequency, Acceptance Parameters

Quality Control Test	Frequency of Test	Acceptance Parameters	Performed on Mobile Equipment
Automatic collimation	Semiannual	± 3% of the SID	No
Light field/beam alignment	Semiannual	± 2% of SID	Yes
Beam perpendicularity	Semiannual	The image of the upper bead should fall within 5 mm of the lower bead	Yes
Bucky/light field alignment	Semiannual	± 2% of SID	No
Bucky/beam perpendicularity	Semiannual	The image of the upper bead should fall within 5 mm of the lower bead	No
Grid image receptors, etc.	Semiannual	Uniform film density of 1.2 ± 0.10	No
AEC reproducibility	Annual	± 0.1 of each image or ±5%	No
AEC mA consistency	Annual	± 0.2 of each image	No
AEC kVp consistency	Annual	± 0.2 of each image	No
AEC sensor consistency	Annual	± 0.2 of each image	No
AEC exposure consistency with varying patient thickness	Annual	± 0.3 of each image	No
AEC exposure consistency with varying field size	Annual	± 0.1 of each image	No
AEC backup time	Annual	6 seconds or 600 mAs, whichever comes first	
Light field illuminance	Annual	160 lux or 15 footcandles	
Focal spot size: star test	Annual	< 0.8 mm up to 50% greater 0.8 mm to 1.5 mm up to 40% greater > 1.5 mm up to 30% greater	Yes
mA linearity	Annual	± 10% over clinical range	Yes
Exposure reproducibility	Annual	± 5%	Yes
mAs reciprocity	Annual	± 10%	Yes
mAs reciprocity (stepwedge)	Annual	± 0.10 OD	Yes
Exposure time: single phase	Annual	Refer to manual spin top test	No
Exposure time: three phase	Annual	± 5%	No
Source-to-image distance	Annual	± 2%	No
Kilovoltage accuracy	Annual	± 4 kVp	Yes
mR/mAs output	Annual	± 10%	Yes
Timer linearity	Annual	± 10%	No
Grid uniformity (Bucky)	Annual	Uniform films; no grid lines, density of 1.20 ± 0.10	No
Grid alignment	Annual	Uniform films; optical density of 1.0 ± 0.10	No
Tomography: section level	Annual	± 5 mm	No
Tomography: spatial resolution	Annual	40 mesh or better	No
Tomography: exposure uniformity and beam path	Annual	Per manufacturer's specifications	No
Visual checks	Annual	Pass/fail	Yes

trons, a means of accelerating the electrons, and some way to suddenly stop the electrons. This is achieved by having an anode and cathode enclosed in a glass tube that has had all of the air removed. The source of the electrons is the cathode, which generally has two filaments. The electrons are boiled off the filament when a current heats the filament. When a voltage is applied to the cathode the speed of the electrons is increased and they are accelerated at or near the speed of light across a very short distance (less than 1 inch) toward the anode. Upon reaching the anode, the high-speed electrons are suddenly stopped and x-rays are produced. The electron to x-ray energy conversion is an inefficient process because less than 1% of the resulting energy is in the form of x-rays. The remaining energy conversion is in the form of heat (>99%). The x-rays that are produced are Bremsstrahlung and characteristic. **Bremsstrahlung x-rays** are the result of the incident electrons interacting with the nuclei of the target atoms. **Characteristic x-rays** are produced when incident electrons interact with the inner shell (K shell) electrons of the atom. The x-rays produced by this interaction will be characteristic of the target material. The type of target material used influences both the **discrete** (characteristic) and the **continuous** (Bremsstrahlung) portions of the x-ray emission spectrum. As the atomic number of the target material increases, there is a shift in the discrete portion of the x-ray emission spectrum to the right. Therefore, more x-rays will be produced per unit of energy and the energy of the characteristic x-rays will be higher. The continuous portion of the x-ray emission spectrum will increase in quantity but there will be no change in quality (energy).

Focal spot size is determined by several factors (Fig. 4-1), but it is important to remember that x-rays originate from a point source on the anode. When the **focal spot** is projected onto the image receptor, its actual shape is rectangular. All of the factors identified in Fig. 4-1 are of great importance in determining focal spot size, but the steepness of the anode angle plays an important role in determining the size. It is important to keep in mind that anode angle is measured from the perpendicular. The standard anode angle for most

◆ **Filament size and shape**

◆ **Filament position within the focusing cup**

◆ **Physical dimensions of the focusing cup**

◆ **Distance between the anode and cathode**

◆ **Anode angle**

Figure 4-1 Factors that determine focal spot size.

diagnostic applications is approximately 12°. A steep anode angle will result in a smaller focal spot size, which will produce greater resolution but will have a heat loading limitation. In other words, the x-ray tube will need to cool longer before additional exposures can be made and lower mA techniques should be used. An x-ray tube with a target angle that is less steep will have a larger apparent focal spot that can accept more of a heat load, but has a decrease in resolution (Fig. 4-2). This trade off will allow more heat loading and therefore the use of higher mA techniques.

The variable aperture collimator of the x-ray tube is designed to provide the radiographer with a variety of field sizes. The collimator consists of first stage

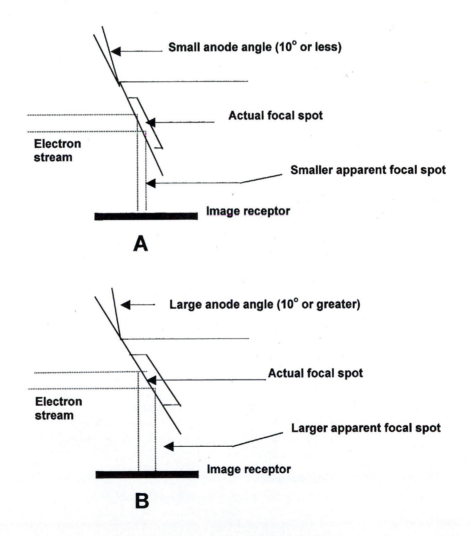

Figure 4-2 The relationship between anode angle and focal spot.

entrance shutters, a set of longitudinal shutters, a set of transverse shutters, a light source, and a mirror. The first stage shutters are located at the top of the collimator; these shutters protrude into the x-ray tube housing and function to reduce the off-focus radiation produced by the anode. The longitudinal and transverse shutters are located within the collimator housing and can be varied to obtain the desired field size. This is achieved by adjusting two knobs or levers on (the front of the) collimator housing or by automatic sensing devices that are located in the bucky tray and result in positive beam limitation (PBL). The selected field size is made visible by a light and mirror in the upper part of the collimator housing. The mirror is angled approximately 45° and is used to project the light down onto the patient. When the collimator light burns out, it will be necessary to replace the bulb. Replacing the bulb will require great care because it is easy to accidentally knock the mirror out of alignment. After replacing the bulb, a light field test must be performed. When replacing the collimator light source, it is important to remember to turn off the machine. Failure to turn off the machine could result in electrical shock and serious injury.

There are a variety of QC tests that should be performed on the tube and collimator to ensure that they are within acceptance parameters. When either the tube or collimator is not within acceptance parameters, service must be called immediately. The tests performed are focal spot size, light field/beam alignment, beam perpendicularity, light field/beam alignment/beam perpendicularity, and source-to-distance indicator.

Focal Spot Size: Star Test Pattern

Rationale

This procedure is designed to confirm that the small and large focal spots are within the tube manufacturers stated specifications.

Testing Frequency

Focal spot size should be checked annually, when the x-ray tube has been replaced, or as workload dictates.

Equipment

- 2° star test pattern (Fig. 4-3)
- Tape
- 8 × 10 mammography image receptor
- Ruler (clear plastic) with centimeter markings
- A lead "A" and "C" to indicate the anode and cathode or some other markers
- 6-inch carpenter's level

Procedure

A. Place the image receptor on the tabletop.
B. Tape the star test pattern to the faceplate of the collimator.
C. Use the 6-inch carpenter's level to check that the tube and the tabletop are level.

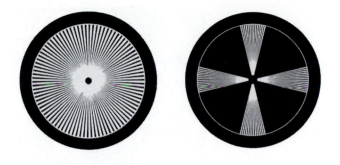

Figure 4-3 Star test patterns used to measure focal spot size. *(Courtesy of Nuclear Associates, used with permission.)*

D. The central ray should be perpendicular to the star test pattern. The central ray should pass through the center of the test pattern.
E. The tube should be set at a 24-inch SID.
F. Collimate the beam to include the image on the image receptor. Within the collimated area, indicate the anode side of the tube with a marker and the cathode side of the tube with a marker (i.e., "A" and "C" or a penny and nickel).
G. Select the small focal spot and exposure factors that will provide an optical density of approximately 1.0.
H. The technique selected should use one-half the maximum operating mA at 70 kVp.
I. Expose the film and process the film (Fig. 4-4).
J. For the large focal spot, repeat steps H and I.
K. Calculate the size of the small and large focal spots.
- Calculate the magnification using the following formula:

$$M = \frac{\text{Image Size (mm)}}{\text{Object Size (mm)}}$$

- Find the zero contrast area (the area of blur) on the film. The zero contrast area is found by visually scanning the image from the outer edge inward to the area where blur is detected.
- Measure both the parallel and perpendicular diameter of the zero contrast area across its greatest extent.
- The parallel diameter will be called D_1 and the perpendicular diameter will be called D_2.
- The actual size of the focal spot (length and width) can be determined by using the following formula:

$$\text{FSS}_{\text{Length}} = \frac{N}{57.3} \times \frac{D_1}{(M-1)} \text{ and FSS}_{\text{Width}} = \frac{N}{57.3} \times \frac{D_2}{(M-1)}$$

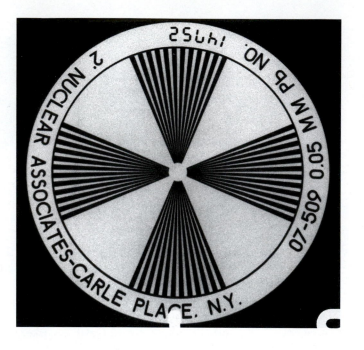

Figure 4-4 Star test pattern image of the small focal spot.

where FSS is the focal spot size in mm; N is the angle of the star test pattern (i.e., 2°, 1.5°, 1°, etc.); D_1 and D_2 are the diameters of the parallel and perpendicular zero contrast areas in mm; and M is the magnification.

    L. Record the results.

Acceptance Parameters

The National Electrical Manufacturers Association (NEMA) standards for new tubes are listed in the chart below.

Focal Spot Size	Allowance Parameters
<0.8 mm	Up to 50% greater
0.8 mm to 1.5 mm	Up to 40% greater
>1.5 mm	Up to 30% greater

Record Keeping

A record should be kept that documents the date of the test, who performed the test, the results of the test, and the corrective action taken.

    Note: When corrective action is taken, the before and after films should be kept on file.

Potential Problems

- If the tube or table is not level there is a remote possibility that image will be affected.
- Motion of the tube due to vibrations will the cause image blurring.
- Bucky vibration may cause image blurring.

Points to Ponder

- For smaller focal spots that are less than 0.5 mm, a 0.5° star, 1° star, or 1.5° star should be used to measure the focal spot size.

- It is important to use the same kVp for both small and large focal spots. Using an extremely high kVp may result in **filament bloom** (expansion of the filament).

- NEMA standards are based on the use of direct exposure film. For preliminary tests, single emulsion film and single screen image receptors are acceptable.

BRAIN TEASER 1

The stated focal spot sizes for a conventional tomography tube are 0.4 and 0.8 millimeters. After performing the focal spot test using the star test pattern, you determine that the small focal spot is actually 0.9 millimeter and the large focal spot is actually 1.8 millimeters. Are the focal spots within acceptance parameters? What would be your recommendations?

EXAMPLE 1

Calculate the focal spot size for Fig. 4-4.

1. The diameter of the image is 112 millimeters and the diameter of the object is 55 millimeters.

2. $\text{Magnification} = \dfrac{\text{Image Diameter}}{\text{Object Diameter}} = \dfrac{112 \text{ mm}}{55 \text{ mm}} = 2.04$

3. For the parallel diameter (anode to cathode):

$$\text{FSS} = \frac{N}{57.3} \times \frac{D_1}{(M-1)} = \frac{2}{57.3} \times \frac{55 \text{ mm}}{(2.04-1)} = .035 \times \frac{55 \text{ mm}}{1.04} = .035 \times 52.9 = 1.9$$

$N = 2 \quad M = 2.04 \quad D_1 = 55 \text{ mm}$

4. For the perpendicular diameter:

$$\text{FSS} = \frac{N}{57.3} \times \frac{D_2}{(M-1)} = \frac{2}{57.3} \times \frac{77 \text{ mm}}{(2.04-1)} = .035 \times \frac{77 \text{ mm}}{1.04} = .035 \times 74 = 2.6$$

$N = 2 \quad M = 2.04 \quad D_2 = 77$

5. At the mA and kVp setting used the focal spot size is 1.9×2.6 millimeters.
6. The stated large focal spot of this tube is 1.2 millimeters. The measured focal spot of 1.9 millimeters is in compliance with NEMA standards.

Light Field/Beam Alignment Test

Rationale

This procedure is designed to confirm that the x-ray field and **light field** are the same.

Testing Frequency

The light field and x-ray field should be checked semiannually, when the collimator has been replaced, a light bulb has been replaced, or when the x-ray tube has been replaced.

Equipment

- 8×10 image receptor
- Collimator test template (see to Fig. 4-8)
- 6-inch carpenter's level
- Ruler with centimeter and inch markings

Procedure

A. Place the image receptor on the tabletop.
B. Center the tube to the image receptor and set the tube at a 40-inch SID.
C. Use the 6-inch carpenter's level to check that the tube and the tabletop are level.
D. Place the template on top of the image receptor. The dot in the corner of the template should correspond to the patient's right shoulder. The dot helps to determine the direction of collimator error later.
E. Collimate the x-ray beam to the rectangular outline on the template. This area is approximately 7×5 inches.
F. Set an approximate technique of 10 mAs at 60 kVp for single-phase units and 2.5 mAs at 60 kVp for three-phase units. The selected technique depends on the speed of the image receptor system.
G. Expose the film.
H. Open the collimator shutters to an 8 x 10 size and expose the film again using a technique of 0.4 mAs at 45 kV.
I. Process the film.
J. Measure the image (Fig. 4-5).
K. Record the results.

Acceptance Parameters

National Council on Radiation Protection and Measurements (NCRP) Report #99 makes the following recommendations.

- The collimator light to x-ray field must be within ±2% of the SID.

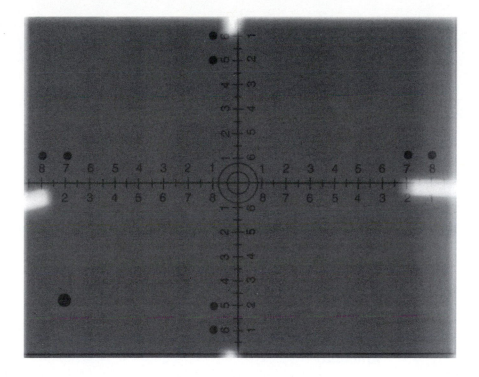

Figure 4-5 Template image.

- At a 40-inch SID, the light field to should be within ±0.8 inches.
- At a 100-centimeter SID, the light field should be within ±2 centimeters.

Record Keeping

A record should be kept that documents the date of the test, who performed the test, the results of the test, and the corrective action taken.

Note: When corrective action is taken, the before and after films should be kept on file.

Potential Problems

- Failure to level the table could provide the radiographer with inaccurate measurements.
- Failure to have the x-ray tube perpendicular could provide the radiographer with inaccurate measurements.

Points to Ponder

- The light field/beam alignment and beam perpendicularity test may be combined when the collimator test tool and beam alignment test tool are used in conjunction.
- This test should be performed whenever the collimator light bulb is replaced.

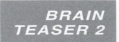

The light field/beam alignment indicates that the light field is greater on the longitudinal axis and half as much on the vertical axis of the film. Can you identify the possible cause or causes for this finding?

Light Field/Beam Alignment: The Nine-Cent Test

Rationale

This procedure is designed to confirm that the x-ray field and light field are the same.

Testing Frequency

The light field and x-ray field should be checked semiannually, when the collimator or a light bulb has been replaced, or when the x-ray tube has been replaced.

Equipment

- 10 × 12 image receptor
- 9 pennies
- Ruler with centimeter and inch markings
- 6-inch carpenter's level

Procedure

A. Place the image receptor on the tabletop.
B. Center to the tube to the image receptor and set the tube at a 40-inch SID.
C. Collimate to a 6- × 6-inch field size.
D. Use the 6-inch carpenter's level to check that the tube and the tabletop are level.
E. At the center of each edge of the light field place two pennies side by side; one penny is placed in the light field and the other penny is placed outside the light field (Fig. 4-6).
F. Place the ninth penny within the light field to indicate the anode side of the tube and the Bucky handle side of the table.
G. Set a technique comparable to a hand technique and expose the film.
H. Open the collimators to the size of the film and expose the film again using an approximate technique of 0.4 mAs at 45 kVp. The technique selected depends on the type of film used and the speed of the imaging system.
I. Process the film.
J. Measure the image (Fig. 4-7).
K. Record the results.

Acceptance Parameters

NCRP Report #99 makes the following recommendations.
- The collimator light to x-ray field must be within ±2% of the SID.

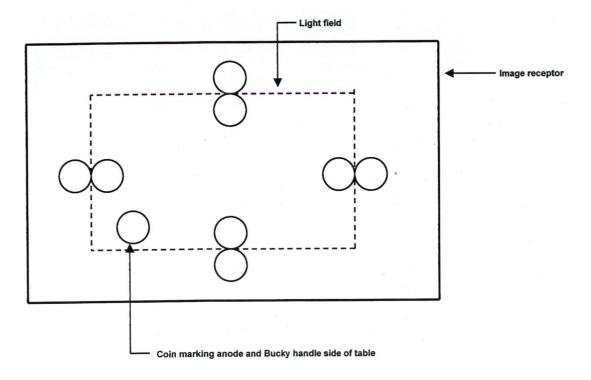

Figure 4-6 Diagram of the layout for the nine penny test.

- At a 40-inch SID, the light field should be within ±0.8 inches.
- At a 100-centimeter SID, the light field should be within ±2 centimeters (about 1 penny).

  Note: The width of a penny is approximately 0.8 inches or 2 centimeters.

Record Keeping

A record should be kept that documents the date of the test, who performed the test, the results of the test, and the corrective action taken.

  Note: When corrective action is taken, the before and after films should be kept on file.

Potential Problems

- Failure to level the table could provide the radiographer with inaccurate measurements.
- Failure to have the x-ray tube perpendicular could provide the radiographer with inaccurate measurements.

Points to Ponder

- This test should be performed whenever the collimator light bulb is replaced.

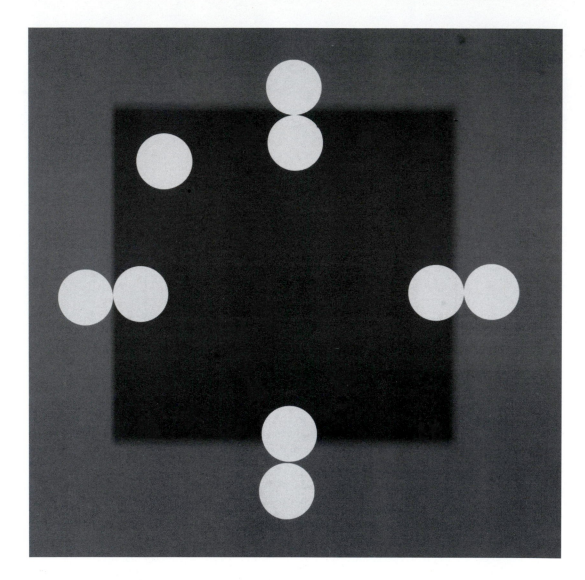

Figure 4-7 Image of the nine penny test.

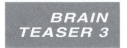

The light field/beam alignment indicates that the light field is greater on both the longitudinal axis and vertical axis of the film. Can you identify the possible cause or causes for this finding?

Light Field/Beam Alignment/Beam Perpendicularity Test

Rationale

This procedure is designed to confirm that the x-ray field, light field, and beam perpendicularity are the same.

Testing Frequency

The light field and x-ray field and **beam perpendicularity** should be checked semiannually, when the collimator or a light bulb has been replaced, or when the x-ray tube has been replaced.

Equipment

- 8 × 10 image receptor
- Collimator test template and beam alignment test tool (Fig. 4-8)
- 6-inch carpenter's level
- Ruler with centimeter and inch markings

Procedure

A. Place the image receptor on the tabletop.
B. Center the tube to the image receptor and set the tube at a 40-inch SID.
C. Use the level to assure that the tabletop and x-ray tube are level.
D. Place the template on top of the image receptor. The dot in the corner of the template should correspond to the patient's right shoulder. The dot helps determine the direction of collimator error later.

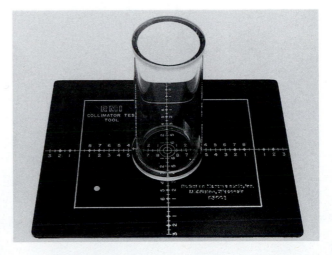

Figure 4-8 Beam alignment test tool and collimator template. *(Courtesy of Nuclear Associates, used with permission.)*

E. Place the beam alignment test tool in the middle of the template.
F. Collimate the x-ray beam to the rectangular outline on the template. This is an area approximately 7 × 5 inches.
G. Set an approximate technique of 10 mAs at 60 kVp for single-phase units and 2.5 mAs at 60 kVp for three-phase units. The type of film used and the imaging system speed will determine the technique used.
H. Expose the film.
 I. Open the collimator shutters to an 8 × 10 size and expose the film again using a technique of 0.4 mAs at 45 kV. The type of film used and the imaging system speed will determine the technique used.
J. Process the film.
K. Measure the image (Fig. 4-9A and B).
L. Record the results.

Acceptance Parameters

NCRP Report #99 makes the following recommendations.

• The collimator light to x-ray field must be within ±2% of the SID.

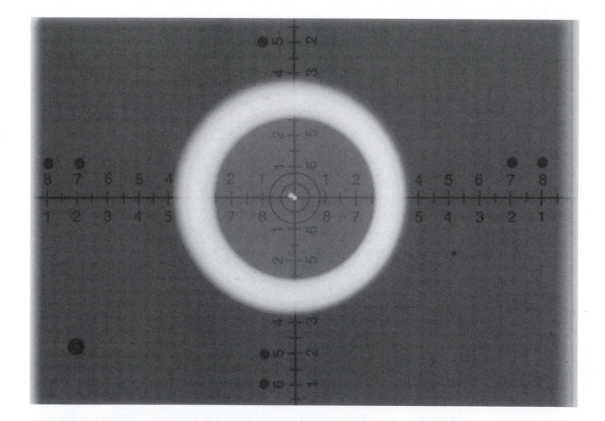

Figure 4-9 *A*. Radiograph demonstrating satisfactory beam alignment.

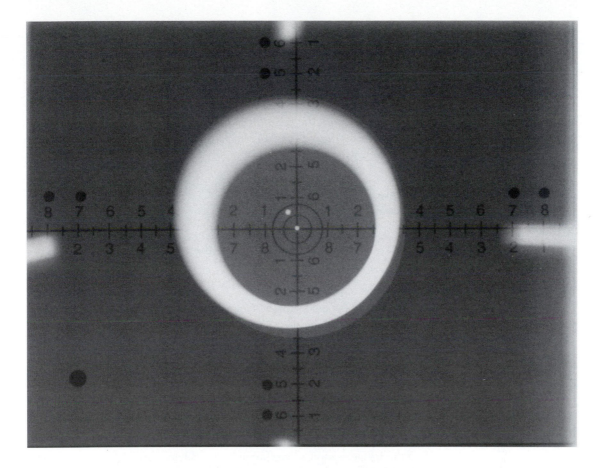

Figure 4-9 *B.* Radiograph demonstrating beam alignment being off by 1.5°.

- At a 40-inch SID, the light field to should be within ±0.8 inches.
- At a 100-centimeter SID, the light field should be within ±2 centimeters.
- For beam alignment, the upper bead should be within 5 millimeters of the lower bead.
  - If the image of the magnified (upper) bead intersects the first ring, the beam is approximately 1.5° away from perpendicular.
  - If the image of the magnified (upper) bead intersects the second ring the beam is approximately 3.0° away from perpendicular.

Record Keeping

It is important to record all information in the room and master QC logs. A record should be kept that documents the date of the test, who performed the test, the results of the test, and the corrective action taken.

Note: When corrective action is taken, the before and after films should be kept on file.

Potential Problems

- Failure to level the table could provide the radiographer with inaccurate measurements.
- Failure to have the x-ray tube perpendicular could provide the radiographer with inaccurate measurements.

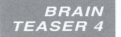

The radiograph from the beam perpendicularity test demonstrates that the upper bead is outside the second ring. Can you identify the possible cause or causes for this finding?

Bucky/Light Field Alignment Test

Rationale

This procedure is designed to confirm that the x-ray field and light field are the same.

Testing Frequency

The light field and x-ray field should be checked semiannually, when the collimator or a light bulb has been replaced, or when the x-ray tube has been replaced.

Equipment

- 8 × 10 image receptor
- Collimator test template (see Fig. 4-8)
- 6-inch carpenter's level
- Ruler with centimeter and inch markings

Procedure

A. Place the image receptor lengthwise in the Bucky tray.

B. Center the tube to the image receptor and set the tube at a 40-inch SID.

C. Use the 6-inch carpenter's level to check that the tube and the tabletop are level.

D. Place the template on top of the table with the dot in the lower left corner of the template corresponding to the patient's right shoulder. The dot helps to determine the direction of collimator error later.

E. Disengage the automatic collimation and collimate the x-ray beam to the rectangular outline on the template. This area is approximately 7 × 5 inches.

F. Set an approximate technique of 20 mAs at 60 kVp for single-phase units and 10 mAs at 60 kVp for three-phase units. The actual technique will be determined by the speed of the image receptor system.

G. Expose the film.

H. Open the collimator shutters to an 8 × 10 size and expose the image receptor again using a technique of 5 mAs at 60 kV. The actual technique will be determined by the speed of the image receptor system.

I. Process the film.
J. Measure the image.
K. Record the results.

Acceptance Parameters

NCRP Report #99 makes the following recommendations.
- The collimator light to x-ray field must be within ±2% of the SID.
  - At a 40-inch SID, the light field to should be within ±0.8 inches.
  - At a 100-centimeter SID, the light field should be within ±2 centimeters.

Record Keeping

A record should be kept that documents the date of the test, who performed the test, the results of the test, and the corrective action taken.

   Note: When corrective action is taken, the before and after films should be kept on file.

Potential Problems

- Failure to level the table could provide the radiographer with inaccurate readings.
- Failure to have the x-ray tube perpendicular could provide the radiographer with inaccurate readings.
- Failure to have the tube centered to the table will provide inaccurate measurements.
- Failure to have the Bucky tray completely in will result in inaccurate measurements.

Points to Ponder

- The light field/beam alignment and beam perpendicularity test may be combined when the collimator test tool and beam alignment test tool are used at the same time.

Bucky/Light Field/Beam Alignment/Beam Perpendicularity Test

Rationale

This procedure is designed to confirm that the x-ray field, light field, and beam perpendicularity are the same.

Testing Frequency

The light field and x-ray field and beam perpendicularity should be checked semiannually, when the collimator or a light bulb has been replaced, or when the x-ray tube has been replaced.

Equipment

- 8 × 10 image receptor
- Collimator test template and beam alignment test tool (see Fig. 4-8)
- 6-inch carpenter's level
- Ruler with centimeter and inch markings

Procedure

A. Place the image receptor on the tabletop.
B. Center the tube to the image receptor and set the tube at a 40-inch SID.
C. Use the 6-inch carpenter's level to check that the tube and the tabletop are level.
D. Place the template on top of the image receptor with the dot in the lower left corner of the template corresponding to the patient's right shoulder. The dot help determines the direction of collimator error later.
E. Place the beam alignment test tool in the middle of the template.
F. Collimate the x-ray beam to the rectangular outline on the template. This area is approximately 7×5 inches.
G. The technique used depends on the speed of the image receptor system being used. A suggested starting technique would be 20 mAs at 60 kVp for single-phase units and 10 mAs at 60 kVp for three-phase units.
H. Expose the film.
I. Open the collimator shutters to an 8×10 size and expose the film again using a technique of 5 mAs at 60 kV.
J. Process the film.
K. Measure the image.
L. Record the results.

Acceptance Parameters

NCRP Report #99 makes the following recommendations.
- The collimator light to x-ray field must be within ±2% of the SID.
  - At a 40-inch SID, the light field to should be within ±0.8 inches.
  - At a 100-centimeter SID, the light field should be within ±2 centimeters.
- For **beam alignment** the upper bead should be within 5 millimeters of the lower bead.
  - If the image of the magnified (upper) bead intersects the first ring the beam is approximately 1.5° away from perpendicular.
  - If the image of the magnified (upper) bead intersects the second ring the beam is approximately 3.0° away from perpendicular.

Record Keeping

A record should be kept that documents the date of the test, who performed the test, the results of the test, and the corrective action taken.

Note: When corrective action is taken, the before and after films should be kept on file.

Potential Problems

- Failure to level the table could provide the radiographer with inaccurate measurements.
- Failure to have the x-ray tube perpendicular could provide the radiographer with inaccurate measurements.

Bucky/Beam Perpendicularity Test (Washer Method)

Rationale
This procedure is designed to confirm that the x-ray beam is perpendicular to the Bucky.

Testing Frequency
Beam perpendicularity should be checked semiannually or when the x-ray tube has been replaced.

Equipment
- Lead zero or steel washer
- 6-inch carpenter's level
- 8 × 10 image receptor
- A nickel
- Fine point felt marker
- A clear ruler with centimeter markings

Procedure
A. Place the image receptor in the Bucky tray.
B. Center the tube to the image receptor and set the tube at a 40-inch SID.
C. Use the 6-inch carpenter's level to check that the tube and tabletop are level.
D. Place the lead zero or washer in the center of the cross hairs of the central ray.
E. To indicate the Bucky side of the table, place the nickel within the light field. The nickel is used as a point of reference if the central ray and Bucky are not perpendicular.
F. The technique used depends on the speed of the image receptor system being employed. A suggested starting technique would be 2 mAs at 50 kVp. The background density should be light enough to perform Step I.
G. Expose and process the film.
H. Evaluate the film by making an "X" from corner to corner.
I. Measure the image (Fig. 4-10 A and B).
J. Record the results.

Acceptance Parameters
The zero or washer should be within 1 centimeter of the center of the film.

Record Keeping
A record should be kept that documents the date of the test, who performed the test, the results of the test, and the corrective action taken.

    Note When corrective action is taken, the before and after films should be kept on file.

Potential Problems
- Failure to level the table could provide the radiographer with inaccurate measurements.

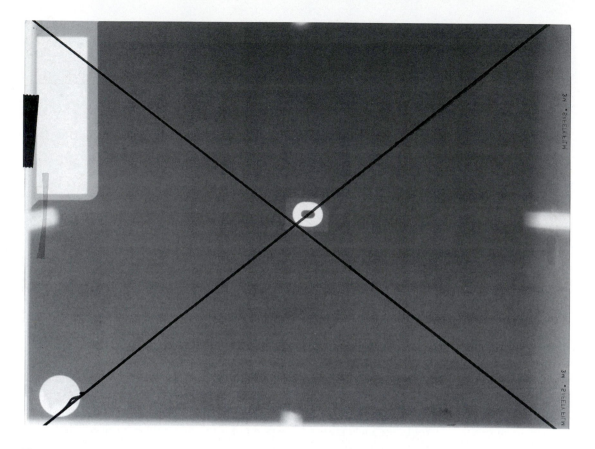

Figure 4-10 *A*. Radiograph demonstrating satisfactory beam alignment (Washer Method).

- Failure to have the x-ray tube perpendicular could provide the radiographer with inaccurate measurements.
- Failure to have the tube centered to the table will provide inaccurate measurements.
- Failure to have the Bucky tray completely in will result in inaccurate measurements.

Bucky/Beam Perpendicularity Test (Ragins Method)*

Rationale

This procedure is designed to confirm that the x-ray beam is perpendicular to the Bucky.

*Developed by Travis Ragins, RT(R) as a senior student QA project.

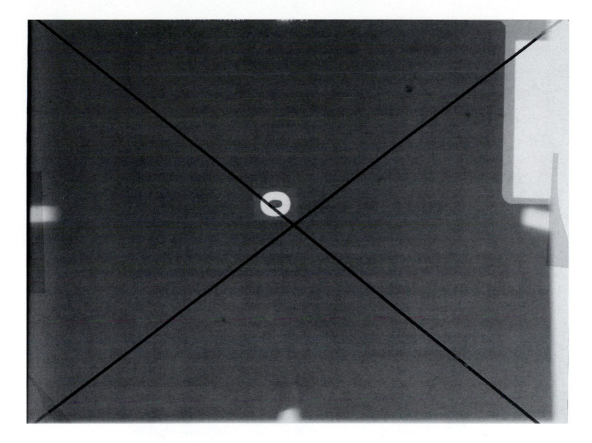

Figure 4-10 *B.* Radiograph demonstrating unsatisfactory beam alignment (Washer Method).

Testing Frequency
Beam perpendicularity should be checked semiannually or when the x-ray tube has been replaced.

Equipment
- Two fender washers (1/8 × 1 inch) (Fig. 4-11)
- 6-inch carpenter's level
- 8 × 10 image receptor
- China marker
- Clear tape
- A coin
- Fine point felt marker
- A clear ruler with centimeter markings

Procedure
A. Prior to doing the test, perform the following steps.

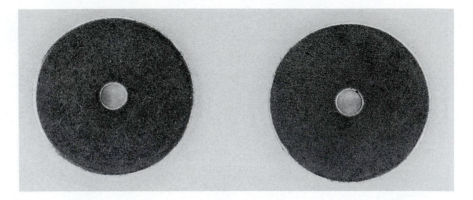

Figure 4-11 Fender washers.

- Using the china marker draw a transverse and longitudinal line on the image receptor front that intersects in the middle of the image receptor.
- Tape one of the fender washers to front of the image receptor where the lines intersect.

B. Place the image receptor longitudinally in the Bucky tray.

C. Center the tube to the image receptor and set the tube at a 40-inch SID.

D. Use the 6-inch carpenter's level to check that the tube and the tabletop are level.

E. Place the second fender washer on the tabletop in the center of the cross hairs of the central ray.

F. To indicate the Bucky handle side of the table, place the coin within the light field. The nickel is used as a point of reference if the central ray and Bucky are not perpendicular.

G. The technique used depends on the speed of the image receptor system being employed. A suggested starting technique would be 2 mAs at 50 kVp. The background density should be light enough to perform Step I.

H. Expose and process the film.

I. Evaluate the film by making an "X" from corner to corner.

J. Measure the distance between the holes of the fender washer images (Fig. 4-12).

K. Record the results.

Acceptance Parameters

The fender washers should be within 1 centimeter of each other.

Record Keeping

A record should be kept that documents the date of the test, who performed the test, the results of the test, and the corrective action taken.

Note: When corrective action is taken, the before and after films should be kept on file.

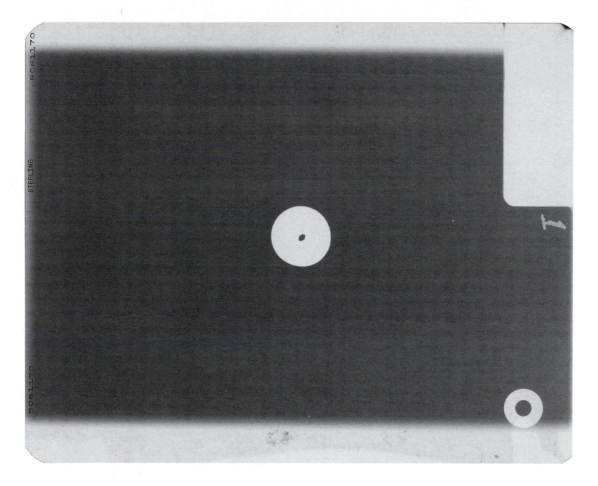

Figure 4-12 Radiograph demonstrating satisfactory beam alignment using fender washer.

Potential Problems

- Failure to level the table or have the x-ray tube perpendicular will provide the radiographer with inaccurate measurements.
- Failure to have the tube centered to the table will provide inaccurate measurements.
- Failure to have the Bucky tray completely in will result in inaccurate measurements.

Automatic Collimation (Positive Beam Limitation) Test

Rationale

This procedure is designed to confirm that the PBL is functioning properly.

Testing Frequency

The automatic collimation should be checked semiannually, when the collimator or a light bulb has been replaced, or when the x-ray tube has been replaced.

Equipment

- 8 × 10 image receptor
- Collimator test template (see Fig. 4-8)
- 6-inch carpenter's level
- Ruler with centimeter and inch markings

Procedure

A. Place the image receptor in the Bucky tray. Confirm that the automatic collimation is engaged.
B. Center the tube to the image receptor and set the tube at a 40-inch SID.
C. Use the 6-inch carpenter's level to check that the tube and tabletop are level.
D. Place the template on top of the table with the dot in the lower left corner of the template corresponding to the patient's right shoulder. The dot helps to determine the direction of collimator error later.
E. Set an approximate technique of 10 mAs at 60 kVp for single-phase units and 5 mAs at 60 kVp for three-phase units. The technique selected depends on the speed of the imaging system being used.
F. Expose and process the film.
G. Measure the image.
H. Record the results.

Acceptance Parameters

NCRP Report #99 makes the following recommendations.
- The positive beam limitation must be within ±3% of the SID.
  - At a 40-inch SID, the light field to should be within ±1.2 inches.
  - At a 100-centimeter SID, the light field should be within ±3 centimeters.

Record Keeping

A record should be kept that documents the date of the test, who performed the test, the results of the test, and the corrective action taken.

   Note: When corrective action is taken, the before and after films should be kept on file.

Potential Problems

- Failure to level the table could provide the radiographer with inaccurate readings.
- Failure to have the x-ray tube perpendicular could provide the radiographer with inaccurate readings.
- Failure to have the tube centered to the table will provide inaccurate measurements.

- Failure to have the Bucky tray completely in will result in inaccurate measurements.

Light Field Illumination Test

Rationale

This procedure is designed to confirm that the illumination level of the collimator light is visible in the lighting conditions that are routinely used during positioning.

Testing Frequency

- The illumination level of the collimator light field is checked when a piece of equipment is installed, removed, and reinstalled in another location.
- The illumination level of the collimator light field should be checked annually or as often as the management of the Medical Imaging Department deems it necessary.

Equipment

- Photometer or photographic light meter (see Figs. 3-23 and 3-24)

Procedure

A. Adjust the ambient lighting to levels that would be used during a routine radiographic procedure.
B. Set the tube at a distance of 40 inches (100 centimeters) or at the maximum SID, whichever is less.
C. Adjust the collimator to an appropriate field size (i.e., 10 × 12 inches).
D. Divide the light field at the image receptor into four equal quadrants.
E. Turn the photometer on and take a reading in the center of each quadrant.
F. Average the readings and record the results (Fig. 4-13).

Acceptance Parameters

The Code of Federal Regulations 21 1020.31 (2) requires that the light field illuminance be no less than 160 lux or 15 footcandles at an SID of 40 inches.

Record Keeping

A record should be kept that documents the date of the test, who performed the test, the results of the test, and the corrective action taken.

Potential Problems

- Low batteries in either the light meter or photometer may lead to inaccurate readings.
- Failure to have the photometer set on the correct units will be a source of error.

    Note: A photographic light meter can be used but the EV reading will have to be converted to footcandles.

Light Field Illumination Record Form

Room _____   **Unit** _____   **Single phase** ☐   **Three phase** ☐

Quadrant	Reading
1	
2	
3	
4	
Average	

Comments:

_____   _____
Signature   **Date**

Figure 4-13 Light field illuminance record form.

Source-to-Image Distance Indicator

Rationale
This procedure is designed to confirm that the tube to tabletop SID is accurate and to confirm that the tube to Bucky SID is accurate.

Testing Frequency
This test should be done annually or as needed.

Equipment
- Tape measure

Procedure
A. Set the tube at a 40-inch SID.
B. Determine exactly where the focal spot is. On most x-ray tubes this will be easy to determine by checking the anode end of the tube housing. Most manufacturers place some sort of mark on the end of the housing to indicate where the focal spot is located.
C. Use the tape measure to determine the distance from the focal spot to the tabletop.
D. Pull the Bucky tray out and center the tube to the Bucky tray.
E. Use the tape measure to determine the distance from the focal spot to the Bucky tray.
F. Record the results.

Acceptance Parameters
NCRP Report #99 recommends that the SID be within ±2% of the established SID.

Record Keeping
- A record should be kept that documents the date of the test, who performed the test, the results of the test, and the corrective action taken.

Potential Problems
- SID to Bucky readings will be inaccurate if the type of tabletop is not taken into consideration.
  - For stationary tabletops there is an approximate 2 inch difference between the tabletop and Bucky tray.
  - For floating tabletops there is approximately 3 to 4 inch difference between the tabletop and the Bucky tray.

Points to Ponder
- When an x-ray machine is installed, the 40-inch SID will be established by the service engineer. The primary SID will be based on either the tube to tabletop distance or the tube to Bucky distance.
- It is important that the technologist responsible for performing this test find out either from the service engineer or check the equipment specifications manual included with the equipment.

THE GENERATOR

In the United States there are three types of x-ray generators available for producing x-rays—single-phase, three-phase, and high frequency. As the power of an x-ray generator increases there is a corresponding affect on the x-ray emission spectra (Table 4-2). This affect can be readily seen in the quality of films produced in the Medical Imaging Department. The advantages that are obtained from increasing generator power include more efficient x-ray production, reduction of radiation exposure to the patient, the selection of higher mA techniques, and the selection of faster exposure times.

Generally the medical physicist or equipment service engineers perform the QC tests discussed in this section. However, any competent medical radiographer can do the QC tests performed on the generator. There is a variety of test equipment available on the market to perform the tests described in this chapter. This equipment may be purchased as a single device, which has the capability of performing multiple tests, or as individual devices that perform one type of test. One such multi-test instrument is the Non-invasive Evaluator of Radiation Outputs (NERO mAx) Model 8000 (Fig. 4-14). This particular instrument has the capability of measuring kilovoltage, mAs, mA, exposure time, HVL, radiation exposure, and radiation rate. The data obtained from the various tests can is placed directly in a spread sheet (e.g., Microsoft Excel) for easy access and report generation. In the atmosphere of managed healthcare and cost reductions, most institutions avoid purchasing this type of equipment because of its cost.

Table 4-2
How the Generator and Tube Affect the X-Ray Emission Spectra (Quality and Quantity)

As Factor Increases	Affect on Quality and Quantity	Change in the Continuous Spectrum	Change in the Discrete Spectrum
Generator phase (voltage waveform)	Increase in quality and quantity	Amplitude increases	Shift to right
kVp	Increase in quality and quantity	Amplitude increases	Shift to right
mA	Increase in quantity; no change in quality	Amplitude increases	No shift
mAs	Increase in quantity; no change in quality	Amplitude increases	No shift
Added filtration	Increase in quality; decrease in quantity	Amplitude increases	No shift
Target material	Increase in quantity and quality	Amplitude increases slightly	Shift to right
SID	No change	No change	No change

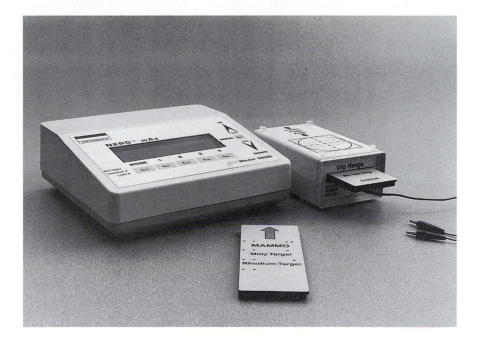

Figure 4-14 NERO-max. *(Courtesy of Nuclear Associates, used with permission.)*

The QC tests discussed in this section include exposure time accuracy, kVp accuracy, **mAs reciprocity, mA linearity, timer linearity, exposure reproducibility,** mR/mAs Output, a variety of automatic exposure control (AEC) tests, and half value layer (HVL). When possible, the author has tried to provide alternate tests for the radiographer that does not have access to the proper test equipment.

Exposure Time Accuracy: Spin Top Test (Single Phase Only)

Rationale
This procedure is designed to confirm that the generator is producing the exposure time that has been set on the control panel.

Testing Frequency
Exposure time should be checked annually, when a generator has been worked on, or when there are light and dark films.

Equipment
- Manual spin top test tool (Fig. 4-15)
- 10 × 12 image receptor
- Two lead mats

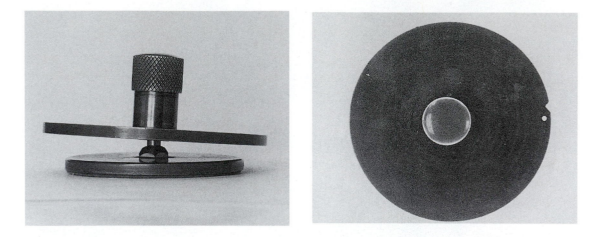

Figure 4-15 Manual spin top used for determining timer accuracy in single-phase generators.

Procedure

A. Place the image receptor on the table.
B. Place the spin top on the upper left quarter of the image receptor, center the tube to the spin top, collimate to the section of film, and use a 40-inch SID.
C. Four exposures will be made using:
    - 50 mA, 1/5 sec at 70 kV to expose the upper left quarter of the image receptor.
    - 100 mA, 1/10 sec at 70 kV to expose the upper right quarter of the image receptor.
    - 200 mA, 1/20 sec at 70 kV to expose the lower right quarter of the image receptor.
    - 300 mA, 1/30 sec at 70 kV to expose the lower left quarter of the image receptor.
    - The spin top must be rotating prior to each exposure.
    - It is important to cover each exposed quarter of the image receptor with lead mats.
D. Process the film.
E. Mark each image with the correct exposure time and then count the dots (Figs. 4-16A and B).
F. Record the results (Fig. 4-17).

Acceptance Parameters

NCRP Report #99 recommends the following guidelines for single-phase full-wave rectified generators.

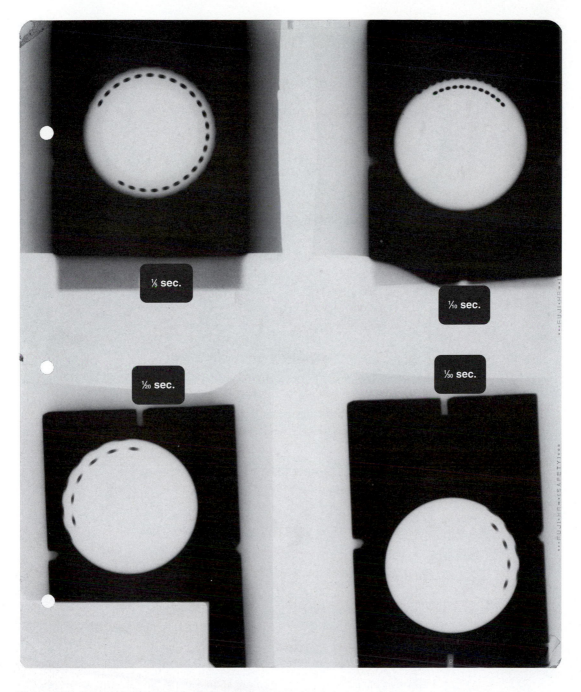

Figure 4-16 *A.* Image of a normal spin top test.

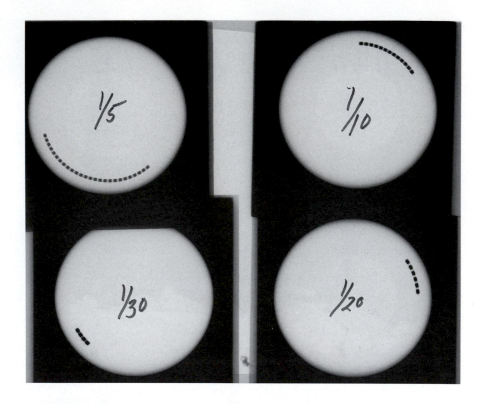

Figure 4-16 *B.* Spin top image demonstrating a timer malfunction.

Exposure Time (sec)	Acceptance Limits
1/5	24 dots ± 1 dot
1/10	12 dots ± 1 dot
1/20	6 dots ± 0 dot
1/30	4 dots ± 0 dot

Record Keeping

A record should be kept that documents the date of the test, who performed the test, the results of the test, and the corrective action taken.

Note: When corrective action is taken, the before and after films should be kept on file.

Potential Problems

- Failure to have the spin top spinning at an acceptable rate will result in an inadequate number of dots in the image and misinterpretation of results.
- Spinning the manual spin at too fast a rate will result in the dots running together in an arc, which prohibits the evaluation of the timer.

Exposure Time Record Form

Room _____   Unit _____   Single phase ☐   Three phase ☐

Timer Accuracy (Spin Top)	
Exposure Time	Number of Dots
1/5 sec	
1/10 sec	
1/20 sec	
1/30 sec	

Comments:

Room _____   Unit _____   Single phase ☐   Three phase ☐

Timer Accuracy (Mechanized Spin Top)	
Exposure Time	Number of Degrees
1/5 sec	
1/10 sec	
1/20 sec	
1/30 sec	

Comments:

Room _____   Unit _____   Single phase ☐   Three phase ☐

Timer Accuracy (Digital Device)			
Selected		Measured	

Comments:

_____
Signature

Figure 4-17 Exposure time record form.

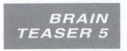

BRAIN TEASER 5

You have just completed a manual spin top test in a single-phase radiographic room. All four of your images demonstrate the appropriate number of dots, but in each image you observe that every other dot is light. Can you identify the cause of this anomaly?

You have just completed a manual spin top test in a single-phase radiographic room. All of the images demonstrate half the expected number of dots. Can you identify the probable cause for this?

Exposure Time Accuracy: Mechanized Spin Top Test (Single Phase and Three Phase)

Rationale

This procedure is designed to confirm that the generator is producing the exposure time that has been set on the control panel.

Testing Frequency

Exposure time should be checked annually, when a generator has been worked on, or when there are light and dark films.

Equipment

- Mechanized timing test tool (Fig. 4-18)
- Protractor

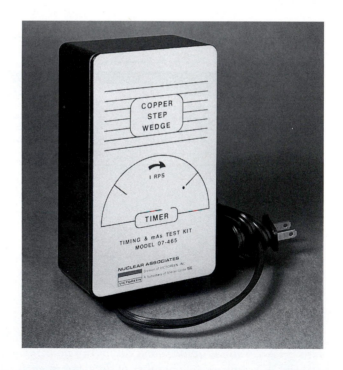

Figure 4-18 Mechanized spin top. *(Courtesy of Nuclear Associates, used with permission.)*

- 10×12 image receptor
- Two lead mats

Procedure

A. Place the image receptor on the table and place the lead mats on the image receptor so that the upper left quarter of the image receptor is uncovered.

B. Plug in the test tool and place it on the upper left quarter of the image receptor.

C. Center the tube to the device, collimate to the section of film, and use a 40-inch SID.

D. Four exposures will be made using:
   - 50 mA, 1/5 sec at 70 kV to expose the upper left quarter of the image receptor.
   - 100 mA, 1/10 sec at 70 kV to expose the upper right quarter of the image receptor.
   - 200 mA, 1/20 sec at 70 kV to expose the lower right quarter of the image receptor.
   - 300 mA, 1/30 sec at 70 kV to expose the lower left quarter of the image receptor.

E. Process the film.

F. After processing the film perform the following tasks:
   - Mark each image with the correct exposure time.
   - Use the protractor to measure the angle of each arc in degrees.
   - Calculate the exposure time for each image using the following formula:

$$\text{Measured Exposure Time} = \frac{\text{Number of Degrees}}{360}$$

   - For examples refer to Fig. 4-19.

G. Record the results (see Fig. 4-17).

Acceptance Parameters

- NCRP Report #99 states that acceptance criteria for three-phase full-wave rectified generators is ±5% of the established exposure time.
- When using a protractor the following table may be used to determine if the timer is within acceptable limits.

Exposure Time (sec)	Angle in Degrees
1/5	72° ± 3°
1/10	36° ± 2°
1/20	18° ± 2°
1/30	12° ± 2°

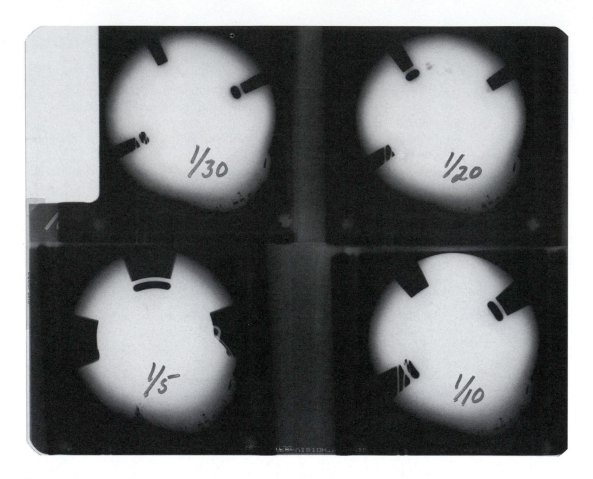

Figure 4-19 Mechanized spin top image.

Record Keeping

A record should be kept that documents the date of the test, who performed the test, the results of the test, and the corrective action taken.

Note: When corrective action is taken, the before and after films should be kept on file.

Potential Problems

Failure to use the protractor correctly may result in inaccurate results.

BRAIN TEASER 7

You have just completed a mechanized test tool in a three-phase radiographic room. The image for the 1/5 second timer station indicates an angle of 80°. Is the time station accurate? If the timer is not accurate, is the exposure time too short or too long?

Exposure Time Accuracy: Digital Timer Test (All Generator Types)

Rationale

This procedure is designed to confirm that the generator is producing the exposure time that has been set on the control panel.

Testing Frequency

Exposure time should be checked annually, when a generator has been worked on, or when there are light and dark films.

Equipment

- Digital x-ray timer (Fig. 4-20)

Procedure

A. Before performing the test, it is important to follow the appropriate tube warm up procedure.
B. Turn the digital timer on and allow it to warm as recommended by the manufacturer.
C. Place the digital timer on the tabletop.
D. Use a 40-inch SID, center the central ray to the middle of the timer, and collimate to the timer.
E. Readings should be taken in the 10 millisecond to half-second range.
F. At the time settings selected it is important to do a minimum of five exposures for each selected time station.

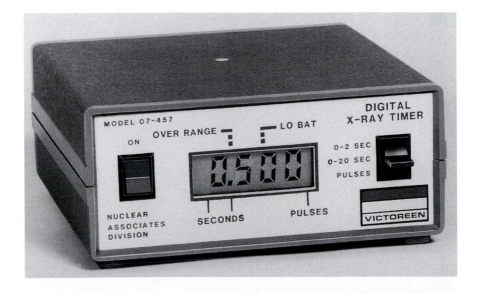

Figure 4-20 Digital x-ray timer. *(Courtesy of Nuclear Associates, used with permission.)*

G. Multiple exposures will allow for any variations in line voltage.

H. On a sheet of paper record the timer readings for each selected time station. Average the readings and record the results (see Fig. 4-17).

Acceptance Parameters

NCRP Report #99 states that acceptance criteria for all generators is ±5% of the established exposure time.

Record Keeping

A record should be kept that documents the date of the test, who performed the test, the results of the test, and the corrective action taken.

Potential Problems

Failure to warm up the digital timer may result in inaccurate results.

Kilovoltage Accuracy

Rationale

This test is designed to confirm that the generator is producing the kVp as indicated on the control panel.

Testing Frequency

The kilovoltage should be checked annually or when there is an indication that the generator is not producing the kilovoltage selected.

Equipment

• Digital kVp meter (Fig. 4-21)

Procedure

A. Before performing the test, it is important to follow the appropriate tube warm up procedure.

B. Turn the kVp meter on and allow it to warm as recommended by the manufacturer.

C. Place the kVp meter on the tabletop.

D. Use a 40-inch SID, center the central ray to the middle of the kVp meter, and collimate to the meter.

E. Readings should be taken in the 50 kV to 140 kV range. The readings may be taken in either 10 or 20 kV increments.

F. At the kV ranges selected it is important to do a minimum of five exposures for each selected kV. Multiple exposures will allow for any variations in line voltage.

G. On a sheet of paper record the kVp readings for each selected kV. Average the readings and record the results (Fig. 4-22).

Acceptance Parameters

• The NCRP recommends that the kilovoltage be within ±4 kVp of the selected kVp.

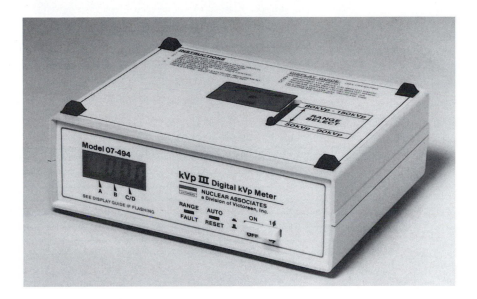

Figure 4-21 Digital kVp meter. *(Courtesy of Nuclear Associates, used with permission.)*

- The NCRP further states that in the 60 kV to 100 kV range, it is possible that generators can be better calibrated to a ±2 kV tolerance.

Record Keeping

A record should be kept that documents the date of the test, who performed the test, the results of the test, and the corrective action taken.

Potential Problems

- Inaccurate readings may be obtained during times of high electrical power demand.
- Inaccurate readings may be obtained if the incoming power supply is constantly fluctuating.

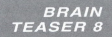

You have just completed testing the 60 kVp to 100 kVp range in 10 kVp increments with the digital kVp meter. You determined that you were obtaining 62 kVp, 68 kVp, 81 kVp, 90 kVp, and 100 kVp at the designated kVp selections. Are the kVp selections within accepted parameters?

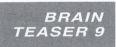

You have just completed testing the 60 kVp to 100 kVp range in 10 kVp increments. The results you obtained were 57 kVp, 74 kVp, 85 kVp, 95 kVp, and 95 kVp. Are the kVp selections within accepted parameters? If they are not what are the possible causes for this?

kVp Record Form

Room _____   **Unit** _____

Single phase ☐   **Three phase** ☐

Acceptance Parameters:

Exposure	50 kVp	60 kVp	70 kVp	80 kVp	90 kVp	100 kVp
#1						
#2						
#3						
#4						
#5						
#6						
Average						

Comments:

_____   _____
Signature   **Date**

Figure 4-22 kVp record form.

mAs Reciprocity Test: R-Meter Method

Rationale

This procedure is designed to confirm that similar exposures are obtained for the same mAs and kVp, regardless of the exposure time and mA used.

Testing Frequency

This test should be done annually or when the generator has been worked on.

Equipment

- R-meter with an ionization chamber (Fig. 4-23)
- Lead apron

Procedure

A. Place the lead apron on the tabletop. The apron will help reduce the effect of backscatter.
B. Place the ionization chamber on the lead apron and connect it to the R-meter.
C. Turn the R-meter on and allow it to warm up for approximately 2 minutes.
D. Center the x-ray tube to the ionization chamber and collimate to area slightly larger then the device. The SID should be 40 inches.
E. Make four exposures using the following factors:
- 100 mA at 1/10 second at 80 kVp.
- 200 mA at 1/20 second at 80 kVp.
- 300 mA at 1/30 second at 80 kVp.
- 400 mA at 1/30 second at 80 kVp.
F. After each exposure, measure and record the mR readings. Reset the R-meter after the exposure.
G. For each exposure, calculate the **mR/mAs ratio** and record the data. The following formula should be used:

$$\text{mR/mAs Ratio} = \frac{\text{mR}}{\text{mAs}}$$

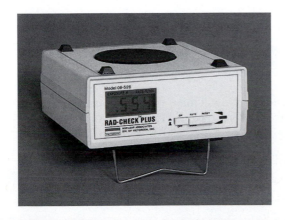
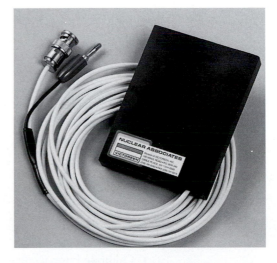

Figure 4-23 Digital R-meter and ionization chamber. *(Courtesy of Nuclear Associates, used with permission.)*

H. Calculate the average mR/mAs. The following formula should be used:

$$\text{Average mR/mAs} = \frac{\text{Sum of the mR/mAs Ratios}}{\text{Number of mA Stations Tested}}$$

I. Determine the variation in reciprocity using the following formula:

$$\text{Percent Reciprocity Variation} = \frac{(\text{mR/mAs}_{max} - \text{mR/mAs}_{min})/2}{\text{Average mR/mAs}} \times 100$$

J. Record the results (Fig. 4-24).

Acceptance Parameters
NCRP Report #99 states that mAs reciprocity should be ±10%.

Record Keeping
A record should be kept that documents the date of the test, who performed the test, the results of the test, and the corrective action taken.

Potential Problems
- If the R-meter is not warmed up, inaccurate readings may be obtained.
- Failure to reset the R-meter may result in inaccurate readings.
- Failure to convert R to mR may cause problems.

Points to Ponder
- The reading on the R-meter will be in R and that number will have to be multiplied by 1000 to obtain mR.

BRAIN TEASER 10

It was found that the mAs reciprocity variation was 12%. What would be the probable cause for this?

mAs Reciprocity Test: Step-Wedge Method

Rationale
This procedure is designed to confirm that similar exposures are obtained for the same mAs and kVp, regardless of the exposure time and mA used.

Testing Frequency
This test should be done annually or when the generator has been serviced.

Equipment
- Densitometer
- Calibrated step wedge (Fig. 4-25)
- One 11 × 14 image receptor
- Three lead mats

mAs Reciprocity Record Form

Room _____   Unit _____   Single Phase ☐   Three Phase ☐

kVp _____

mA	Exp. Time	mAs	mR	mR/mAs
100				
200				
300				
400				
			Percent Variation	

Comments:

_____   _____
Signature   Date

Figure 4-24 mAs reciprocity record form.

Procedure

A. Place the image receptor on the tabletop.
B. Cover three-fourths of the image receptor with the lead masks.
C. Place the step wedge on the remaining one-fourth of the image receptor.

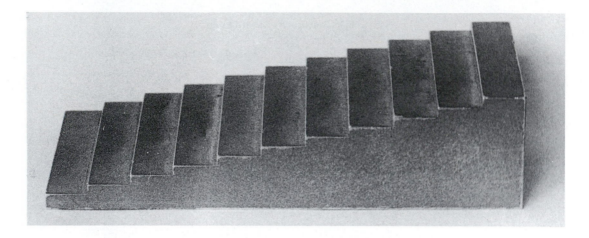

Figure 4-25 Calibrated step wedge.

D. Center the x-ray tube to the step wedge and collimate to the device. The SID should be 40 inches.
E. Make four exposures using the following factors:
- 100 mA at 1/10 second at 70 kVp.
- 200 mA at 1/20 second at 70 kVp.
- 300 mA at 1/30 second at 70 kVp.
- 400 mA at 1/40 second at 70 kVp.
- It is important to cover each exposed section of the image receptor with lead mats.
F. Expose and process the film (Fig. 4-26).
G. Use the densitometer to measure each step.
H. Record the results (Fig. 4-27).

Acceptance Parameters

The density of each step should be within a density of ±0.1.

Record Keeping

A record should be kept that documents the date of the test, who performed the test, the results of the test, and the corrective action taken.

Note: When corrective action is taken, the before and after films should be kept on file.

Potential Problems

Failure to adequately use lead masking may lead to increased density and readings that are inaccurate.

Points to Ponder

- This particular method has been widely replaced by the method using the digital R-meter, which is more accurate and reliable.

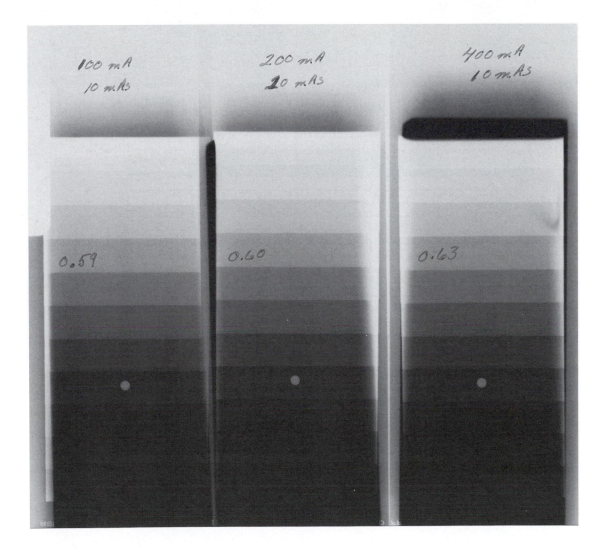

Figure 4-26 Stepwedge image.

mA/mAs Linearity Test

Rationale
This procedure is designed to confirm that mA or mAs is linear with exposure.

Testing Frequency
This test should be performed annually or when service has been performed on the generator.

mAs Reciprocity Record Form (Stepwedge Method)

Room _____   Unit _____   Single phase ☐   Three phase ☐

Exposure time _____   kVp _____

Acceptance Parameters:

| Step | Densitometer Readings at | | | |
	100 mA	200 mA	300 mA	400 mA
1				
2				
3				
4				
5				
6				
7				
8				
9				
10				
11				
12				
13				
14				
15				
16				
17				
18				
19				
20				
21				

Comments:

_____   _____
Signature   Date

Figure 4-27 mAs reciprocity (step wedge) record form.

Equipment
- Ionization chamber and R-meter (see Fig. 4-23)
- Lead apron

Procedure
A. Place the lead apron on the tabletop. The apron will help reduce the effect of backscatter.
B. Place the ionization chamber and R-meter on the lead apron.
C. Turn the R-meter on and allow it to warm up for approximately 2 minutes.
D. Center the x-ray tube to the ionization chamber and collimate to an area slightly larger than the device. A 40-inch SID should be used.
E. The following factors are to be used:
  - 80 kVp
  - 0.1 second (100 milliseconds)
  - mA values of 50, 100, 200, 300, 400, and 600
F. Measure the exposure (mR) for each set of exposure factors and record the data. After the exposure reset the R-meter.
G. For each exposure, calculate the mR/mAs ratio and record the data. The following formula should be used:

$$mR/mAs = \frac{mR}{mAs}$$

H. Calculate the average mR/mAs. The following formula should be used:

$$Average\ mR/mAs = \frac{Sum\ of\ the\ mR/mAs\ Ratios}{Number\ of\ mA\ Stations\ Tested}$$

I. Determine the variation in linearity using the following formula:

$$Percent\ mA\ Linearity\ Variation = \frac{(mR/mAs_{max} - mR/mAs_{min})/2}{Average\ mR/mAs} \times 100$$

J. Record the results (Fig. 4-28).

Acceptance Parameters
NCRP Report #99 states that mA/mAs linearity should be ±10% over the clinical range.

Record Keeping
A record should be kept that documents the date of the test, who performed the test, the results of the test, and the corrective action taken.

Potential Problems
- If the R-meter is not warmed up, inaccurate readings may be obtained.
- Failure to reset the R-meter may result in inaccurate readings.

mA/mAs Linearity Record Form

Room _____   Unit _____   Single phase ☐   Three phase ☐

mA/mAs Linearity						
80 kVp	.	Factor adjacent				
	.	Factor any				
mA		Measured Seconds	mAs	kVp		mR	mR/mAs

Comments:

Signature   Date

Figure 4-28 mA linearity record form.

- Variations in electrical power may cause problems.
- Failure to convert R to mR may cause problems.

> ### Points to Ponder
>
> - Milliamperage is assumed to be linear; as mA doubles, the number of x-rays produced doubles, and as a result of this so does exposure.
> - The reading on the R-meter will be in R and that number will have to be multiplied by 1000 to obtain mR.

BRAIN TEASER 11

It was found that the exposure in mR from the 100 mA station to the 200 mA station tripled. Is this acceptable? What would cause this?

Timer Linearity Test

Rationale

This procedure is designed to confirm that exposure time is linear with exposure.

Testing Frequency

This test should be performed annually, when service has been performed on the generator, or when the timer has been recalibrated.

Equipment

- R-meter with an ionization chamber (see Fig. 4-23)
- Lead apron

Procedure

A. Place the lead apron on the tabletop. The apron will help reduce the effect of backscatter.
B. Place the ionization chamber on the lead apron.
C. Turn the R-meter on and allow it to warm up for approximately 2 minutes.
D. Center the x-ray tube to the ionization chamber and collimate to an area slightly larger than the device. The SID should be 40 inches.
E. The following factors are to be used:
  - 80 kVp
  - 0.1 second (100 milliseconds)
  - mA values of 50, 100, 200, 300, 400, and 600
F. Measure the exposure (mR) for each set of exposure factors and record the data. After each exposure reset the R-meter.
G. For each exposure, calculate the mR/mAs ratio and record the data. The following formula should be used:

$$mR/mAs = \frac{mR}{mAs}$$

H. Calculate the average mR/mAs. The following formula should be used:

$$\text{Average mR/mAs} = \frac{\text{Sum of the mR/mAs Ratios}}{\text{Number of mA Stations Tested}}$$

I. Determine the variation in linearity using the following formula:

$$\text{Percent mA Linearity Variation} = \frac{(\text{mR/mAs}_{max} - \text{mR/mAs}_{min})/2}{\text{Average mR/mAs}} \times 100$$

J. Record the results (Fig. 4-29).

Acceptance Parameters

NCRP Report #99 states that timer linearity should be ±10% over the clinical range.

Record Keeping

A record should be kept that documents the date of the test, who performed the test, the results of the test, and the corrective action taken.

Potential Problems

- If the R-meter is not warmed up, inaccurate readings may be obtained.
- Failure to reset the R-meter may result in inaccurate readings.
- Variations in electrical power may cause problems.
- Failure to convert R to mR may cause problems.

Points to Ponder

- Exposure time is assumed to be linear; as exposure time doubles, so does exposure.
- The reading on the R-meter will be in R and that number will have to be multiplied by 1000 to obtain mR.

Exposure Reproducibility Test

Rationale

This procedure is designed to confirm that the exposure produced for the same mA, time, and kVp is the same from exposure to exposure.

Testing Frequency

This test should be done annually, when there is an indication that exposures are not consistent, or when the generator has been calibrated.

Equipment

- Ionization chamber and R-meter (see Fig. 4-23)
- Lead apron

Procedure

A. Place the lead apron on the tabletop. The apron will help reduce the effect of backscatter.

Timer Linearity Record Form

Room Number: _____   Generator Phase: _____   Date: _____

mA	Exp. Time	mAs	kVp	mR	mR/mAs
50	0.1	.05	80		
100	0.1	.10	80		
200	0.1	.20	80		
300	0.1	.30	80		
400	0.1	.40	80		
600	0.1	.60	80		
				Percent Variation	

Comments:

Signature   Date

Figure 4-29 Timer linearity record form.

      B. Place the R-meter on the apron.

      C. Turn the R-meter on and allow it to warm up for approximately 2 minutes.

      D. Center the x-ray tube to the ionization chamber and collimate to an area slightly larger than the device. A 40-inch SID should be used.

      E. Make six exposures using 40 mAs and 80 kVp. The same technical factors should be used for each exposure.

F. Record the mR value for each exposure.
G. Determine the percent of variation using the following formula:

$$\text{Reproducibility Percent of Variation} = \frac{mR_{max} - mR_{min}}{mR_{max} + mR_{min}} \times 100$$

H. Record the results (Fig. 4-30).
 I. If exposure reproducibility is greater than 5% at the selected mA and mAs, it is suggested that other mA stations at the same mAs be checked.

Acceptance Parameters

NCRP Report #99 recommends that exposure reproducibility be maintained within ±5%.

Record Keeping

A record should be kept that documents the date of the test, who performed the test, the results of the test, and the corrective action taken.

Potential Problems

• If the R-meter is not warmed up, inaccurate readings may be obtained.
• Failure to reset the R-meter may result in inaccurate readings.
• Variations in electrical power may cause problems.
• Failure to convert R to mR may cause problems.

> #### Points to Ponder
>
> • The exposure reproducibility test can be used to confirm the mAs reciprocity and mA linearity results.
>
> • The reading on the R-meter will be in R and that number will have to be multiplied by 1000 to obtain mR.

BRAIN TEASER 12

It was found that the exposure reproducibility for a single-phase generator was 6%. What would cause this?

Coefficient of Variation

Rationale

This procedure is designed to confirm that the exposure produced for the same mA, time, and kVp is the same from exposure to exposure.

Testing Frequency

This test should be done annually, when there is an indication that exposures are not consistent, or when the generator has been calibrated.

Equipment

NERO mAx Model 8000 and detector assembly (see Fig. 4-15)

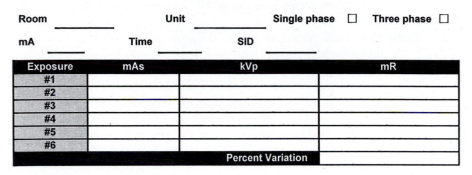

Comments:

Signature   Date

Figure 4-30 Exposure reproducibility record form.

Procedure

A. Place the detector assembly on the x-ray table and connect it to the readout display console.

B. Turn the display console on and follow the manufacturer's specified warm-up procedure.

C. Center the x-ray tube to the detector assembly and collimate to the detector assembly. A 40-inch SID should be used.

D. Make three to six exposures using 100 mAs at 80 kVp.

   A. To prevent tube damage, a large focal spot should be used.

   B. Suggested exposure factors are 400 mA at 0.25 second.

E. After each exposure record the mR, kVp, and time measurements (see Fig. 4-26).

F. Calculate the mean, standard deviation, and coefficient of variation for the mR, kVp, and time.

G. Record the results (Fig. 4-31).

Acceptance Parameters

For any specific combination of exposure factors, the estimated coefficient of variation shall be no greater than 0.05.

Record Keeping

A record should be kept that documents the date of the test, who performed the test, the results of the test, and the corrective action taken.

Potential Problems

- If the test device is not warmed up, inaccurate readings may be obtained.
- Variations in electrical power may cause problems.

Radiation Output Test in Air (mR/mAs Output)

Rationale

- This procedure is designed to confirm that the average radiation output of different generators is consistent.
- This procedure is designed to confirm that the average radiation output of like generators is consistent from room to room.

Testing Frequency

This test should be performed annually, or when the generator is producing exposures that result in over- and underexposed films, or when the tube has been replaced.

Equipment

- Ionization chamber and R-meter (see Fig. 4-23)
- Lead apron

Procedure

A. Place the lead apron on the tabletop. The apron will help reduce the effect of backscatter.

Room _____ **Unit** _____ **Single phase** ☐ **Three phase** ☐

Coefficient of Variation						
Selected -	kVp		mA	sec	mAs	
Measured -	mR		kVp		seconds	
Mean						
Std Dev (σ)						
COV						

Comments:

_____ _____
Signature **Date**

Figure 4-31 Coefficient of variation record form.

B. Place the ionization chamber on the lead apron; turn the R-meter on and allow it to warm up for approximately 2 minutes.

C. Center the x-ray tube to the ionization chamber and collimate to area just slightly larger then the device. A 40-inch SID should be used.

D. Assessment of mR/mAs output requires that the same mAs and kVp be used and that all mA stations be tested.

E. The following factors are to be used:
- 80 kVp

- 0.1 second (100 milliseconds)
- 100 mA
- Large focal spot

F. Make three or four exposures at the selected mA and time and measure the exposure in mR.

G. Record each exposure in the mR/mAs record form. After each exposure reset the R-meter.

H. For each exposure, calculate the average mR using the following formula:

$$\text{Average mR} = \frac{\text{Sum of the mR Values}}{\text{Number of Exposures}}$$

I. Determine the variation in mR/mAs consistency using the following formula:

$$\text{Percent mR/mAs Variation} = \frac{(\text{mR}_{max} - \text{mR}_{min})/2}{\text{Average mR}} \times 100$$

J. Record the results (Fig. 4-32).

Acceptance Parameters

- NCRP Report #99 states that mR/mAs for a single unit should not vary more than ±10% over time at 80 kVp.
- NCRP Report #99 states that for rooms having the same types of generators, tubes, and tables the mR/mAs should not vary more than ±10% at 80 kVp.
- At 80 kVp the expected mR/mAs output for single phase generators should be 8.96 and for three phase generators it should be 13.44.

Record Keeping

A record should be kept that documents the date of the test, who performed the test, the results of the test, and the corrective action taken.

Potential Problems

Failure to follow the test protocol will lead erroneous results.

Points to Ponder

- When the mR/mAs for like rooms varies by more than 10% it will be necessary to provide individual technique charts for each room.

- The reading on the R-meter will be in R and that number will have to be multiplied by 1000 to obtain mR.

- This test can also be performed using a patient equivalent phantom.

mR/mAs Output Record Form

Room _____ Unit _____ Single phase ☐ Three phase ☐

Radiation Output		
Selected kVp	Measured kVp	Free-in-air mR/mAs

kVp	Single phase (mR/mAs)	Three phase (mR/mAs)
60	5.12	7.68
80	8.96	13.44
100	14.08	20.48
125	22.40	30.72

Technique: _____ mA

_____ mAs

@ _____ " SCD

Comments:

Signature   Date

Figure 4-32 mR/mAs output record form.

AUTOMATIC EXPOSURE CONTROL

There are two types of **automatic exposure control (AEC)** devices, and both operate on the principle of sensing the amount of radiation passing through the patient and terminating the exposure when a predetermined exposure has been reached. The devices used to accomplish this are the photomultiplier tube and ionization chamber. The photomultiplier tube is an obsolete process for controlling the exposure. The photomultiplier tube is located below the Bucky tray assembly and the radiation actually passes through the film before the exposure is terminated. The ionization chamber form of automatic exposure control places three ionization chambers in a wafer thin holder between the Bucky assembly and tabletop. The actual exposure is terminated when the radiation has passed through the ionization chamber. The primary advantage of AEC is that it provides consistent film densities over a wide range of kVp and patient thicknesses.

It is important to remember that, when using AEC, the most common cause of repeat films is the failure to correctly position the anatomic area over the ionization chamber. When this occurs the resulting radiograph will be light due to early termination of the exposure.

The QC tests performed on an AEC device require a minimum of equipment. The most important piece of equipment is the phantom, which must be homogenous and patient equivalent. Water or four Lucite slabs are the most commonly used materials for the phantom. If water is used, the water must be at least 10 inches deep and placed in a 5-gallon plastic bucket. The Lucite slabs must be 25 × 25 centimeters × 5.08 centimeters (~10 × 10 × 2 inches) thick. Figure 4-33 shows a commercially available AEC test phantom.

The tests performed on the AEC include back-up time (maximum exposure time) function, mA exposure consistency, kVp exposure consistency, ion chamber (sensor cell) consistency, exposure reproducibility, consistency of exposure with varying field sizes, and consistency of exposure with varying patient thicknesses.

Automatic Exposure Control (AEC): Back-up Time Test

Rationale
This test is designed to ensure that the back-up time is functioning satisfactorily.

Testing Frequency
This test should be performed annually or when the AEC has been serviced.

Equipment
- Lead apron
- Stopwatch

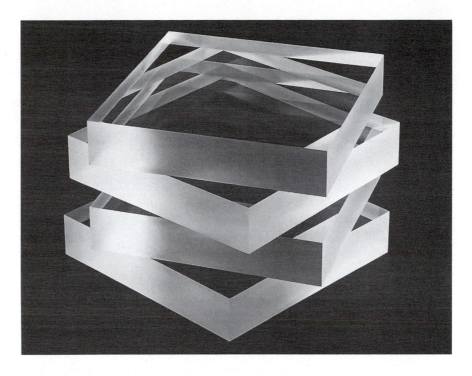

Figure 4-33 AEC test phantom. *(Courtesy of Nuclear Associates, used with permission.)*

Procedure
A. Place the lead apron on the table over the ionization chambers of the AEC device.
B. Center the tube over lead apron. A 40-inch SID should be used.
C. Perform the following tasks:
  - On the control panel set a technique of 200 mA at 70 kVp.
  - Make an exposure.
  - Watch the mAs meter or LED readout on the control to see if the exposure is terminated within 600 mAs.
  - Use the stopwatch to time the length of the exposure.
D. Record the results as a pass or fail (Fig. 4-34).

Acceptance Parameters
NCRP Report #99 states that the backup timer test should terminate the exposure within 6 seconds or 600 mAs, whichever comes first.

Record Keeping
A record should be kept that documents the date of the test, who performed the test, the results of the test, and the corrective action taken.

Potential Problems

- If the back-up timer does not terminate the exposure within 6 seconds or 600 mAs, there is a possibility that the x-ray tube may be damaged.
- Improper use of the stopwatch may result erroneous results.

Automatic Exposure Control: mA Exposure Consistency Test

Rationale

This test is designed to ensure that the AEC device adjusts exposure time and maintain optical density with changes in mA.

Testing Frequency

This test is performed annually or when the AEC device is malfunctioning.

Equipment

- AEC phantom (see Fig. 4-33)
- Four 10×12 image receptors
- Densitometer

Procedure

A. Place the AEC phantom on the table over the center cell of the AEC device.
B. Center the x-ray tube to the phantom and collimate the beam to the phantom. A 40-inch SID should be used.
C. Make four exposures using the following exposure factors:
   - 100 mA and 70 kVp.
   - 200 mA and 70 kVp.
   - 300 mA and 70 kVp.
   - 400 mA and 70 kVp.
D. Prior to each exposure, place an image receptor in the Bucky tray.
E. Process each image.
F. Use the densitometer to measure the optical density in the center of each image.
G. Record the results (see Fig. 4-34).

Acceptance Parameters

The optical density for each image should be the same or within ±0.2 OD of each image.

Record Keeping

A record should be kept that documents the date of the test, who performed the test, the results of the test, and the corrective action taken.

Potential Problem

Failure to follow the test protocol will lead to erroneous results.

Automatic Exposure Control Record Form

Room _____   Unit _____   Single phase ☐   Three phase ☐

mA Exposure Consistency		
Acceptance: ±0.2 O.D.		
mA	kVp	O.D.
100	70	
200	70	
300	70	
400	70	

kVp Exposure Consistency		
Acceptance: ±0.3 O.D.		
mA	kVp	O.D.
200	60	
200	70	
200	80	
200	90	

Sensor Chamber Consistency		
Acceptance: ±0.2 O.D.		
Exposure	Cm of Attenuation	O.D.
One		
Two		
Three		

Exposure Reproducibility		
Acceptance: ±0.1 O.D.		
mA	kVp	O.D.
200	80	
200	80	
200	80	

Consistency of Exposure with Varying Field Size	
Acceptance: ±0.1 O.D.	
Field Size	O.D.
6 x 6	
10 x 10	
14 x 14	

Consistency of Exposure with Varying Patient Thicknesses	
Acceptance: ±0.1 O.D.	
Phantom Size	O.D.
10 cm	
20 cm	
30 cm	

Backup Exposure Time	
mAs	
Sec	
Pass	
Fail	

Comments:

_____
Signature

Figure 4-34 Automatic exposure control record form.

Automatic Exposure Control: kVp Exposure Consistency Test

Rationale
This test is designed to ensure that the AEC device adjusts exposure time and maintains optical density with changes in kVp.

Testing Frequency
This test is performed annually or when the AEC device is malfunctioning.

Equipment
- AEC phantom (see Fig. 4-33)
- Densitometer
- Four 10×12 image receptors

Procedure
A. Place the AEC phantom on the table over the center cell of the AEC device.
B. Center the x-ray tube to the phantom and collimate the beam to the phantom. A 40-inch SID should be used.
C. Make four exposures using the following exposure factors:
- 200 mA and 60 kVp.
- 200 mA and 70 kVp.
- 200 mA and 80 kVp.
- 200 mA and 90 kVp.
D. Prior to each exposure place an image receptor in the Bucky tray.
E. Process each image.
F. Use the densitometer to measure the optical density in the center of each image.
G. Record the results (see Fig. 4-34).

Acceptance Parameters
NCRP Report #99 states the optical density for each image should be the same or within ±0.3 OD of each image.

Record Keeping
A record should be kept that documents the date of the test, who performed the test, the results of the test, and the corrective action taken.

Potential Problem
Failure to follow the test protocol will lead to erroneous results.

Automatic Exposure Control: Sensor Chamber Consistency Test

Rationale
This test is designed to assure that each ionization chamber of the AEC device produces consistent exposures.

Testing Frequency
This test is performed annually or when the AEC device is malfunctioning.

Equipment
- AEC phantom (see Fig. 4-33)
- Densitometer
- Three 10 × 12 image receptors

Procedure
A. Make three exposures using the following information.
- First exposure
  Place the AEC phantom on the table over the center cell of the AEC device.
  Center the x-ray tube to the phantom and collimate the beam to the phantom. A 40-inch SID should be used.
  Place the image receptor in the Bucky tray and expose it using 200 mA and 70 kVp.
- Second exposure
  Place the AEC phantom on the table over the left cell of the AEC device.
  Center the x-ray tube to the phantom and collimate the beam to the phantom. A 40-inch SID should be used.
  Place the image receptor in the Bucky tray and expose it using 200 mA and 70 kVp.
- Third exposure
  Place the AEC phantom on the table over the right cell of the AEC device.
  Center the x-ray tube to the phantom and collimate the beam to the phantom. A 40-inch SID should be used.
  Place the image receptor in the Bucky tray and expose it using 200 mA and 70 kVp.
B. Process each image.
C. Use the densitometer to measure the optical density in the center of each image.
D. Record the results (see Fig. 4-34).

Acceptance Parameters
The optical density for each image should be the same or within ±0.2 OD of each image.

Record Keeping
A record should be kept that documents the date of the test, who performed the test, the results of the test, and the corrective action taken.

Potential Problem
Failure to follow the test protocol will lead to erroneous results.

Automatic Exposure Control: Exposure Reproducibility Test

Rationale
This test is designed to ensure that the AEC device produces the same density when exposures using the same kVp and mA are used.

Testing Frequency
This test is performed annually or when the AEC device is malfunctioning.

Equipment
- AEC phantom (see Fig. 4-33)
- Densitometer
- Three 10 × 12 image receptors

Procedure
A. Place the AEC phantom on the table over the center cell of the AEC device.
B. Center the x-ray tube to the phantom and collimate the beam to the phantom. A 40-inch SID should be used.
C. Make three exposures using 200 mA and 80 kVp.
D. Prior to each exposure, place an image receptor in the Bucky tray.
E. Process each image.
F. Use the densitometer to measure the optical density in the center of each image.
G. Record the results (see Fig. 4-34).

Acceptance Parameters
The optical density should be within ±0.1 of each image.

Record Keeping
A record should be kept that documents the date of the test, who performed the test, the results of the test, and the corrective action taken.

Potential Problem
Failure to follow the test protocol will lead to erroneous results.

Automatic Exposure Control: Exposure Reproducibility Test (R-Meter Method)

Rationale
This test is designed to ensure that the AEC device produces the same density when exposures using the same kVp and mA are used.

Testing Frequency
This test is performed annually or when the AEC device is malfunctioning.

Equipment
- AEC phantom (see Fig. 4-33)
- Ionization chamber with R-meter (see Fig. 4-23)

Procedure
A. Perform the following tasks.
- Place the ionization chamber over cell of the AEC device.
- Place the AEC phantom over the ionization chamber.
- Turn the R-meter on and allow the R-meter to warm up according to the manufacturer's specifications.
- Center the x-ray tube to the phantom and collimate the beam to the phantom. A 40-inch SID should be used.
B. Make four exposures using 200 mA and 80 kVp.
- After each exposure, record the reading from the R-meter.
C. Determine the percent of variation using the following formula:

$$\text{Reproducibility Percent of Variation} = \frac{mR_{max} - mR_{min}}{mR_{max} + mR_{min}} \times 100$$

D. Record the results (Fig. 4-35).

Acceptance Parameters
NCRP Report #99 states that the exposure reproducibility variance for an AEC device should be ±5%.

Record Keeping
A record should be kept that documents the date of the test, who performed the test, the results of the test, and the corrective action taken.

Potential Problems
- If the R-meter is not warmed up, inaccurate readings may be obtained.
- Failure to reset the R-meter may result in inaccurate readings.
- Variations in electrical power may cause problems.
- Failure to convert R to mR may cause problems.

Automatic Exposure Control: Consistency of Exposure with Varying Field Sizes

Rationale
This test is designed to ensure that the AEC device is able to adjust exposure for changes in field size.

Testing Frequency
This test is performed annually.

AEC Exposure Reproducibility Record Form (R-Meter)

Room _____ Unit _____ Single phase ☐ Three phase ☐

Exposure	Sensor Location	mR	mR/mAs
#1			
#2			
#3			
		Percent Variation	

Comments:

_____   _____
        Signature   Date

Figure 4-35 Automatic exposure control: exposure reproducibility record form (R-meter method).

Equipment
- AEC phantom (see Fig. 4-33)
- Three image receptors (8×10, 10×12, and 14×17)
- Densitometer

Procedure
A. Place the AEC phantom on the table over the center cell of the AEC device.
B. Center the x-ray tube to the phantom. A 40-inch SID should be used.
C. Set a technique of 200 mA at 70 kVp on the generator.
D. Make three exposures using the
- 8×10 image receptor and a 6×6 field size.
- 10×12 image receptor and a 10×10 field size.
- 14×17 image receptor and a 14×14 field size.
E. Prior to each exposure place an image receptor in the Bucky tray.

F. Process each image.
G. Use the densitometer to measure the optical density in the center of each image.
H. Record the results (see Fig. 4-34).

Acceptance Parameters

NCRP Report #99 states the optical density should be within ±0.1 of each image.

Record Keeping

A record should be kept that documents the date of the test, who performed the test, the results of the test, and the corrective action taken.

Potential Problem

Failure to follow the test protocol will lead to erroneous results.

Automatic Exposure Control: Consistency of Exposure with Varying Patient Thicknesses

Rationale

This test is designed to ensure that the AEC device is able to adjust exposure for changes in patient thickness.

Testing Frequency

This test is performed annually.

Equipment

- AEC phantom (see Fig. 4-33)
- Densitometer
- Three 10 × 12 image receptors

Procedure

A. Make three exposures using the following information.
  - First exposure
    Place the 10-centimeter portion of the AEC phantom on the table over the center cell of the AEC device.
    Center the x-ray tube to the phantom and collimate the beam to the phantom. A 40-inch SID should be used.
    Place the image receptor in the Bucky tray and expose it using 200 mA and 70 kVp.
  - Second exposure
    Place the 20-centimeter portion of the AEC phantom on the table over the center cell of the AEC device.
    Center the x-ray tube to the phantom and collimate the beam to the phantom. A 40-inch SID should be used.
    Place the image receptor in the Bucky tray and expose it using 200 mA and 70 kVp.

- Third exposure

  Place the 30-centimeter portion of the AEC phantom on the table over the center cell of the AEC device.

  Center the x-ray tube to the phantom and collimate the beam to the phantom. A 40-inch SID should be used.

B. Place the image receptor in the Bucky tray and expose it using 200 mA and 70 kVp.

C. Process each image.

D. Use the densitometer to measure the optical density in the center of each image.

E. Record the results (see Fig. 4-34).

Acceptance Parameters

NCRP Report #99 states the optical density should be within ±0.3 of each image.

Record Keeping

A record should be kept that documents the date of the test, who performed the test, the results of the test, and the corrective action taken.

Potential Problem

Failure to follow the test protocol will lead to erroneous results.

HALF VALUE LAYER

When x-rays are produced, they exit the tube as a polyenergetic beam. The beam consists of different wavelengths and frequencies. The x-ray beam is often described as having "soft" and "hard" rays. The "soft" rays of the beam have are low energy and are absorbed in the soft tissues, which result in increased exposure to the patient. These low energy x-rays can be eliminated or reduced by placing an absorbing material in the path of the x-ray beam that attenuates the beam and makes it more homogenous.

The amount of material (usually aluminum) needed to reduce the intensity of an x-ray beam by 50% is called the **half value layer (HVL).** The HVL provides information about the penetrating ability (quality) of the x-ray beam. It is also used to determine that the filtration placed in the path of the x-ray beam is sufficient. Information regarding the minimum HVLs required is found in Table 4-3.

Half Value Layer Measurement

Rationale

This procedure is designed to confirm that the filtration installed at the x-ray tube is kept at a suitable level to help minimize exposure to the patient.

Table 4-3
Minimum Half-Value Layers (mm Al) for Single- and Three-Phase Units and Minimum Total Filtration at Various Tube Potentials.

Tube Potential (kVp)	30	50	70	90	110	130	150
HVL 1 phase	0.3	1.2	1.6	2.6	3.1	3.6	3.9
HVL 3 phase	0.4	1.5	2.0	3.1	3.6	4.2	4.8
Required minimum total filtration	0.5 mm Al 0.3 mm Mo for molybdenum target tubes	1.5 mm Al		2.5 mm Al			

From NCRP Report No. 102 page 13.

Testing Frequency

This test should be performed annually or when the x-ray tube has been replaced.

Equipment

- Digital R-meter with ionization chamber attachment (see Fig. 4-20)
- Lead sheet or lead vinyl
- Six pieces of 1-millimeter aluminum (Fig. 4-36)
- Support stand for the aluminum
- HVL record form

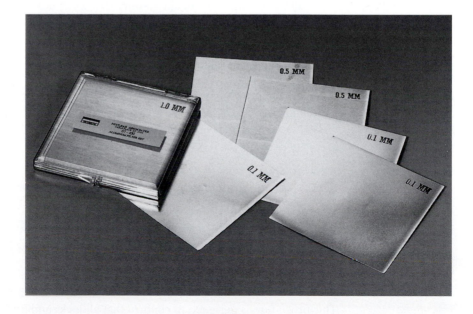

Figure 4-36 Half value layer attenuators. *(Courtesy of Nuclear Associates, used with permission.)*

Procedure

A. Place the lead sheet on the tabletop. The lead sheet will help reduce the effect of backscatter.
B. Place the support stand on the lead sheet.
C. Place the ionization chamber on the lead sheet directly under the support stand and attach it to the R-meter.
D. Turn the R-meter on and allow it to warm up for approximately 2 minutes.
E. Center the x-ray tube to the center of the ionization chamber and collimate to area just slightly larger then the device. The SID should be ~24 to ~30 inches.
F. Set a technique of 80 kVp at 200 mA and 1 second.
G. Perform the following tasks:
    • Make an exposure with no aluminum in the beam and record the results on the HVL record form (Fig. 4-37).
    • Place 1 millimeter of aluminum in the x-ray beam; make an exposure and record the results.
    • Place 2 millimeters of aluminum in the x-ray beam; make an exposure and record the results.
    • Place 3 millimeters of aluminum in the x-ray beam; make an exposure and record the results.
    • Place 4 millimeters of aluminum in the x-ray beam; make an exposure and record the results.
    • Place 5 millimeters of aluminum in the x-ray beam; make an exposure and record the results.
    • Place 6 millimeters of aluminum in the x-ray beam; make an exposure and record the results.

Acceptance Parameters

• NCRP Report #99 states that the minimum HVL at 80 kVp is 2.3 millimeters of Al.
• NCRP Report #99 suggests that increasing the HVL from 2.3 to 3 millimeters of Al at 80 kVp will reduce the exposure to the patient by 25%. This increase will have a minimal effect on contrast and density.

Record Keeping

A record should be kept that documents the date of the test, who performed the test, the results of the test, and the corrective action taken.

Potential Problem

Failure to follow the test protocol will lead erroneous results.

Visual Checks

Rationale

This procedure is designed to confirm that all locks and cables are functioning properly.

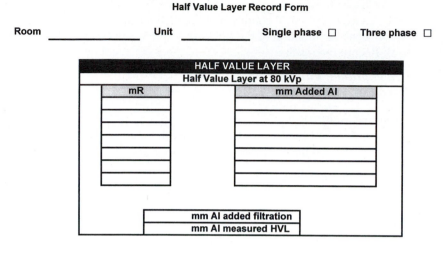

Half Value Layer Record Form

Room _____ Unit _____ Single phase ☐ Three phase ☐

HALF VALUE LAYER	
Half Value Layer at 80 kVp	
mR	mm Added Al
mm Al added filtration	
mm Al measured HVL	

Comments:

_____   _____
Signature   Date

Figure 4-37 Half value layer record form.

Testing Frequency
Visual checks are performed annually.

Equipment
No equipment is needed.

Procedure
A. Check all tube and table locks.
B. Check the angulation indicator.

C. Check the ease of overhead crane movement.

D. Check the physical condition of the high tension cables.

E. Check the function of the Bucky tray and image receptor locks.

F. Record the results.

Acceptance Parameters

Pass/fail

Record Keeping

A record should be kept that documents the date of the test, who performed the test, the results of the test, and the corrective action taken.

Potential Problems

None

GRIDS

The primary purpose of a grid is to improve radiographic contrast by absorbing the scatter radiation produce during an exposure before it reaches the film. Grids may be either focused or nonfocused and have different grid ratios. Grids are found in the Bucky assembly, grid image receptors, grid caps, and slide on grids. After a grid is manufactured, test radiographs are made of the grid to ensure that it is functioning properly. Once the grid has been sold to a Medical Imaging Department, the test films are enclosed with the grid and they become part of the department's records. When a grid reaches the Medical Imaging Department, it is very important that, prior to use, comparison films be made to ensure that the grid has not been damaged during shipment. This is also a quick test that can be performed when one suspects that a grid has been damaged. Figure 4-38 is an example of grid cap that was damaged through improper use.

The technique selected for the initial check will depend on the speed of the imaging system. The author has found from experience that an approximate technique of 4 mAs at 60 kVp provides adequate density for rare earth imaging systems. There are essentially two tests that can be performed on grids that are used in medical radiography—grid uniformity and grid alignment.

Grid Uniformity Test

Rationale

This procedure is designed to confirm that the lead strips of the grid are uniform and not producing any type of artifact in the image.

ULTRA-VISION™ RAPID BACK

Figure 4-38 Image of a damaged grid.

Testing Frequency

This test should be conducted annually on all grids in the department and when the Bucky has been worked on.

Equipment

- Homogenous phantom (aluminum or lucite) or water phantom (~10 to 15 cm H_2O in a plastic container)
- Image receptor (will be determined by the size of the grid being checked)
- Grid (Bucky, grid image receptor, grid cap, slide on grid)
- Densitometer

Procedure

A. Image receptor placement:
  - When checking a Bucky grid, place the image receptor in the Bucky tray.
  - When checking a grid image receptor, place the grid image receptor on the tabletop.

- When checking a grid cap, place the image receptor on the tabletop and the grid cap over the image receptor.
- When checking a slide on grid, slide the image receptor into the image receptor track and then place the entire device on the tabletop.

B. Place the homogenous phantom or water phantom on top of the grid to be tested.

C. Center the x-ray tube to the grid and film. The tube should be set at a 40-inch SID.

D. Select a technique that is appropriate for the grid ratio and that would produce a density of 1.5.

E. Expose and process the film.

F. After processing the film, use the densitometer to take readings from the center of the film and all four quadrants. Compare the density readings.

G. Record the results (Fig. 4-39).

Acceptance Parameters

NCRP Report #99 makes the following recommendation: Films should be uniform with an optical density of ±0.10.

Record Keeping

A record should be kept that documents the date of the test, who performed the test, the results of the test, and the corrective action taken.

Note: When corrective action is taken, the before and after films should be kept on file.

Potential Problems

- Failure to have the proper technique set could provide inaccurate results.
- Failure to have the x-ray tube perpendicular could provide the radiographer with inaccurate readings.
- The grid movement mechanism is not functioning properly.

Points to Ponder

- If there is a lack of uniform density in the films produced using the Bucky, the grid alignment test should performed immediately.
- If there is a lack of density in the films produced using grid image receptors, grid caps, or slide on grids, the specific grid should be removed from service.
- A damaged grid may cause a lack of uniform density.

Grid Alignment Test

Rationale

This procedure is designed to confirm that the grid is aligned with the tabletop and x-ray beam.

Testing Frequency

This test should be conducted annually or when the Bucky has been worked on.

Grid Uniformity Record Form

Type of grid: _____ **Grid ratio:** _____

_____ **mA** _____ **Exposure time** ____ **kVp** ____ **SID**

Grid Uniformity	
Area	Density Reading
Upper Right Quadrant	
Upper Left Quadrant	
Lower Right Quadrant	
Lower Left Quadrant	
Center	

Comments:

_____ _____

Signature **Date**

Figure 4-39 Grid uniformity record form.

Equipment

- 8 × 10 image receptor
- Grid alignment test tool (Fig. 4-40)
- Two small lead squares
- Four 2-inch pieces of tape

Procedure

A. The grid alignment test tool has five large holes that are spaced approximately 1 inch from the center of each hole. There are five smaller holes on the device that are used for referencing the orientation of the test tool.

B. Place the grid alignment test tool in the center of the table, perpendicular to the short axis of the tabletop.
  - The hole with one small hole on each side should be in the center of the table.
  - The three remaining small holes of test should be facing the front or Bucky handle side of the table.

C. Tape the test tool to the tabletop to ensure that it does not move during the test.

D. Cover the other holes with the two lead squares.

E. Center the x-ray tube to the hole with one small hole on each side. The tube should be set at a 40-inch SID.

F. Collimate the beam to an approximate 2.5- × 2.5-inch area.

G. Place the 8- × 10-inch image receptor crosswise in the Bucky tray and lock it securely in place. Center the Bucky tray to the central ray and close the Bucky tray.
  - For three-phase generators a technique of 2 mAs at 60 kVp should be sufficient.
  - For single-phase generators a technique of 4 mAs at 60 kVp should be sufficient.
  - The technique used depends on the speed of the imaging system.

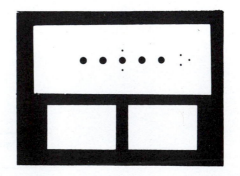

Figure 4-40 Grid alignment test tool.

H. Make the first exposure.
I. For the next four exposures, move the tube laterally and cover all holes that are not being used.
J. After the last exposure, process the film (Fig. 4-41).
K. Read the density of each hole with the densitometer. Write the density reading of each hole on the film.
L. Record the data in the QC log.

Acceptance Parameters

If the grid is properly aligned, the center hole should have the highest optical density with decreasing densities to either side.

Record Keeping

A record should be kept that documents the date of the test, who performed the test, the results of the test, and the corrective action taken.

Note: When corrective action is taken, the before and after films should be kept on file.

Potential Problems

- Failure to have the proper technique set could provide inaccurate results.
- Failure to have the x-ray tube perpendicular could provide the radiographer with inaccurate readings.
- Failure to have long enough exposure for the test could provide inaccurate results.
- The grid movement mechanism is not functioning properly.

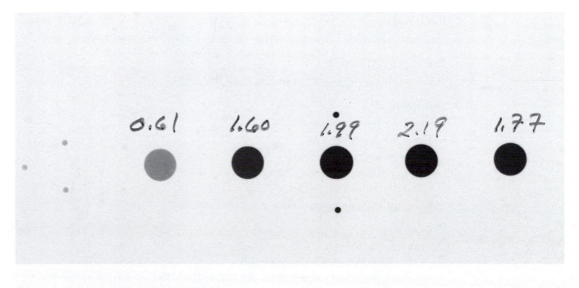

Figure 4-41 Image of the grid alignment test.

CONVENTIONAL TOMOGRAPHIC EQUIPMENT

Over the last three decades many of the procedures that required conventional tomography have been replaced with the use of computed tomography (CT) and magnetic resonance imaging (MRI). It is not within the scope of this text to discuss tomographic theory. However, it is important to remember that there are two types of tomographic systems commercially available. They are adjustable fulcrum and fixed fulcrum tomographic systems. The adjustable fulcrum system operates on the principle of moving the film either up or down to the selected level. The fixed fulcrum system moves the patient either up or down to the selected level. When working with both systems there are simple (i.e., linear) and complex (i.e., circular, elliptical, hypocycloidal, and trispiral) tomographic motions that can be used to image the desired anatomy. It is critical that tomographic equipment be tested routinely to ensure that it is functioning properly.

Typically the tests performed on conventional tomographic equipment are section level, spatial resolution, exposure uniformity, and beam path. There are several tomographic test tools commercially available. The two most commonly used are the Model 76-400 Tomographic Phantom/Test Tool manufactured by Nuclear Associates (Fig. 4-42) and the Model 132 Tomographic Test Tool manufactured by GAMMEX-RMI (Fig. 4-43). Both of these devices have a place and use in the Medical Imaging Department, but the simplest device to use is the Model 132. The following tests are based on the Model 132.

Section Level

Rationale
This test is designed to confirm that the selected fulcrum level is accurate.

Testing Frequency
Tomographic equipment should be tested annually.

Equipment
- 8 × 10 image receptor
- Tomographic test tool
  - 4-centimeter spacer disk
  - 1.5-centimeter number helix disk (Fig. 4-44)
  - 2-centimeter spacer disk
  - 1-centimeter spacer disk

Procedure
A. Initially perform the following tasks.
  - Prepare the unit for tomography.
  - Place the image receptor in the Bucky tray. The image receptor may be placed in the tray either lengthwise or crosswise.

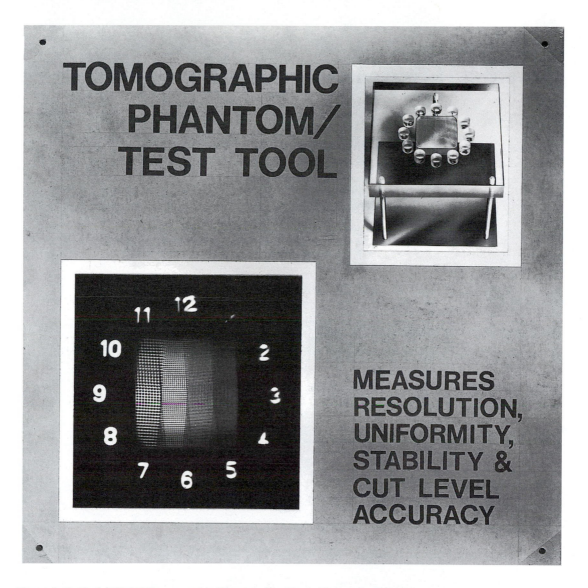

Figure 4-42 Model 76-400 Tomographic Phantom/Test Tool. *(Courtesy of Nuclear Associates, used with permission.)*

- Select a technique commonly used for an extremity (i.e., elbow, ankle, etc.). The technique selected will be determined by the speed of the imaging system, exposure angle, and tomographic mode.

B. Perform the following tasks.
- Turn on the collimator light and place the 4-centimeter spacer disk on the tabletop in the center of the crosshairs.
- Place the 1.5-centimeter disk containing the number helix on top of the 4-centimeter disk.

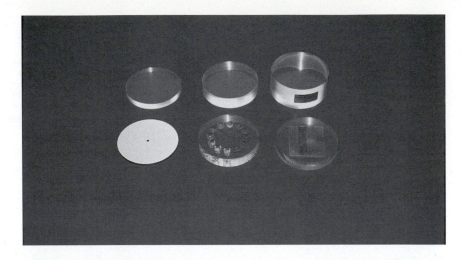

Figure 4-43 Model 132 Tomographic Test. *(Courtesy of GAMMEX-RMI, used with permission.)*

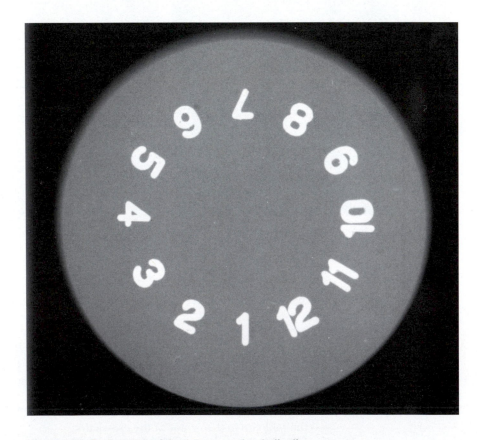

Figure 4-44 Radiograph of the 1.5 cm number helix disc.

  • Set the fulcrum for 4.5 centimeters.
  • Select a tomographic angle that will produce a thin cut.
C. Expose and process the film.
D. Repeat Steps B and C for the other tomographic modes.
E. Analyze the images and record the results.
  • The number 5 should be the clearest, which is 4.5 centimeters above the tabletop; the numbers 4 and 6 should be partially blurred; and the numbers 3 and 7 should be completely blurred.

Acceptance Parameters

NCRP Report #99 makes the following recommendations: The section level should be within ±5 millimeters.

Record Keeping

A record should be kept that documents the date of the test, who performed the test, the results of the test, and the corrective action taken.

Potential Problems

Failure to follow the test protocol could lead to erroneous results.

IMPORTANT REMINDER

• To achieve various section levels the 1- and 2-centimeter spacer disks are used in conjunction with the 4-centimeter disk to provide a variety of section levels from 1 millimeter to 8.2 centimeters.
• Successful tomographic images are achieved by selecting a low mA and a long exposure time.

Spatial Resolution

Rationale

This test is designed to confirm that the resolution of the tomographic unit is optimal.

Testing Frequency

Spatial resolution of tomographic equipment should be tested annually.

Equipment

• 8 × 10 image receptor
• Ruler with metric markings
• Tomographic test tool
  • 4-centimeter spacer
  • 1.3-centimeter mesh pattern (contains wire mesh segments of 20, 30, 40, and 50) [Fig. 4-45]
  • 2-centimeter spacer
  • 1-centimeter spacer

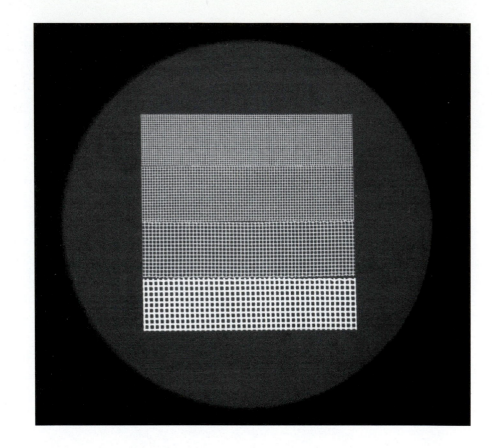

Figure 4-45 Radiograph of the 1.3 cm mesh pattern.

Procedure

A. Initially perform the following tasks.
  - Prepare the unit for tomography.
  - Place the image receptor in the Bucky tray. The image receptor may be placed in the tray either lengthwise or crosswise.
  - Select a technique commonly used for an extremity (i.e., elbow, ankle, etc.). The technique selected will be determined by the speed of the imaging system, exposure angle, and tomographic mode.
B. Perform the following tasks.
  - Turn on the collimator light and place the 4-cm spacer disk on the tabletop in the center of the crosshairs.
  - Place the 1.3-cm disk containing the wire mesh on top of the 4-cm disk. Arrange the disk so that the long axis of the wire mesh is parallel to the direction of tube movement.
  - Set the fulcrum for 4.5 cm.
  - Select a tomographic angle that will produce a thin cut.

C. Expose and process the film.
D. Repeat steps B and C for the other tomographic modes.
E. Analyze the images and record the results.
   - The 40-mesh portion should be clearly seen for at least 3 mm of the strip length.

Acceptance Parameters

NCRP Report #99 makes the following recommendation: 40 mesh or better should be visualized.

Record Keeping

A record should be kept that documents the date of the test, who performed the test, the results of the test, and the corrective action taken.

Potential Problems

Failure to follow the test protocol could lead to erroneous results.

> **IMPORTANT REMINDER**
>
> - Successful tomographic images are achieved by selecting a low mA and a long exposure time.

Exposure Uniformity and Beam Path

Rationale

This test is designed to confirm that exposure uniformity and beam path of the tomographic unit are optimal.

Testing Frequency

Exposure uniformity and beam path of tomographic equipment should be tested on an annual basis.

Equipment

- 8 × 10 image receptor
- Densitometer
- Tomographic test tool
  - 4-cm spacer
  - 2-cm spacer
  - 1-cm spacer
  - lead aperture blocker

Procedure

A. Initially perform the following tasks.
   - Prepare the unit for tomography.
   - Place the image receptor in the Bucky tray. The image receptor may be placed in the tray either lengthwise or crosswise.

- Select a technique commonly used for an extremity (i.e., elbow, ankle, etc.). The technique selected will be determined by the speed of the imaging system, exposure angle, and tomographic mode.

B. Perform the following tasks.
- Turn on the collimator light and stack the 4-, 2-, and 1-centimeter spacer disks on top of each other and place them on the tabletop in the center of the crosshairs.
- Place the lead blocker on top of the three disks.
- Set the fulcrum at 4.5 centimeters.
- Select a tomographic angle that will produce a thin cut.

C. Expose and process the film.

D. Repeat steps A and B for the other tomographic modes.

E. Analyze the images and record the results.
- The line image produced should have an optical density of 1.0.
- The width of the line should be approximately 4 millimeters.

Acceptance Parameters
- NCRP Report #99 states that this is a qualitative assessment.
- Test results should be compared with the manufacturer's specifications.

Record Keeping
A record should be kept that documents the date of the test, who performed the test, the results of the test, and the corrective action taken.

Potential Problem
Failure to follow the test protocol could lead to erroneous results.

IMPORTANT REMINDER
- Successful tomographic images are achieved by selecting a low mA and a long exposure time.

CHAPTER REVIEW

- The radiographic systems of the Medical Imaging Department are an important component of the overall QA program. Failure to have all systems properly calibrated will result in increased film costs, increased exposure to the patient and personnel, and suboptimal diagnosis on the part of the radiologist.
- The x-ray emission spectrum is greatly affected by changes in target material, kVp, mA, mAs, filtration, and voltage waveform.
- Focal spot size is determined by several factors. It is important to remember that focal spot size may exceed the manufacturers stated size by as much as 30% to 50%.
- Light field/beam alignment is a simple test that determines how effective beam collimation is. Failure to have the beam properly collimated results in

increased exposure to the patient. Collimation of the x-ray beam needs be within ±2% of the SID.

- Beam perpendicularity is a QC test that can be done individually or inconjunction with the light field/beam alignment test. Failure to have the beam perpendicular to the film may result in errors in diagnosis and potentially an increase in repeat films. The upper bead of the beam perpendicularity needs to be within 5 millimeters of the lower bead.
- Bucky/light field alignment is a simple test that determines how effective beam collimation is when the PBL is not engaged. Failure to have the beam properly collimated results in increased exposure to the patient. Collimation of the x-ray beam needs be within ±2% of the SID.
- Bucky/beam perpendicularity is a QC test that can be done individually or in conjunction with the Bucky/light field alignment test. Failure to have the beam perpendicular to the film may result errors in diagnosis and potentially an increase in repeat films. The upper bead of the beam perpendicularity should be within 5 millimeters of the lower bead.
- The NCRP states that, when automatic collimation (positive beam limitation) is engaged, the collimated light field should be within ±3% of the SID.
- Light field illuminance should be checked annually and the illuminance level should be no less than 160 lux or 15 footcandles.
- Checking the SID is a simple procedure and requires only a few minutes. It is important to check both the SID to tabletop distance and the SID to bucky distance. Failure to have the correct SID may lead to films that are either overexposed or underexposed. The SID indicator must be within ±2% of the stated SID.
- Exposure time for single phase generators may be checked using either the manual spin top or mechanized spin top. Typically the times of 1/30 second, 1/20 second, 1/10 second, and 1/5 second are checked.
- Exposure times for three phase generators are checked using the mechanized spin top. Exposure times of 1/5 second or less may be checked. The images produced are measured in degrees of arc, using a timing protractor.
- Kilovoltage is measured over the 50 kVp to 140 kVp range using a digital kVp meter. The kilovoltage of a particular generator may be measured in either 10 or 20 kVp increments. Kilovoltage over this range must be within ±4 kVp of the set kVp. According to the NCRP, in the 60 kVp to 100 kVp range it is possible to have a tolerance of ±2 kVp.
- The ability of a generator to reproduce the same mAs at different mA and exposure times is called millamperage-seconds (mAs) reciprocity. mAs has an acceptance tolerance of ±10% of the established mAs.
- It is assumed that when milliamperage is doubled, the quantity of x-rays produced will double, and exposure will double. This concept is called linearity. Over the clinical range mA linearity should be within ±10% of the established mA.

- It is assumed that when exposure time is doubled, exposure also doubles. This concept is called linearity. Timer linearity has an accepted tolerance of ±10%.
- The ability of a specified generator to consistently produce exposures is called exposure reproducibility. Exposures for a specified generator need to be reproducible within ±5%.
- An alternate test for exposure reproducibility is coefficient of variation, which measures mR, kVp, and time. The coefficient of variation for each factor should be no greater than 0.05.
- mR/mAs output determines that the average radiation output of different and like generators is consistent. The NCRP recommends that both different and like generators have an average radiation output of ±10% at 80 kVp.
- AEC devices operate on the principle of sensing the amount of radiation passing through the patient and terminating the exposure when a predetermined exposure has been reached.
- The primary advantage of AEC is that it provides consistent film densities over a wide range of kVp and patient thicknesses.
- The most common cause of repeat films is the failure to correctly position the anatomic area over the ionization chamber.
- The amount of material (usually aluminum) needed to reduce the intensity of an x-ray beam by 50% is the HVL. The HVL provides information about the penetrating ability (quality) of the x-ray beam. It is also used to determine that the filtration placed in the path of the x-ray beam is sufficient. The HVL should be checked for the 50 to 130 kVp ranges. The minimum HVL for 50 to 70 kVp is 1.5 mm Al and 2.5 mm Al for 90 kVp and higher. At 80 kVp the HVL should be 2.3 mm Al.
- The primary purpose of a grid is to improve radiographic contrast by removing scatter radiation.
- When new grids are purchased, it is important to take test radiographs to ensure that they are not damaged or have imperfections.
- It is important to check the grids in the Medical Imaging Department for uniformity. Density readings must be taken in the center and all four quadrants. When measured with a densitometer, test films should have an optical density of 1.0 ± 0.10.
- Proper grid alignment is critical for image quality. The NCRP states that when girds are used, the resulting films should be uniform.
- Visual checks of the radiographic systems are done annually and are either pass or fail.
- The section level, spatial resolution, exposure uniformity, and beam path are aspects of conventional tomographic systems that need to be checked annually.

DISCUSSION QUESTIONS

1. What information can the staff radiographer assigned to a particular room provide the QC technician?
2. What are the responsibilities of the staff radiographer in the QA and QC program?
3. Where should QC results be recorded?
4. How often should QC tests be performed on a specific radiographic system?
5. Which QC tests are of critical importance?

REVIEW QUESTIONS

1. The spinning top test can be used to evaluate
   1. Timer accuracy
   2. Effect of kVp on contrast
   3. Rectifier failure
   a. 1 only
   b. 1 and 2 only
   c. 1 and 3 only
   d. 1, 2, and 3
2. PBL devices must be accurate to within
   a. ±5% of the SID
   b. ±4% of the SID
   c. ±3% of the SID
   d. ±2% of the SID
3. What are the accepted mAs reciprocity parameters?
   a. ±5%
   b. ±10%
   c. ±15%
   d. ±20%
4. What are the accepted exposure reproducibility parameters?
   a. ±5%
   b. ±10%
   c. ±15%
   d. ±20%
5. What are the acceptable mR/mAs output parameters?
   a. ±5%
   b. ±10%
   c. ±15%
   d. ±20%

6. It was determined that the x-ray field size was off by 1 centimeter on three of four sides at 100 centimeters. Is the collimator within acceptable parameters?
   a. Yes
   b. No
   c. Not enough information has been given

7. A comprehensive quality control program includes the testing and/or monitoring of the
   1. kVp
   2. Focal spot size
   3. Exposure time accuracy
   a. 1 only
   b. 1 and 2 only
   c. 1 and 3 only
   d. 1, 2, and 3

8. What mAs should be duplicated for the mAs reciprocity test?
   a. 5 mAs
   b. 10 mAs
   c. 15 mAs
   d. 20 mAs

9. Which of the following test results is within the range of tolerance for the component evaluated?
   a. A selected kVp of 80 yields a measured kVp of 86.
   b. A spinning top test yields eight dots for selected exposure time of 0.05 seconds.
   c. X-ray/light field alignment varies by 3 centimeters toward the head of the table at SID of 40 inches.
   d. A stated focal spot of 0.6 millimeters measures 0.9 millimeters.

10. A properly functioning exposure timer on a three-phase radiographic unit would demonstrate an
    a. arc of 6° for an exposure of 0.017 seconds.
    b. arc of 9° for an exposure of 0.05 seconds.
    c. arc of 12° for an exposure time of 0.25 seconds.
    d. arc of 16° for an exposure time of 0.5 seconds.

11. If an x-ray beam is created using exposure factors of 80 kV, 600 mA, and 0.016 seconds and yields an exposure output of 240 mR, what would the mR/mAs be?
    a. 2.5
    b. 25
    c. 250
    d. 2500

12. Radiographs from a particular single-phase, full-wave rectified unit were underexposed, using known correct exposures. A spinning top test was performed at 100 mA, 1/20 second, and 70 kVp, and four dots (dashes)

were visualized on the finished film. Which of the following is indicated?

   a. The 1/20-second time station is inaccurate.

   b. The 100-mA station is inaccurate.

   c. A rectifier is not functioning.

   d. The processor needs servicing.

13. What is the NEMA allowance parameter for x-ray tubes that have a stated focal spot size greater than 1.5 millimeters?

   a. The stated focal spot size may be to 50% greater.

   b. The stated focal spot size may be up to 40% greater.

   c. The stated focal spot size may be up to 30% greater.

   d. The stated focal spot size may be up to 20% greater.

14. What is the acceptance criterion for exposure time when using a digital timer?

   a. ±5%

   b. ±10%

   c. ±15%

   d. ±20%

15. Which of the following statements is correct about grid uniformity?

   a. Films should be uniform with an optical density of ±0.4.

   b. Films should be uniform with an optical density of ±0.3.

   c. Films should be uniform with an optical density of ±0.2.

   d. Films should be uniform with an optical density of ±0.1.

16. Which of the following statements is correct?

   a. Characteristic radiation is produced when incident electrons interact with an inner shell electron.

   b. Characteristic radiation is produced when incident electrons interact with the nucleus.

   c. Characteristic radiation is produced when incident electrons interact with an outer shell electron.

   d. Characteristic radiation is produced when incident electrons interact with an inner shell electron and the nucleus.

17. Bremsstrahlung radiation is associated with the

   a. continuous x-ray emission spectrum

   b. discrete x-ray emission spectrum

   c. both a and b

   d. neither a nor b

18. When using a calibrated stepwedge for mAs reciprocity the density of each step should be within a density of

   a. ±0.1

   b. ±0.2

   c. ±0.3

   d. ±0.4

19. Characteristic radiation is associated with the

   a. continuous x-ray emission spectrum

   b. discrete x-ray emission spectrum

    c. both a and b

    d. neither a nor b

20. Which of the following statements is correct?

    a. As kVp increases, there is a corresponding increase in quality and quantity.

    b. As kVp increases, there is a corresponding decrease in quality and no change in quantity.

    c. As kVp increases, there is a corresponding decrease in quality and quantity.

    d. As kVp increases, there is a corresponding increase in quality and no change in quantity.

21. Which of the following factors affects the x-ray emission spectrum?

        1. Added filtration

        2. Anode angle

        3. Voltage waveform

        4. Source-to-image distance

    a. 1 and 3 only

    b. 2 and 4 only

    c. 1, 2, and 3 only

    d. 1, 2, 3, and 4

22. Which of the following statements is correct?

    a. Bremsstrahlung radiation is produced when incident electrons interact with an inner shell electron.

    b. Bremsstrahlung radiation is produced when incident electrons interact with the nucleus.

    c. Bremsstrahlung radiation is produced when incident electrons interact with an outer shell electron.

    d. Bremsstrahlung radiation is produced when incident electrons interact with an inner shell electron and the nucleus.

23. Which of the following determines focal spot size?

        1. Anode angle

        2. Filament size

        3. Filament shape

        4. Distance between the anode and cathode

    a. 1 and 3 only

    b. 2 and 4 only

    c. 1, 2, and 3 only

    d. 1, 2, 3, and 4

24. At 80 kVp the HVL should be

    a. 2.1 mm Al

    b. 2.3 mm Al

    c. 2.5 mm Al

    d. 2.7 mm Al

25. For any combination of selected technique factors, the estimated coefficient of variation of radiation exposures shall be no greater than
    a. 0.05
    b. 0.07
    c. 0.10
    d. 0.20
26. Which of the following statements is correct?
    a. The AEC shall maintain a constant film density to within ±0.05 of the average OD while varying kVp.
    b. The AEC shall maintain a constant film density to within ±0.1 of the average OD while varying kVp.
    c. The AEC shall maintain a constant film density to within ±0.2 of the average OD while varying kVp.
    d. The AEC shall maintain a constant film density to within ± 0.3 of the average OD while varying kVp.

5

Fluoroscopic Systems

KEY WORDS

Anode	Image intensifer
Electrostatic lenses	Input screen
Half value layer (HVL)	Photocathode
Imaging chain	Output screen

GOALS

1. To learn the required and optional quality control (QC) tests for fluoroscopic equipment.
2. To understand the findings from fluoroscopic QC tests.
3. To understand the required procedures for performing fluoroscopic QC tests.
4. To learn the required QC tests for mobile fluoroscopic equipment.

OBJECTIVES

1. Identify the routine QC tests performed on fluoroscopic equipment.
2. State the rationale for performing each QC test.
3. Explain the rationale behind testing frequency.
4. Identify and discuss how often each test is performed.
5. Identify and describe the equipment used for all QC tests.
6. Describe and discuss the procedure for performing each test.
7. State the acceptance parameters for each test.
8. Identify and discuss potential problems that might arise during or after each test.
9. Discuss problems that might result in erroneous findings for each test.
10. Discuss and explain the importance of record keeping.

11. Analyze and interpret test results.
12. Identify and discuss the tests performed on mobile fluoroscopic equipment.

INTRODUCTION

Historically, fluoroscopy has been a part of the imaging sciences for over one hundred years. In February of 1896, Enrico Salvoni described a device where the internal structures of an object could be viewed through direct observation. This device was called a cryptoscope (Eisenberg, 1992). Thomas Edison, in March of 1896, discovered that calcium tungstate would fluoresce when stimulated by x-rays. Edison developed a calcium tungstate screen that was used with his vitascope for viewing the internal structures of an object. Both the cryptoscope and vitascope were the precursors of the modern fluoroscope (Eisenberg, 1992). The cryptoscope and vitascope were hand-held devices and were used well into the 1920s. In 1900 and 1901, the open fluoroscopic screen was introduced and would continue be used as the primary method for viewing of internal structures into the 1960s. In 1953, Westinghouse introduced the first commercially available image intensifier. It should be stressed that practical image intensification did not occur until 1962 with the introduction of a compact, 6-inch **image intensifier.** In the 1980s and 1990s, digital fluoroscopy was developed and introduced in medical imaging. Figure 5-1 illustrates the development of fluoroscopy in medical imaging.

As a result of the changes and progress made in fluoroscopy, it has become an important component of the medical imaging department. The same diligence that is demonstrated in the maintenance and quality control (QC) testing of radiographic systems should be extended to the fluoroscopic systems of the medical imaging department.

When discussing fluoroscopic imaging, it is important to outline the fluoroscopic imaging chain as it presently exists (Fig. 5-2). There are several excellent texts available that discuss the major components of the **imaging chain.** This text will review only the image intensifier and requirements for the x-ray tube.

THE X-RAY TUBE AND IMAGE INTENSIFIER

The fluoroscopic x-ray tube is similar to a radiographic tube but it is designed to function at a much lower mA for a longer period of time. Fluoroscopic x-ray tubes generally operate in the range of 0.5 to 5 mA. The typical mA used for

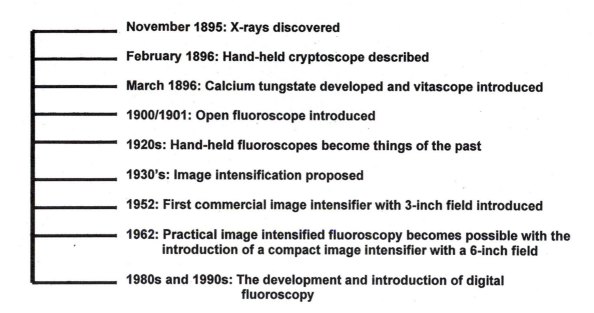

November 1895: X-rays discovered

February 1896: Hand-held cryptoscope described

March 1896: Calcium tungstate developed and vitascope introduced

1900/1901: Open fluoroscope introduced

1920s: Hand-held fluoroscopes become things of the past

1930's: Image intensification proposed

1952: First commercial image intensifier with 3-inch field introduced

1962: Practical image intensified fluoroscopy becomes possible with the introduction of a compact image intensifier with a 6-inch field

1980s and 1990s: The development and introduction of digital fluoroscopy

Figure 5-1 Fluoroscopy timeline.

fluoroscopic procedures is between 1 and 3 mA. The tube is mounted under the table and has a fixed source-to-object distance (SOD) of at least 15 inches (38 centimeters). On mobile fluoroscopic units the SOD is at least 12 inches (30 centimeters). These distances have been established as a radiation safety measure for the patient. The fluoroscopic tube may be operated from a foot switch or a hand control that is located on the image intensifier tower.

The **image intensifier** (II) consists of an input phosphor, photocathode, electrostatic lenses, anode, and output screen surrounded by an evacuated glass envelope. Table 5-1 describes each component.

All of the components work together to amplify electronically the brightness of the fluoroscopic image by an average of 5000 to 20,000 times. The enhancement of the image begins as the primary beam exits the patient and interacts with the input screen of the II. The x-rays are absorbed by the **input screen** and converted to light. The light then interacts with the **photocathode** and this interaction results in the production of electrons. The electrons are then accelerated by the potential difference that exists between the photocathode and **anode.** The **electrostatic lenses** focus and accelerate the electrons toward the output screen of the II. Upon reaching the output screen the electrons are converted to light and the image may be viewed or recorded or both.

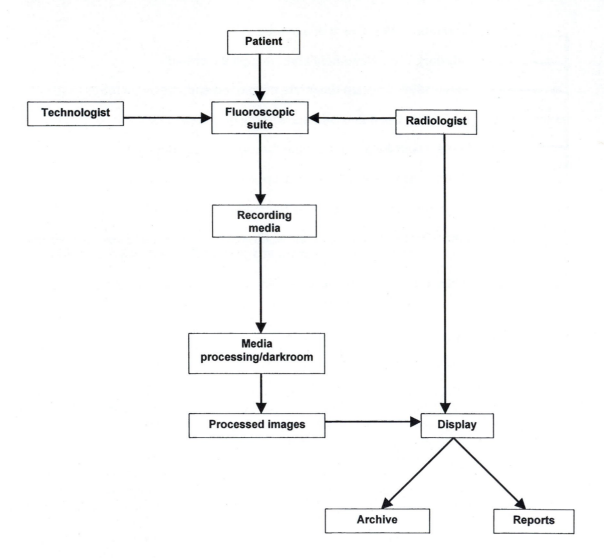

Figure 5-2 Fluoroscopic imaging chain.

FLUOROSCOPIC QUALITY CONTROL TESTS

There are a variety of QC tests performed on fixed and mobile fluoroscopic systems. QC testing of both fixed and mobile fluoroscopic systems should be carried out on a routine schedule by the person assigned. The QC tests that are performed on fluoroscopic equipment are listed in Table 5-2. QC testing of digital fluoroscopy equipment will not be discussed because, at the present time, there are no guidelines for testing of the equipment. However, the ma-

Table 5-1
Components of the Image Intensifier Tube

Component	Description
Input screen	Sodium activated cesium iodide
	~0.1–0.2 mm thick
	Between 6 and 23 inches in diameter
	Use of cesium iodide reduces patient dose
	A 50 keV x-ray photon produces ~2000 light photons
Photocathode	Antimony and cesium compound
	Converts ~2000 light photons to ~100 photoelectrons
	Separated from the input screen by a protective coating
Electrostatic lenses	Positively charged electrodes
	Located on the sides of the imaging tube
	Focuses and accelerates the electrons
	A higher or lower voltage is applied to change field size
Anode	Attracts the photoelectrons
	Carries a positive charge of ~25,000 volts (25 kV)
	Has a small hole in center to permit passage of photoelectrons
Output screen	Silver activated zinc cadmium sulfide phosphor
	Converts ~100 photoelectrons to ~200,000 light photons

jority of tests conducted on regular fluoroscopic systems can be applied to digital systems.

There is nothing written that says the technical staff assigned to rotate through a particular fluoroscopic room cannot assist in the testing program. In fact, it is an excellent idea because the technical staff can provide valuable information to the quality control technologist. The tests performed on fluoroscopic equipment are image size, beam limitation (field size), beam alignment, half value layer, maximum exposure rate, standard exposure levels, fluoroscopic resolution (TV), fluoroscopic resolution (spot film device), image quality (high and low contrast), exposure reproducibility, automatic brightness stabilization (ABS), and automatic gain control (AGC).

Fluoroscopic Image Size

Rationale

This procedure is designed to confirm that the fluoroscopic system is imaging the entire area it was designed to image.

Testing Frequency

Fluoroscopic image size is checked on a semi-annual basis.

Table 5-2
Fluoroscopic Equipment: Testing Frequency, Acceptance Parameters

Quality Control Test	Frequency of Test	Acceptance Parameters	Performed on Mobile Equipment
Fluoroscopic image size	Semiannual	Not < 1 cm smaller than specified diameter	Yes
Fluoroscopic beam limitation	Semiannual	No greater than 3% of SID	Yes
Maximum fluoroscopic exposure rate	Semiannual	Manual: ≤ 1.3 mC/kg/min or ≤ 5 R/min AEC systems: ≤ 2.6 mC/kg/min or ≤ 10 R/min	Yes
Standard fluoroscopic exposure levels	Semiannual	6-inch mode without grid: 0.5–0.8 mC/kg/min	Yes
		9-inch mode without grid: 0.4–0.7 mC/kg/min	
		Exposure values should be between 1 and 3 R/min	
		AEC should set 80–90 kV	
Exposure reproducibility	Semiannual	<0.05	Yes
mA linearity	Semiannual	Within 0.1 of set mA	Yes
kVp accuracy	Semiannual	± 5%	Yes
Fluoroscopic resolution (TV)	Semiannual	6-inch intensifier: should not be <30 mesh/in at the center and not <24 mesh/in at the edge	Yes
		9-inch intensifier: should not be <20 mesh/in at the center and edge	
Fluoroscopic resolution (spot film)	Semiannual	6-inch intensifier: should be 40 mesh/in at the center and 35 mesh/in at the edge	Yes
		9-inch intensifier: should be 35 mesh/in at the center and 30 mesh/in at the edge	
Low contrast fluoroscopic test	Semiannual	The 1/4-inch and 3/16-inch holes should be seen clearly and the 1/8-inch holes should be barely seen	Yes
ABC and AEC controls	Semiannual	These systems should function similar to same installations and systems	Yes

Equipment
- Collimator template (see Fig. 4-8)
- Direct exposure film holder
  - Use an 8×10 for the 6-inch mode
  - Use a 10×12 for the 9-inch mode
- Nongumming tape (i.e., masking)
- Patient equivalent phantom

Procedure

A. Initially perform the following tasks.
  - Turn on the fluoroscopic unit.
  - Raise the fluoroscopic tower to its maximum height and remove the grid.
  - Open the collimator shutters to their maximum dimension.
  - Set the mA and kVp at the lowest settings possible and record the values.
B. Under fluoroscopy, center and tape the template underneath the fluoroscopic tower, as close as possible to the input end of the II tube.
C. Perform the following tasks.
  - Measure and record the distance from the template to the tabletop.
  - From the TV monitor, measure the vertical and longitudinal dimensions.
  - Carefully slip the direct exposure film holder between the template and the II.
D. Expose the film; the amount of time required for exposure will vary from 15 seconds to 2 minutes. If overexposure occurs, a patient equivalent phantom may need to be placed on the tabletop.
E. Process the film.
F. Measure and record the vertical and longitudinal axis of the film.
G. Repeat Steps A through F for the remaining film size.

Acceptance Parameters

NCRP Report #99 recommends that fluoroscopic image should not be less than 1 centimeter smaller than the specified diameter.

Record Keeping

A record should be kept that documents the date of the test, who performed the test, the results of the test, and the corrective action taken.

Potential Problem

Failure to follow the procedure will result in erroneous results.

Fluoroscopic Beam Limitation

Rationale

This procedure is designed to confirm that the shutters of the collimator are within in specified standards.

Testing Frequency

Fluoroscopic beam limitation is performed semiannually.

Equipment

- Template (see Fig. 4-8)
- Direct exposure film holder
  - Use an 8 × 10 for the 6-inch mode
  - Use a 10 × 12 for the 9-inch mode

Procedure

A. Initially perform the following tasks.
  - Turn on the fluoroscopic unit.
  - Raise the fluoroscopic tower to its maximum height and remove the grid.
  - Set the mA and kVp at the lowest settings possible and record the values.
B. Open the collimator shutters as follows:
  - For the 6-inch mode, approximately 6×6 inches.
  - For the 9-inch mode, approximately 9×9 inches.
C. Under fluoroscopy, center and tape the template underneath the fluoroscopic tower, as close as possible to the input end of the II tube.
D. Perform the following tasks.
  - Measure and record the distance from the template to the tabletop.
  - From the TV monitor, measure the vertical and longitudinal dimensions
  - Carefully slip the direct exposure film holder between the template and the II.
E. Measure the image size on the TV monitor and record it.
F. Carefully slip the direct exposure film holder between the template and the II.
G. Expose the film; the amount of time required for exposure will vary from 15 seconds to 2 minutes. If overexposure occurs, a patient equivalent phantom may need to be placed on the tabletop.
H. Process the film.
I. Measure and record the vertical and longitudinal axis of the film.
J. Repeat Steps B through I for the remaining film size.
K. Repeat this procedure for the minimum SID.
L. Make the following comparisons.
  - Compare the minimum SID film with the monitor measurement
  - Compare the maximum SID film with the monitor measurement

Acceptance Parameters

- NCRP Report #99 recommends that fluoroscopic beam limitation be no greater than 3% of the SID at any tower height.
- The difference between the fluoroscopic image and the spot film image should be no greater than 3% of the SID.

Record Keeping

A record should be kept that documents the date of the test, who performed the test, the results of the test, and the corrective action taken.

Potential Problems

Failure to follow the procedure will result in erroneous results.

Fluoroscopic Beam Alignment

Rationale
This procedure is designed to confirm that the x-ray field and image receptor are aligned.

Testing Frequency
The light field and x-ray field and beam perpendicularity should be checked semiannually.

Equipment
- Nonscreen film
- Fluoroscopic beam alignment device (Fig. 5-3)
- Ruler with centimeter and inch markings

Procedure
A. Initially perform the following tasks.
- Turn on the fluoroscopic unit.
- Raise the fluoroscopic tower to its maximum height and remove the grid.
- Set the mA and kVp at the lowest settings possible and record the values.
- Place the test device on the table.
  One set of brass strips will be along the center line of table.
  Push the four strips toward the center of the device.
B. Perform the following tasks.
- Under fluoroscopy, center and lock the imaging tower.
- Lower the imaging tower to its lowest limit.
- Open the collimator to its fullest extent.
C. Under fluoroscopy, withdraw the brass strips so that the inner end of each strip corresponds to the four edges of the visual field.

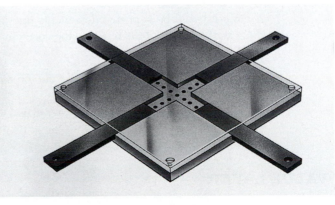

Figure 5-3 Fluoroscopic beam alignment device. *(Courtesy of Nuclear Associates, used with permission.)*

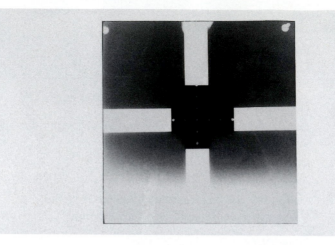

Figure 5-4 Image of the fluoroscopic beam alignment device taken by a misaligned fluoroscope with a defective collimator. *(Courtesy of Nuclear Associates, used with permission.)*

D. To determine the visual field size, record the spacing distribution of the four brass strips.
E. Place a film on top of the test device and expose it.
F. Process the film.
G. Measure the image and record the results (Fig. 5-4).
H. Repeat steps B through G for the maximum height of the II.

Acceptance Parameters
The ends of the brass strips should correspond with the edges of the field.

Record Keeping
A record should be kept that documents the date of the test, who performed the test, the results of the test, and the corrective action taken.

Potential Problems
- Failure to level the table could provide the radiographer with inaccurate measurements.
- Failure to have the x-ray tube perpendicular could provide the radiographer with inaccurate measurements.

HALF VALUE LAYER

When x-rays are produced, they exit the tube as a polyenergetic beam. The beam consists of different wavelengths and frequencies. The x-ray beam is of-

Table 5-3
Minimum Half-Value Layers (mm Al) for Single- and Three-Phase Units and Minimum Total Filtration at Various Tube Potentials

Tube Potential (kVp)	Minimum HVL (mm of Al)
80	2.3
90	2.5
100	2.7
110	3.0
120	3.2
130	3.5
140	3.8
150	4.1

From NCRP Report #99 page 62.

ten described as having "soft" and "hard" rays. The "soft" rays of the beam are low energy and are absorbed in the soft tissues, which results in increased exposure to the patient. These low energy x-rays can be eliminated or reduced by placing an absorbing material in the path of the x-ray beam to attenuate the beam and make it more homogenous.

The amount of material (usually aluminum) needed to reduce the intensity of an x-ray beam by 50% is called the **half value layer (HVL).** The HVL provides information about the penetrating ability (quality) of the x-ray beam. It is also used to determine whether the filtration placed in the path of the x-ray beam is sufficient. Information regarding the minimum HVLs required can be found in Table 5-3.

Half-Value Layer Measurement

Rationale
This procedure is designed to confirm that the filtration installed at the fluoroscopic x-ray tube is kept at a suitable level to help minimize exposure to the patient.

Testing Frequency
This test should be performed semiannually or when the x-ray tube has been replaced.

Equipment
- Digital R-meter with ionization chamber attachment (Fig. 5-5)
- Support stand for the ionization chamber
- Six pieces of 1-millimeter aluminum (see Fig. 4-36)
- HVL record form

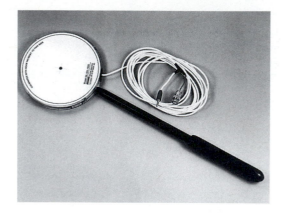
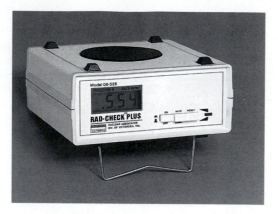

Figure 5-5 Direct readout R-meter and ionization chamber. *(Courtesy of Nuclear Associates, used with permission.)*

Procedure
A. Initially perform the following tasks.
- Raise the image intensifier tower to its maximum height.
- Place the support stand on the table.
- Place the ionization chamber on the support stand.
- Raise the support stand so the ionization chamber is halfway between the tower and tabletop.
- Under fluoroscopy, center the ionization chamber to the center of beam.
- Collimate the beam to an area just slightly smaller than the a 6 × 6 aluminum sheets.
- Turn the R-meter on and allow it to warm up.
- Attach the ionization chamber to the R-meter.
- Select the kVp that is most commonly used for fluoroscopy (i.e., 100 kVp).

B. Perform the following tasks.
- Make an exposure with no aluminum in the beam and record the results on the HVL record form.
- Place 1 millimeter of aluminum in the x-ray beam; make an exposure and record the results.
- Place 2 millimeters of aluminum in the x-ray beam; make an exposure and record the results.
- Place 3 millimeters of aluminum in the x-ray beam; make an exposure and record the results.
- Place 4 millimeters of aluminum in the x-ray beam; make an exposure and record the results.
- Place 5 millimeters of aluminum in the x-ray beam; make an exposure and record the results.

- Place 6 millimeters of aluminum in the x-ray beam; make an exposure and record the results.

Acceptance Parameters
- NCRP Report #99 states that the minimum HVL at 100 kVp is 2.7 mm Al.
- Refer to Table 5-3 for other HVL information.

Record Keeping
A record should be kept that documents the date of the test, who performed the test, the results of the test, and the corrective action taken.

Potential Problem
Failure to follow the test protocol will lead to erroneous results.

Maximum Fluoroscopic Exposure Rate (Manual Mode)

Rationale
This procedure is designed to confirm that the maximum fluoroscopic rate for manual systems does not exceed Federal regulations.

Testing Frequency
Maximum fluoroscopic rates are performed semiannually.

Equipment
- Direct readout R-meter and ionization chamber
- Two 3-millimeter-thick sheets of lead
- Support structure for lead sheets

Procedure
A. Prior to starting this procedure, a concise written plan should be established for repeating this procedure. The plan should include the following information.
- Operating mA
- Operating kVp
- Collimation
- Tower height
- Position of the ionization chamber
- Position of the phantom
B. Initially perform the following tasks.
- Turn the fluoroscopic unit on.
- Place the unit in the manual exposure mode.
- Select the maximum mA and kVp.
- Place the ionization chamber on the tabletop and attach it to the R-meter.
- Turn on the R-meter and ensure that it is in the exposure rate mode.
C. Under fluoroscopic control, position the ionization chamber in the radiation field.

D. Place the support structure over the ionization chamber.
E. Place the lead sheets on the support structure over the ionization chamber.
F. Place the II tower over the test equipment.
G. Fluoroscope the ionization chamber long enough for the automatic exposure controls (AECs) to stabilize.
H. Read and record the exposure rate.

Acceptance Parameters
NCRP Report #99 recommends that the maximum fluoroscopic rate for manual systems should be ≤5 R/min (1.3 mC/kg/min).

Record Keeping
A record should be kept that documents the date of the test, who performed the test, the results of the test, and the corrective action taken.

Potential Problem
Failure to accurately record all systems parameters could lead to inconclusive results.

Maximum Fluoroscopic Exposure Rate (Automatic Mode)

Rationale
This procedure is designed to confirm that the maximum fluoroscopic rate for manual systems and automatic exposure control systems does not exceed Federal regulations.

Testing Frequency
Maximum fluoroscopic rates are performed semiannually.

Equipment
- Direct readout R-meter and ionization chamber
- Two 3-millimeter-thick sheets of lead
- Support structure for lead sheets

Procedure
A. Prior to starting this procedure, a concise written plan should be established for repeating this procedure. The plan should include the following information.
   - Operating mA
   - Operating kVp
   - Collimation
   - Tower height
   - Position of the ionization chamber
   - Position of the phantom
B. Initially perform the following tasks.
   - Turn the fluoroscopic unit on.

- Place the unit in the automatic exposure mode.
- If mA and kVp controls are available, select the maximum mA and kVp.
- Place the ionization chamber on the tabletop and attach it to the R-meter.
- Turn on the R-meter and ensure that it is in the exposure rate mode.

C. Under fluoroscopic control, position the ionization chamber in the radiation field.
D. Place the support structure over the ionization chamber.
E. Place the lead sheets on the support structure over the ionization chamber.
F. Place the II tower over the test equipment.
G. Fluoroscope the ionization chamber long enough for the automatic exposure controls to stabilize.
H. Read and record the exposure rate.

Acceptance Parameters
NCRP Report #99 recommends that the maximum fluoroscopic rate for AEC systems ≤10 R/min (2.6 mC/kg/min).

Record Keeping
A record should be kept that documents the date of the test, who performed the test, the results of the test, and the corrective action taken.

Potential Problem
Failure to accurately record all systems parameters could lead to inconclusive results.

Standard Fluoroscopic Exposure Levels

Rationale
This procedure is designed to confirm the normal operating exposure rate for fluoroscopic systems.

Testing Frequency
Standard fluoroscopic exposure rates should be done semiannually.

Equipment
- Homogeneous patient equivalent phantom
- Direct readout R-meter and ionization chamber
- Support apparatus for the phantom

Procedure
A. Prior to starting this procedure, a concise written plan should be established for repeating this procedure. The plan should include the following information.
  - Operating mA
  - Operating kVp

- Collimation
- Tower height
- Position of the ionization chamber
- Position of the phantom

B. Initially perform the following tasks.
  - Turn the fluoroscopic unit on.
  - Place the unit in the manual exposure mode.
  - Select the maximum mA and kVp.
  - Place the ionization chamber on the tabletop and attach it to the R-meter.
  - Turn on the R-meter and ensure that it is in the exposure rate mode.

C. Place the support apparatus and the patient equivalent phantom over the ionization chamber.

D. Place the fluoroscopic tower directly over the test equipment.

E. In the 6-inch mode, fluoroscope the equipment for an adequate amount of time for the dosimeter reading to stabilize.
  - Record the exposure rate with the grid and without the grid.

F. In the 9-inch mode, fluoroscope the equipment for an adequate amount of time for the dosimeter reading to stabilize.
  - Record the exposure rate with the grid and without the grid.

Acceptance Parameters

- NCRP Report #99 recommends that entrance exposures for the 6-inch mode without a grid should be 2 to 3 R/min (0.5 to 0.8 mC/kg/min) for a 21-centimeter patient equivalent phantom.
- NCRP Report #99 recommends that entrance exposures for the 9-inch mode without a grid should be 1.5 to 2.5 R/min (0.4 to 0.7 mC/kg/min) for a 21-centimeter patient equivalent phantom.

Record Keeping

A record should be kept that documents the date of the test, who performed the test, the results of the test, and the corrective action taken.

Potential Problem

Failure to accurately record all systems parameters could lead to inconclusive results.

Fluoroscopic Exposure Reproducibility

Rationale

To confirm that the generator is producing the kVp as indicated on the control panel.

Testing Frequency

The fluoroscopic exposure reproducibility should be checked semiannually.

Equipment
- Digital R-meter and ionization chamber
- Patient equivalent phantom
- Stopwatch

Procedure
A. Initially perform the following tasks.
- Turn the fluoroscopic unit on.
- Place the unit in the manual exposure mode.
- Select the maximum mA and kVp.
- Place the ionization chamber on the tabletop and attach it to the R-meter.
- Turn on the R-meter and ensure that it is in the exposure rate mode.
- Under fluoroscopy, center the tube to the middle of the ionization chamber and collimate to the chamber.
B. Expose the ionization chamber for 10 to 15 seconds.
- Use the stopwatch to determine this.
- Record the results.
C. Repeat Step B for four additional exposures.
D. Perform the following tasks.
- For each exposure, calculate the mR/mAs ratio and record the data. The following formula should be used:

$$\text{mR/mAs Ratio} = \frac{\text{mR}}{\text{mAs}}$$

- Calculate the average mR/mAs. The following formula should be used:

$$\text{Average mR/mAs} = \frac{\text{Sum of the mR/mAs Ratios}}{\text{Number of mA Stations Tested}}$$

- Determine the variance in reproducibility using the following formula:

$$\text{Reproducibility Variance} = \frac{(\text{mR/mAs}_{max} - \text{mR/mAs}_{min})/2}{\text{Average mR/mAs}}$$

Acceptance Parameters
The reproducibility of variance must be less than 0.05.

Record Keeping
A record should be kept that documents the date of the test, who performed the test, the results of the test, and the corrective action taken.

Potential Problem
Failure to follow the protocol may lead to erroneous results.

Fluoroscopic mA Linearity

Rationale
To confirm that the generator is producing the selected mA as indicated.

Testing Frequency
The fluoroscopic mA should be checked semiannually.

Equipment
- Digital R-meter and ionization chamber
- Patient equivalent phantom
- Stopwatch

Procedure
A. Initially perform the following tasks.
  - Turn the fluoroscopic unit on.
  - Place the unit in the manual exposure mode.
  - Select 0.5 mA.
  - Place the ionization chamber on the tabletop and attach it to the R-meter.
  - Turn on the R-meter and ensure that it is in the exposure rate mode.
  - Under fluoroscopy, center the tube to the middle of the ionization chamber and collimate to the chamber.
B. Expose the ionization chamber for 10 to 15 seconds.
  - Use the stopwatch to determine this.
  - Record the results.
C. Repeat Step B for 1, 2, and 3 mA.
D. Perform the following tasks.
  - For each exposure, calculate the mR/mAs ratio and record the data. The following formula should be used:

$$\text{mR/mAs Ratio} = \frac{\text{mR}}{\text{mAs}}$$

  - Calculate the average mR/mAs. The following formula should be used:

$$\text{Average mR/mAs} = \frac{\text{Sum of the mR/mAs Ratios}}{\text{Number of mA Stations Tested}}$$

  - Determine the variance in reproducibility using the following formula:

$$\text{Linearity Variance} = \frac{(\text{mR/mAs}_{max} - \text{mR/mAs}_{min})/2}{\text{Average mR/mAs}}$$

Acceptance Parameters

The fluoroscopic mA linearity variance should be within 0.1.

Record Keeping

A record should be kept that documents the date of the test, who performed the test, the results of the test, and the corrective action taken.

Potential Problem

Failure to follow the protocol may lead to erroneous results.

Fluoroscopic Kilovoltage Accuracy

Rationale

To confirm that the generator is producing the kVp indicated on the control panel.

Testing Frequency

The fluoroscopic kilovoltage should be checked semiannually or when there is an indication that the generator is not producing the kilovoltage selected.

Equipment

• Digital kVp meter (see Fig. 4-21)

Procedure

A. Initially perform the following tasks.
  • Before performing the test, it is important to follow the appropriate tube warm-up procedure.
  • Turn the kVp meter on and allow it to warm up as recommended by the manufacturer.
  • Place the kVp meter on the tabletop facing the direction of the x-ray tube.
  • Readings should be taken in the 80 to 120 kV range in increments of 10 kE.
  • Under fluoroscopy, center the tube to the middle of the kVp meter, and collimate to the meter.
B. At the kV ranges selected it is important to do a minimum of five exposures for each selected kV. Multiple exposures will allow for any variations in line voltage.
C. On a sheet of paper record the kVp readings for each selected kV. Average the readings and record the results.

Acceptance Parameters

The NCRP recommends that the kilovoltage be within ±5% of the selected kVp.

Record Keeping

A record should be kept that documents the date of the test, who performed the test, the results of the test, and the corrective action taken.

Potential Problem

Inaccurate readings may be obtained during times of high electrical power demand.

High Contrast Fluoroscopic Resolution (Optical Viewing)

Rationale

This procedure is designed to confirm that the resolution capability of the imaging system is within accepted parameters.

Testing Frequency

Fluoroscopic resolution tests should be done when new fluoroscopic equipment is installed, and then semiannually or when the imaging system is worked on.

Equipment

- Copper mesh test pattern (Fig. 5-6)
- Nongumming tape (i.e., masking)

Procedure

A. Center and tape the test pattern to the bottom of the II.
   - For TV systems, the test pattern should be placed at a 45° angle to the scan lines of the TV monitor.
   - For mirror optics systems, the test pattern is placed so that the 24 and 40 mesh areas of the template are at the top of the image and the 50 and 30 mesh areas are at the bottom of the image.
B. Collimate the beam to the size of the test pattern.
C. Set the lowest possible kVp level that would be used for making spot films.
D. Observe the test pattern image in both the 6- and 9-inch imaging modes.
E. Record the results.

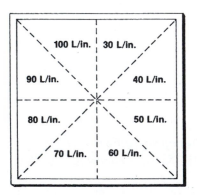

Figure 5-6 Fluoroscopic resolution test tool. (Courtesy of Nuclear Associates, used with permission.)

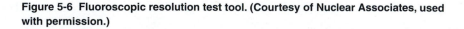

Acceptance Parameters

- NCRP Report #99 states that the acceptance parameters for optical viewing for the
  - 6-inch imaging mode should be 40 mesh/inch at the center of the image and 35 mesh/inch at the edge of the image.
  - 9-inch imaging mode should be 40 mesh/inch at the center of the image and 30 mesh/inch at the edge of the image.
- For the standard TV monitor the acceptance parameters for the
  - 6-inch imaging mode should not be <30 mesh/inch at the center of the image and <24 mesh/inch at the edge of the image.
  - 9-inch imaging mode should not be <20 mesh/inch at the center and edge of the image.

Record Keeping

A record should be kept that documents the date of the test, who performed the test, the results of the test, and the corrective action taken.

Potential Problem

Failure to center the test pattern may lead to inaccurate results.

Points to Ponder

- This test is subjective. Ambient lighting and the settings on the monitor may influence the results.

High Contrast Fluoroscopic Resolution (Spot Films)

Rationale

This procedure is designed to confirm that the resolution capability of the imaging system is within accepted parameters.

Testing Frequency

Fluoroscopic resolution tests should be done when new fluoroscopic equipment is installed and then semiannually.

Equipment

- Copper mesh test pattern
- Nongumming tape (i.e., masking)
- 9.5- × 9.5-inch image receptor and film

Procedure

A. Insert the image receptor in the spot film device.
B. Center and tape the test pattern to the bottom of the II.
C. Collimate the beam to the size of the test pattern.
D. Set the lowest possible kVp level that would be used for making spot films.
E. Observe the test pattern image in both the 6- and 9-inch imaging modes.

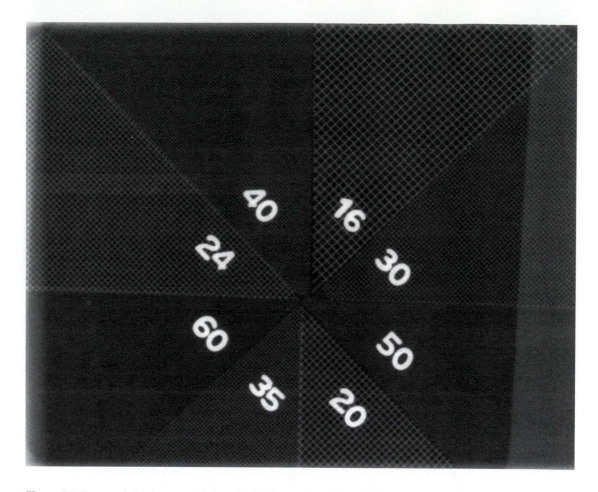

Figure 5-7 Image of the fluoroscopic test tool. *(Courtesy of Michael Biddy, Phoenix Technology.)*

F. Expose the film and process it (Fig. 5-7).
G. Record the results.

Acceptance Parameters
- For spot films the acceptance parameters for the
  - 6-inch imaging mode should be 40 mesh/inch at the center of the image and 35 mesh/inch at the edge of the image.
  - 9-inch imaging mode should be 40 mesh/inch at the center of the image and 30 mesh/inch at the edge of the image.

Record Keeping
A record should be kept that documents the date of the test, who performed the test, the results of the test, and the corrective action taken.

Potential Problem

Failure to center the test pattern may lead to inaccurate results.

Points to Ponder

• This test is subjective. Results may be influenced by ambient lighting conditions.

Low Contrast Fluoroscopic Resolution (Spot Film)

Rationale

This procedure is designed to confirm the ability of the fluoroscopic system to exhibit low contrast information.

Testing Frequency

Low contrast fluoroscopic resolution should be done when new fluoroscopic equipment is installed and then semiannually.

Equipment

• Low contrast resolution test phantom (Fig. 5-8)
    • One sheet of 1/32-inch thick aluminum, 7- × 7-inch with two sets of four holes with diameters of 1/16 inch, 1/8 inch, 3/16 inch, and 1/4 inch.
    • Two sheets of 3/4-inch aluminum, 7 × 7 inches.

Procedure

A. Place the sheet of the 1/32-inch-thick aluminum between the two sheets of 3/4-inch aluminum and then place the test tool on the tabletop.
B. Place the image intensifier 10 to 12 inches above the tabletop and test tool.
C. Collimate the beam to the test tool.

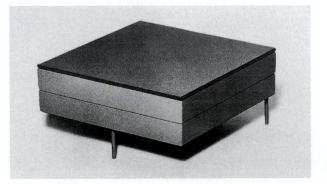

Figure 5-8 Low contrast resolution test tool. *(Courtesy of Nuclear Associates, used with permission.)*

D. Adjust fluoroscopic factors.
E. For manual systems, set the fluoroscopic kV in the 85 to 90 kVp range and adjust the fluoroscopic mA to obtain the best image.
F. For automatic brightness systems, allow the system to adjust exposure factors. The kVp should be between 85 and 90 kVp.
G. Record the results (Fig. 5-9).

Figure 5-9 Image of the low contrast resolution test tool. *(Courtesy of Michael Mandich, BS, RT(R), Samaritan Hospital, Watertown, NY.)*

Acceptance Parameters

- The 1/4-inch and 3/16-inch holes should be seen clearly and the 1/8-inch holes should barely be seen.
- With newer imaging systems, it is possible that the majority of holes may be seen.

Record Keeping

A record should be kept that documents the date of the test, who performed the test, the results of the test, and the corrective action taken.

Potential Problem

Because this test is subjective, failure to adjust the TV controls may lead to an error in interpretation.

Low Contrast Fluoroscopic Resolution (TV Systems)

Rationale

This procedure is designed to confirm the ability of the fluoroscopic system to exhibit low contrast information.

Testing Frequency

Low contrast fluoroscopic resolution should be done when new fluoroscopic equipment is installed and then semiannually.

Equipment

- One sheet of 1/32-inch-thick aluminum, 7 × 7 inches with two sets of four holes with diameters of 1/16-inch, 1/8 inch, 3/16 inch, and 1/4 inch
- Two sheets of 3/4-inch aluminum, 7 × 7 inches

Procedure

A. Place the sheet of 1/32-inch-thick aluminum between the two sheets of 3/4-inch aluminum and then the test tool on the tabletop.
B. Place the image intensifier 10 to 12 inches above the tabletop and test tool.
C. Collimate the beam to the test tool.
D. Allow the automatic brightness system to adjust fluoroscopic factors.
   - The fluoroscopic kV should be the 85 to 90 kVp range.
   - View the image on the TV monitor.
   - If necessary adjust the brightness and contrast controls to obtain the best image.
E. Record the results.

Acceptance Parameters

- The 1/4-inch and 3/16-inch holes should be seen clearly. The 1/8-inch holes should barely be seen.
- With newer imaging systems, it is possible that the majority of holes may be seen.

Record Keeping

A record should be kept that documents the date of the test, who performed the test, the results of the test, and the corrective action taken.

Potential Problem

Because this test is subjective, failure to adjust the TV controls may lead to an error in interpretation.

Fluoroscopic Automatic Brightness Control and Automatic Exposure Control

Rationale

This procedure is designed to confirm that the automatic brightness and exposure controls of the fluoroscopic system is working within accepted criteria.

Testing Frequency

The fluoroscopic automatic brightness and exposure controls should be done semiannually.

Equipment

- Homogeneous patient equivalent phantom
- Direct readout dosimeter
- Support apparatus for the phantom

Procedure

A. Prior to starting this procedure, a concise written plan should be established for repeating this procedure. The plan should include the following information.
   - Operating mA
   - Operating kVp
   - Collimation
   - Tower height
   - Position of the direct readout dosimeter
   - Position of the phantom
B. Turn the fluoroscopic unit on.
C. Place the direct readout dosimeter on the tabletop.
D. Place the support apparatus and the patient equivalent phantom over the direct readout dosimeter.
E. Turn on the direct readout dosimeter and ensure that it is in the exposure rate mode.
F. Place the fluoroscopic tower directly over the test equipment.
G. In the 6-inch mode, fluoroscope the equipment for an adequate amount of time for the dosimeter reading to stabilize.
   - Record the exposure rate with the grid and without the grid.
H. Remove half of the phantom; record the exposure rate for half of the phantom.
I. Repeat Steps G and H for the 9-inch mode.

Acceptance Parameters

NCRP Report #99 recommends that ABC/AEC systems should function similar to same installations and similar systems.

Record Keeping

A record should be kept that documents the date of the test, who performed the test, the results of the test, and the corrective action taken.

Potential Problems

- Failure to accurately record all systems parameters could lead to inconclusive results.
- Comparing ABC/AEC results with dissimilar ABC/AEC units will lead to erroneous results.

CHAPTER REVIEW

- Fluoroscopy has been part of the imaging science since 1896. The basic theory behind fluoroscopy has not changed in over 100 years. The equipment used for fluoroscopic procedures has become more sophisticated over the years.
- The fluoroscopic x-ray tube is designed to operate in the 0.5 to 5 mA range. The typical mA used for fluoroscopy is between 1 and 3 mA.
- The x-ray tube of a fixed fluoroscopic unit has a fixed SOD of ≥15 inches.
- The x-ray tube of a mobile fluoroscopic unit has a fixed SOD of ≥12 inches.
- The image intensifier has five parts: the input screen, the photocathode, the electrostatic lenses, anode, and the output screen.
- All of the components of the image intensifier work together to amplify electronically the brightness of the image by an average of 5000 to 20,000 times.
- All fluoroscopic quality control tests are performed semiannually.
- Fluoroscopic image size is a procedure that determines how large the image is in relationship to the image diameter. Fluoroscopic image size should not less than 1 centimeter of the specified diameter of the imaging field.
- Fluoroscopic beam limitation is an effective procedure that can be used to determine how effective the fluoroscopic shutters are in limiting the amount of radiation reaching the patient. Failure to have the fluoroscopic x-ray beam properly collimated results in increased exposure to the patient. Collimation of the fluoroscopic x-ray beam should not exceed 3% of the SID.
- Maximum fluoroscopic exposure rates are checked in both the manual mode and automatic exposure mode. In the manual mode, the maximum fluoroscopic exposure rate should be ≤1.3 mC/kg/min or ≤5 R/min. The maximum fluoroscopic exposure rate for the AEC mode should be ≤2.6 mC/kg/min or ≤10 R/min.

- Standard fluoroscopic exposure levels are checked without the grid and generally the AEC is set in the 80 to 90 kVp range. The exposure levels for both the 6-inch and 9-inch II modes are checked. The standard fluoroscopic exposure levels for the 6-inch mode should be between 0.5 and 0.8 mC/kg/min and for the 9-inch mode should be between 0.4 to 0.7 mC/kg/min.
- The reproducibility of exposure for fluoroscopic units must be less than 0.05.
- Fluoroscopic mA linearity must be within 0.10 of the set fluoroscopic mA.
- The kV accuracy of fluoroscopic units has been established at ±5% of the established kVp.
- The fluoroscopic resolution should be checked for the TV monitor and the spot film device. How well the fluoroscopic system can resolve an image is based on a minimum number of meshes per inch that are seen.
- The low contrast fluoroscopic test needs to be done for both the TV monitor and spot film device. The number of holes seen on the image determines how well the system can image low level contrast, the more holes that are seen, the better the low contrast resolution of the system.
- The ABC and AEC of a fluoroscopic system can be compared to like systems and should function the same. However, unlike or different systems cannot and should never be compared.

DISCUSSION QUESTIONS

1. How often should QC tests be performed on a specific fluoroscopic system?
2. Which QC tests are of critical importance?
3. Are there any major differences in QC testing between fixed and mobile fluoroscopic systems?
4. Are the same QC tests performed on mobile fluoroscopic systems as fixed systems?
5. Why is it necessary to establish a repeatable test procedure for standard fluoroscopic rates?

REVIEW QUESTIONS

1. What is the minimum spot film fluoroscopic resolution (mesh/inch) for a 9-inch image intensifier?
   a. 20 to 24 at the center and 20 at the edge
   b. 30 to 35 at the center and 24 to 30 at the edge
   c. 35 at the center and 30 at the edge
   d. 40+ at the center and 35+ at the edge

2. In the manual mode maximum fluoroscopic rate *should not* exceed
   a. 5 R/min
   b. 10 R/min
   c. 15 R/min
   d. 20 R/min
3. In the automatic mode maximum fluoroscopic rate shall not exceed
   a. 20 R/min
   b. 15 R/min
   c. 10 R/min
   d. 5 R/min
4. The low contrast fluoroscopic test should permit clear visualization of the
   a. 1/8- and 1/4-inch holes
   b. 1/16- and 1/8-inch holes
   c. 1/8- and 3/16-inch holes
   d. 1/4- and 3/16-inch holes
5. Which of the following statements is correct about fluoroscopic image size?
   a. The size of the fluoroscopic image should not be less than 0.1 centimeter smaller than the specified diameter.
   b. The size of the fluoroscopic image should not be less than 0.5 centimeter smaller than the specified diameter.
   c. The size of the fluoroscopic image should not be less than 1 centimeter smaller than the specified diameter.
   d. The size of the fluoroscopic image should not be less than 2 centimeters smaller than the specified diameter.
6. Fluoroscopic beam limitation should be no greater than
   a. 1% of the SID
   b. 2% of the SID
   c. 3% of the SID
   d. 4% of the SID
7. What are the acceptable standard fluoroscopic exposure levels for a 6-inch II?
   a. 0.4 to 0.7 mC/kg/min
   b. 0.5 to 0.8 mC/kg/min
   c. 0.6 to 0.9 mC/kg/min
   d. 0.7 to 1.0 mC/kg/min
8. Standard fluoroscopic exposure levels are measured
   a. with the grid in place
   b. without the grid in place
   c. both a and b
9. What are the acceptable standard fluoroscopic exposure levels for a nine inch image intensifier?
   a. 0.4 to 0.7 mC/kg/min
   b. 0.5 to 0.8 mC/kg/min

    c. 0.6 to 0.9 mC/kg/min

    d. 0.7 to 1.0 mC/kg/min

10. What is the minimum spot film fluoroscopic resolution (mesh/inch) for a 6-inch II?

    a. 20 to 24 at the center and 20 at the edge

    b. 30 to 35 at the center and 24 to 30 at the edge

    c. 35 at the center and 30 at the edge

    d. 40 at the center and 35 at the edge

11. What is the minimum SOD for a fixed fluoroscopic x-ray tube?

    a. 20 centimeters

    b. 30 centimeters

    c. 38 centimeters

    d. 50 centimeters

12. What mA range is used for fluoroscopy?

    a. <0.05 mA

    b. 0.5 to 5 mA

    c. 5 to 100 mA

    d. >100 mA

13. The acceptance parameters for fluoroscopic exposure reproducibility should be

    a. >0.05

    b. 0.03 to 0.04

    c. 0.01 to 0.02

    d. <0.05

14. Which of the following statements is correct?

    a. The fluoroscopic mA linearity must be within 0.1.

    b. The fluoroscopic mA linearity must be within 0.2.

    c. The fluoroscopic mA linearity must be within 0.5.

    d. The fluoroscopic mA linearity must be within 0.01.

15. Fluoroscopic QC tests are performed

    a. annually

    b. biannually

    c. quarterly

    d. semiannually

16. The components of the II amply electronically the brightness of the image on average

    a. 500 to 2000 times

    b. 5000 to 20,000 times

    c. 50,000 to 200,000 times

    d. 500,000 to 2,000,000 times

17. When a 50 keV x-ray photon interacts with the input screen II, how many light photons are produced?

    a. ~500

    b. ~1000

c. ~1500

d. ~2000

18. Based on the answer from question 17, how many photoelectrons are produced when the light photons interact with the photocathode?

a. ~100

b. ~250

c. ~500

d. ~2000

19. Based on the answer from question 18, how many light photons are produced when the photoelectrons interact with the output screen?

a. ~50,000

b. ~100,000

c. ~200,000

d. ~500,000

20. What is the minimum SOD for a mobile fluoroscopic x-ray tube?

a. 20 centimeters

b. 30 centimeters

c. 38 centimeters

d. 50 centimeters

21. The input screen is made from

a. antinomy and cesium

b. cesium iodide

c. silver activated cesium iodide

d. sodium activated cesium iodide

22. The photocathode is made from

a. antinomy and cadmium

b. antinomy and cesium

c. silver activated cesium

d. sodium activated cesium

23. The anode of the image intensifier has a

a. negative charge of ~15 kV

b. negative charge of ~25 kV

c. positive charge of ~15 kV

d. positive charge of ~25 kV

24. Which of the following statements is correct?

a. The input screen is larger than the output screen

b. The output screen is larger than the input screen

c. The input screen is smaller than the output screen

d. The input screen and output screen are the same size

25. The output screen is made from

a. antinomy and cadmium sulfide

b. cadmium sulfide

c. silver activated zinc cadmium sulfide

d. sodium activated zinc cadmium sulfide

6

Quality Management in Mammographic Services

GOALS

1. To learn about mammography quality management (QM), quality assurance (QA), and quality control (QC).
2. To learn about processor QC.
3. To learn about safelight and darkroom cleanliness checks.
4. To learn about repeat analysis process.
5. To understand the importance of repeat analysis process.

6. To learn about illuminator uniformity checks.
7. To learn about film-screen contact procedures.
8. To learn about the tests performed on mammographic equipment.

OBJECTIVES

1. Differentiate between mammography QM, QA, and QC.
2. Discuss the importance of the medical outcomes audit.
3. Identify and discuss the responsibilities of the radiologist, technologist, and medical physicist in the mammography QM program.
4. Discuss the measures of central tendency.
5. Discuss the measures of dispersion.
6. Identify the QC procedures associated with the darkroom and accessory devices.
7. Discuss the rationale for doing each quality control test.
8. State the testing frequency for each test.
9. Identify the required equipment for each test.
10. Explain the procedure for doing each QC test.
11. Discuss the acceptance parameters for each test.
12. Explain the importance of record keeping.
13. Identify and discuss potential problems that might arise while performing each test.
14. Calculate the speed and contrast indices.
15. Discuss the crossover procedure.
16. Define trend.
17. Given a processor monitoring chart, evaluate the chart for abnormal trends and discuss the impact of elevated processor control parameters on image quality.
18. Explain the rationale for doing a repeat/reject analysis.
19. Identify the key components of a repeat/reject analysis program.
20. Discuss the procedure for doing a repeat/reject analysis.
21. State the accepted range of values for a repeat/reject analysis.
22. Explain why a repeat/reject analysis of less than 3% is not an accurate reflection of a facilities repeat/reject rate.

QUALITY MANAGEMENT IN MAMMOGRAPHY

Quality management (QM) in the Mammography Imaging Facility focuses on performance improvement and image quality improvement. However, **mammography quality management (MQM)** is driven not only by the institution's mission statement, but also the need to personalize services and the Mammography Quality Standards Act (MQSA) of 1999. Many of the topics that were discussed in Chaps. 1 and 2 can be directly applied to mammography imaging services. The goals and outcomes of a comprehensive MQM program are based on the assumptions that the patient and physician are entitled to a certain level of customer service that provides quality images, an accurate diagnosis, and the delivery of results within a reasonable amount of time. This chapter focuses on the responsibilities of the personnel, reporting, record keeping, the medical outcomes audit, consumer complaint mechanism, infection control, radiologist QA, the tracking of suboptimal images, and the QC process that ensures the production of quality images.

Responsibilities

The responsibilities of the lead mammography radiologist, mammography technologist, and medical physicist in the mammography quality control program are outlined and discussed in the American College of Radiology's 1999 edition of the *Mammography Quality Control Manual* (Table 6-1). Failure to ensure that the assigned responsibilities are performed will lead to severe penalties that may result in the termination of mammography performance. It is critical that each individual participating in the MQM program understands their role and specific responsibilities.

Reporting

An integral part of the mammographic process is the reporting of results. As a result of MQSA the mammography report must contain information regarding the facility, patient, examination, and final assessment. The key points pertaining to the facility, patient, and examination are summarized in Table 6-2.

The final report must contain an accurate description of radiologist findings. The final interpretation must state that the mammogram was negative, benign, probably benign, suspicious, highly suggestive of malignancy, or incomplete: needs additional imaging evaluation. Whatever the final findings are they should be expressed in a fashion that leaves no room for doubt.

The final mammography results must be communicated to the health care provider (i.e., physician) and patient within a reasonable amount of time. When mammography results fall into the negative, benign, or probably benign categories, they should be communicated to the physician within 30 days of the examination if not sooner. A mammography examination that results in either a suspicious, highly suggestive of malignancy, or incomplete: needs additional imaging designation must be communicated to the physician within 72 hours. The communication of results may occur via a fax, registered mail, a telephone call, or a face-to-face meeting. Any verbal communication must be followed up with written communication. Talking directly to the physician is the most reliable means for communicating the mammography results because it allows the physician to ask all the necessary questions regarding follow-up options (Bassett et al., 1994).

Table 6-1
Designated Responsibilities

Radiologist	Technologist	Medical Physicist
Ensure that technical staff has adequate mammography training.	On a daily basis monitors darkroom and processor QC.	Ensures that the mammography equipment is functioning properly.
Ensure that technical staff maintains mammography continuing education.	On a weekly basis maintains screen cleanliness, viewboxes and viewing conditions.	Evaluates the mammographic unit assembly, system resolution, and image quality.
Ensures that an orientation program for the technical staff is in place.	On a weekly basis produces and evaluates phantom images.	Assesses uniformity of screen speed, beam quality, and kVp accuracy and reproducibility.
Ensures that an effective mammography QC program exists on site.	On a monthly basis performs a visual check of equipment.	Measures viewbox luminance and room illuminance.
Identifies a single technologist to be the primary QC technologist.	On a quarterly basis performs a repeat analysis and an analysis of fixer retention.	Measures average glandular dose and breast entrance exposure.
Ensures that the appropriate QC equipment and materials are available to perform the required tests.	On a semiannual basis evaluates darkroom fog, screen-film contact, and compression.	Evaluates AEC reproducibility and radiation output rate.
Provides staffing to allow adequate time for performing the QC tests, interpreting, and recording the QC data.		
Ensures that there is a mechanism for the provision of frequent positive and negative feedback for technologists.		
Identifies a medical physicist to perform the required physicist tests and to oversee the equipment-related QC program.		
On a quarterly basis, reviews the technologist's QC test results.		
On an annual basis, reviews the physicist's test results.		
Identifies a qualified individual to oversee the radiation protection program of the mammography department.		
Guarantees records regarding infection control, QC, safety, protection, mammography technique and procedures, and employee qualifications are maintained and updated.		

Table 6-2
Summary of the Mammogram Report

Facility	Patient	Examination
Name	Name	Date
Address	Date of birth	Type
Phone number	Medical record number	Interpreting physician
	Other Options	*Other Options*
	Social security number	Name of technologist
	Address	Second reader
	Phone number	

The report that is communicated to the patient must be written in language that is generally understood by the lay public. After the report has been written, it must be sent directly to the patient. If the patient is given a verbal report, it must be followed up with a written report. The mammography facility is required to send the patient a report within 30 days of the examination when the results are negative, benign, or probably benign. Results that are incomplete, suspicious, or highly suggestive of malignancy must be communicated to the patient within 5 working days.

Record Keeping

Record keeping involves not only maintaining the patient's films and image identification but also the records that pertain to the radiologist, technologist, and the medical physicist. Mammography films must be kept for a minimum of 5 years. However, if state law is more stringent, then the state law supercedes the 5-year federal mandate. Under MQSA, all mammography facilities are required to transfer a patient's original films and copies of reports to the requester.

All mammographic images must be marked in a permanent, legible, and clear fashion that does not obscure anatomic structures. Each image must contain patient information, date of procedure, view, facility information, technologist identification, image receptor (cassette/screen) identification, and mammography unit identification. The patient's name must appear on the film along with one other identifier (i.e., date of birth, social security number, etc.). The date of the procedure must be on the film; it may be either imprinted in the film or a date sticker may be affixed to the film. Each image must include the view (i.e., CC, MLO, etc.) and the view marker must be placed by axilla and follow the American College of Radiology (ACR) guidelines. The information regarding the facility must include the name and location of the facility, plus the city, state, and zip code. By law, the technologist is required to identify each image with their marker, which may be a number or set of initials. Each mammography image receptor must have a number. The mammography unit being used for the procedure must also be evident on the film. The system used to identify a unit is at the discretion of the imaging facility.

Records that must be maintained regarding the interpreting physician are license, certification, evidence of continuing education, documentation of formal training, and evidence of continuing experience criteria. The technologist record requirements include certification in general radiography, certification in mammography, documentation of 40 hours of training, evidence of continuing education (CE) (15 hours in a 3-year period), and evidence of continuing experience (performing 200 mammograms in a 24-month period). This continuing experience requirement must be met by April 28, 2001 and documented by June 30, 2001. Medical physicist records include a state license or certification in an appropriate specialty area, a master's degree or higher in a physical science, and 20 semester hours in physics. In addition, there must be documentation of 20 contact hours in specialized training, evidence in continuing education (15 CEs in mammography within 36 months), and evidence of continuing experience.

Maintaining the records of the radiologist, technologist, and physicist is a critical part the MQM program. The most efficient way to maintain and update the records is by creating a computer data base. A data base allows the periodic updating of all records. Tables 6-3, 6-4, and 6-5 provide examples of acceptable documentation for radiologists, technologists, and physicists.

Medical Outcome Audits

The medical outcomes audit is an essential component of the MQM program whose primary goal is to ensure the reliability, clarity, and accuracy of interpretation. It is a means of demonstrating the success or failure in detecting breast cancers. The audit is a systematic method for comparing results to outcomes data. The outcomes audit consists of a data collection phase and a data analysis phase. Prior to data collection, it is necessary for the lead radiologist to define what constitutes a positive mammogram requiring follow up and the method for following up on positive mammograms. This can be accomplished by using the assessment categories developed by the ACR in their third edition of **Breast Imaging Reporting and Data System (BI-RADS),** which is now required by the ACR and MQSA. The use of the BI-RADS nomenclature organizes the physician's interpretation into universally agreed upon categories. BI-RADS assessment consists of six categories ranging from 0 to 5 (Table 6-6).

The most efficient means for collecting data from the medical outcomes audit is to use a computer program. The data obtained should be categorized in the following manner: true positive (TP), true negative (TN), false positive (FP), and false negative (FN). Once the data have been collected, they can be analyzed. A true positive is a cancer detected within 1 year after a biopsy recom-

Table 6-3
Acceptable Documentation for Radiologists

Requirement	Prior to 10-1-94	10-1-94 to 4-28-99	After 4-28-99

State Licensure	Copy of state license
	Confirming letter from
	  state board
		Copy of state license
		Confirming letter from
		  state board
			Copy of state license
			Confirming letter from
			  state board

Board Certification (ABR,
  AOBR, or RCPSC)
	Original/copy of certificate
	Confirming letter from
	  certifying board
	Confirming letter from
	  ACR
		Original/copy of certificate
		Confirming letter from
		  certifying board
		Confirming letter from
		  ACR
			Original/copy of certificate
			Confirming letter from
			  certifying board
			Confirming letter from
			  ACR

Formal training:
  1. Interim regs:
    2 months
  2. Final regs: 3 months
	Letters/documents from
	  U.S. or Canadian
	  residency programs
	Documentation of formal
	  mammography training
	  courses
	Certificates of
	  Category I CMEs
		Letters/documents from
		  U.S. or Canadian
		  residency programs
		Documentation of formal
		  mammography training
		  courses
		Certificates of Category
		  I CMEs
			Letters/documents from
			  U.S. or Canadian
			  residency programs
			Documentation of formal
			  mammography
			  training courses
			Certificates of Category
			  I CMEs

Initial medical education:
  1. Interim regs: 40 hrs
  2. Final regs:
    60 hrs/15 in last
    3 yrs
	Letter from residency
	  program
	CME certificates
	Letter confirming formal
	  training
		Letter from residency
		  program
		CME certificates
		Letter confirming formal
		  training
			Letter from residency
			  program
			CME certificates
			Letter confirming
			  formal training

Initial experience:
  1. Interim regs: any
    6-month period
  2. Final regs: 2 yrs
    of residency
	Letter from residency
	  program
	Documentation from
	  training program or
	  mammography facility
		Letter from residency
		  program
		Documentation from
		  training program or
		  mammography facility
		  done under direct
		  supervision
			Letter from residency
			  program
			Documentation from
			  training program or
			  mammography facility
			  done under direct
			  supervision

Initial mammographic
  modality specific
  training, final regs:
  8 hrs
	Mammography modality
	  specific CME
	  certificates (category
	  I or II)
	Agendas, outlines, etc.,
	  from CME programs
	Confirming letters from
	  CME granting
	  organizations
		Mammography modality
		  specific CME certificates
		  (category I or II)
		Agendas, outlines, etc.,
		  from CME programs
		Confirming letters from
		  CME granting
		  organizations
			Mammography modality
			  specific CME
			  certificates (category
			  I or II)
			Agendas, outlines, etc.,
			  from CME programs
			Confirming letters from
			  CME granting
			  organizations

Continuing experience:
  960 mammograms/24
  months
	Does not apply	Letter, facility logs, or other
		  documentation from
		  residency program,
		  training program, or
		  mammography facility
			Letter, facility logs, or
			  other documentation
			  from residency
			  program, training
			  program, or
			  mammography facility

(Continued)

Table 6-3
Acceptable Documentation for Radiologists *(continued)*

Requirement	Prior to 10-1-94	10-1-94 to 4-28-99	After 4-28-99

Continuing education:
1. Interim regs:
   15 CMEs/36 months
2. Final regs:
   15 category I
   CMEs/36 months
	Does not apply	CME certificates (category I or II)
		Confirming letters from CME granting organizations
			CME certificates (category I)
			Confirming letters from CME granting organizations

Continuing mammographic modality specific education: Final regs	Does not apply	Mammography modality specific CME certificates (category I or II) Agendas, outlines, etc., from CME programs Confirming letters from CME granting organizations	Mammography modality specific CME certificates (category I) Agendas, outlines, etc., from CME programs Confirming letters from CME granting organizations
Requalification experience: Done under direct supervision	Does not apply	Letter, facility logs, or other documentation from residency program, training program, or mammography facility	Letter, facility logs, or other documentation from residency program, training program, or mammography facility
Requalification education	Does not apply	CME certificates (category I or II) Confirming letters from CME granting organizations	CME certificates (category I) Confirming letters from CME granting organizations

Based on guidelines from Rush, 1999.

mendation based on mammographic examination with abnormal findings (Bassett et al., 1998). A true negative is no known diagnosis of cancer within 1 year of a mammographic examination with normal probably benign findings (Bassett et al., 1998). A false negative is considered to be a diagnosis of cancer within 1 year of a mammographic examination with normal or probably benign findings (Bassett et al., 1998). There are three separate definitions of a false positive finding. They are classified as FP_1, FP_2, and FP_3. A false positive one (FP_1) is defined as no known cancer diagnosis within 1 year of a positive mammographic screening. A false positive two (FP_2) is defined as no known cancer within 1 year after recommendation for biopsy or surgical consultation on the basis of a positive mammogram (Bassett et al., 1998). A false positive three (FP_3) is defined as benign findings at biopsy within 1 year after recommendation for biopsy or surgical consultation on the basis of a positive mammogram (Bassett et al., 1998).

Table 6-4
Acceptable Documentation for Technologists

Requirement	Prior to 10-1-94	10-1-94 to 4-28-99	After 4-28-99
State Licensure	Copy of state license Confirming letter from state board	Copy of state license Confirming letter from state board	Copy of state license Confirming letter from state board
Board Certification (ARRT or ARCRT)	Original/copy of certificate Confirming letter from certifying board	Original/copy of certificate Confirming letter from certifying board	Original/copy of certificate Confirming letter from certifying board
Initial training: 1. Interim regs: ~40 hrs 2. Final regs: 40 hrs with 25 supervised examinations	Letter from training program CE certificates Letter confirming formal training	Letter from training program CE certificates Letter confirming formal training	Letter from training program CE certificates Letter confirming formal training
Initial mammography modality specific training: Final regs 8 hrs	Mammography modality specific CE certificates Agendas, outlines, etc., from CE programs Confirming letters from CE granting organizations	Mammography modality specific CE certificates Agendas, outlines, etc., from CE programs Confirming letters from CE granting organizations	Mammography modality specific CE certificates Agendas, outlines, etc., from CE programs Confirming letters from CE granting organizations
Continuing experience: Final regs 200 examinations/24 months	Does not apply	Does not apply	Letter, facility logs, or other documentation from training program or mammography facility
Continuing education: 15 CE/36 months	Does not apply	CE certificates Confirming letters from CE granting organizations Formal training courses	CE certificates Confirming letters from CE granting organizations Formal training courses
Continuing mammographic modality specific education	Does not apply	Mammography modality specific CE certificates Agendas, outlines, etc., from CE programs Confirming letters from CE granting organizations	Mammography modality specific CE certificates Agendas, outlines, etc., from CE programs Confirming letters from CE granting organizations
Requalification experience: Final regs done under direct supervision	Does not apply	Does not apply	Letter, facility logs, or other documentation from training program or mammography facility done under direct supervision
Requalification education	Does not apply	CE certificates Confirming letters from CE granting organizations	CE certificates Confirming letters from CE granting organizations

Based on guidelines from Rush, 1999.

Table 6-5
Acceptable Documentation for Medical Physicists

Requirement	Prior to 10-1-94	10-1-94 to 4-28-99	After 4-28-99

State Licensure	Copy of state license
	Confirming letter from
	  state board
		Copy of state license
		Confirming letter from
		  state board
			Copy of state license
			Confirming letter from
			  state board

Board Certification
  (ABR or ABMP)
	Original/copy of certificate
	Confirming letter from
	  certifying board
	Confirming letter from
	  ACR
		Original/copy of certificate
		Confirming letter from
		  certifying board
		Confirming letter from
		  ACR
			Original/copy of certificate
			Confirming letter from
			  certifying board
			Confirming letter from
			  ACR

Degree in physical
  science: Final regs
  1. Master's path
  2. Alternative
     Bachelor's path
	Original/copy of diploma
	Confirming letter from
	  college or university
		Original/copy of diploma
		Confirming letter from
		  college or university
			Original/copy of diploma
			Confirming letter from
			  college or university

Initial physics education:
  Final regs
  1. 20 semester hours
  2. Alternative
     10 semester hours
	Transcripts from college
	  or university
	Confirming letter from
	  college or university
		Transcripts from college
		  or university
		Confirming letter from
		  college or university
			Transcripts from college
			  or university
			Confirming letter from
			  college or university

Survey training
  (Final regs):
  1. 20 contact hours
  2. Alternative
     40 contact hours
	Letter from training
	  program
	CE in mammography
	  or medical physics
	Letter confirming in-house
	  training
	Training gained from
	  performing surveys
		Letter from training
		  program
		CE in mammography
		  or medical physics
		Letter confirming in-house
		  training
		Training gained from
		  performing surveys
			Letter from training
			  program
			CE in mammography
			  or medical physics
			Letter confirming in-house
			  training
			Training gained from
			  performing surveys

Initial experience
  (Final regs):
  1. 1 facility 10 units
  2. Alternative 1 facility
     20 units
	Copy or coversheet of
	  survey
	Letter from facility or
	  listing from company
	  providing the physics
	  survey
		Copy or coversheet of
		  survey
		Letter from facility or
		  listing from company
		  providing the physics
		  survey
			Copy or coversheet of
			  survey
			Letter from facility or
			  listing from company
			  providing the physics
			  survey

Initial mammography
  modality specific
  training:
  Final regs 8 hrs
	Mammography modality
	  specific CE certificates
	Agendas, outlines, etc.,
	  from CE programs
	Confirming letters from
	  CE granting
	  organizations
		Mammography modality
		  specific CE certificates
		Agendas, outlines, etc.,
		  from CE programs
		Confirming letters from
		  CE granting
		  organizations
			Mammography modality
			  specific CE certificates
			Agendas, outlines, etc.,
			  from CE programs
			Confirming letters from
			  CE granting
			  organizations

Continuing experience,
  Final regs: 2 facilities
  6 units/24 months
	Does not apply	Does not apply	Copy or coversheet of
			  survey
			Letter from facility or
			  listing from company
			  providing the physics
			  survey

(Continued)

Table 6-5
Acceptable Documentation for Medical Physicists (continued)

Requirement	Prior to 10-1-94	10-1-94 to 4-28-99	After 4-28-99
Continuing education: 15 CE/36 months	Does not apply	CE certificates Confirming letters from CE granting organizations Formal training courses	CE certificates Confirming letters from CE granting organizations Formal training courses
Continuing mammographic modality specific education	Does not apply	Mammography modality specific CE certificates Confirming letters from CE granting organizations Formal training courses	Mammography modality specific CE certificates Confirming letters from CE granting organizations Formal training courses
Requalification experience: Final regs done under direct supervision	Does not apply	Does not apply	Copy or coversheet of survey done under supervision Letter from facility or listing from company providing the physics survey
Requalification education	Does not apply	CE certificates Confirming letters from CE granting organizations Formal training courses	CE certificates Confirming letters from CE granting organizations Formal training courses

Based on guidelines from Rush, 1999.

Table 6-6
BI-RADS Assessment Categories

Category	Description	Recommendation
0	Need additional imaging evaluation	Additional imaging should be done
1	Negative	None required
2	Benign finding	None required
3	Probably benign finding	Short interval follow up
4	Suspicious abnormality	Biopsy should be considered
5	Highly suggestive of malignancy	Appropriate action should be taken

The statistical analysis of the data will be determined by the size of the facility. Areas that are recommend for statistical analysis are sensitivity, specificity, positive predictive value, positive biopsy rate, and the cancer detection rate. Sensitivity is the probability of detecting a cancer when a cancer exists (Bassett et al., 1998). It is determined by the following formula:

$$\text{Sensitivity} = \frac{\text{TP}}{(\text{TP} + \text{FN})}$$

Specificity is the probability of a normal mammogram report when no cancer exists (Bassett et al., 1994). It is determined by the following formula:

$$\text{Specificity} = \frac{\text{TN}}{(\text{FP} + \text{TN})}$$

There are three definitions for positive predictive value (PPV). They are classified as PPV_1, PPV_2, and PPV_3. A PPV_1 is based on an abnormal finding at screening. It is the percentage of all positive screening mammograms that result in a diagnosis of cancer (Bassett et al., 1998). PPV_1 is calculated using the following formula:

$$\text{Positive Predictive Value (PPV}_1) = \frac{\text{TP}}{(\text{TP} + \text{FP}_1)}$$

Alternate method:

$$\text{PPV}_1 = \frac{\text{TP}}{\text{Number of Positive Screening Mammograms}}$$

A PPV_2 is based on a biopsy recommendation. It is the percentage of all screening or diagnostic mammograms recommended for biopsy or surgical consultation (Bassett et al., 1998). PPV_2 is calculated using the following formula:

$$\text{Positive Predictive Value (PPV}_2) = \frac{\text{TP}}{(\text{TP} + \text{FP}_2)}$$

Alternate method:

$$\text{PPV}_2 = \frac{\text{TP}}{\text{Number of Screening or Diagnostic Cases Recommended for Biopsy}}$$

A PPV_3 is based on biopsies performed. It is the percentage of all known biopsies done as result of positive screening, diagnostic mammograms, or additional imaging evaluation of a positive screening mammogram that resulted in the diagnosis of cancer (Bassett et al., 1998). PPV_3 is also referred to as the positive biopsy rate. PPV_3 is calculated using the following formula:

$$PPV_3 = \frac{TP}{(TP + FP_3)}$$

Alternate method:

$$PPV_3 = \frac{TP}{\text{Number of Biopsies}}$$

The cancer detection rate is the number of cancers correctly detected by mammography per 1000 patients examined by mammography. The easiest way to calculate this would be by age group.

The format used for reporting the medical outcomes audit is left entirely up to individual facilities. It would be well worth a facility's time to check the ACR's BI-RADS manual; a variety of reporting formats are provided in the manual.

Consumer Complaints

All mammography facilities are now required to have a mechanism in place for addressing consumer complaints. How this is achieved is up to the facility; the only requirement is that the procedure be written and documented. There are several ways that this can be done, but the easiest and most efficient way is to develop a patient survey that includes this requirement. The guidelines for designing a survey form have been discussed in Chap. 2 and are outlined in Fig. 2-3. A mammography survey should be succinct and as a rule should be no longer than one page. Figure 6-1 is an example of a mammography survey that can be used as a complaint mechanism.

The resolution of a consumer complaint is the sole responsibility of the imaging facility. It should be stressed that the consumer or their representative has the right to lodge a formal complaint directly to the facilities accrediting body or the Food and Drug Administration (FDA). This information should be provided to the patient upon examination. Each patient should be made aware of this prior to the mammography procedure. The imaging facility is required to maintain a record of all serious complaints for a period of 3 years from the date of the complaint. The facility is required to notify the accrediting board of serious complaints that have not been resolved and its attempt to resolve the complaint. When this occurs, the accrediting body will notify the FDA of the complaint.

Infection Control

All mammography facilities are now required by MQSA to have an infection control policy to establish procedures for cleaning and disinfecting mammography equipment that has come into contact with blood or other potentially infectious materials. Facilities are also required to maintain documentation that demonstrates adherence to the policies described in the infection

MAMMOGRAPHY IMAGING SERVICES

Dear Patient,

As stated in our hospitals mission statement, we are committed to proving compassionate patient care of the highest quality. To accomplish this, we need your help. By sharing your opinion, both positive and negative, with us through this survey, you can allow us to see what we are doing right and where we need to improve. Your comments about your experience will be kept confidential. Thank you for taking the time to help us improve.

PLEASE CHECK THE BEST ANSWER FOR EACH QUESTION.

	Excellent	Very Good	Good	Fair	Poor	Does Not Apply
1. The technologist listened closely to my needs.						
2. The technologist took prompt action to meet my needs.						
3. The technologist was friendly and respectful.						
4. The technologist demonstrated caring and concern.						
5. The technologist asked questions about my breast history.						
6. The technologist explained my test to me.						
7. The technologist answered my questions in a way that I could understand.						
8. The technologist demonstrated skill and knowledge.						
9. The exam room was clean and comfortable.						
10. The exam room was quiet and private.						
11. The registration process was simple and wait time was kept to a minimum.						
12. How well were you able to find your way around the Medical Center?						
13. How do you rate the overall quality of the care you received?						
	<20	20-29	30-39	40-49	50-59	60+
14. How old are you?						
					Male	Female
15. What is your gender?						
					Yes	No
16. Have you been a patient at any Medical Center health care facility?						
17. Will you return to the Medical Center the next time you need health care?						
18. Will you recommend the Medical Center to your friends?						
19. Would you like to talk with a manager about a concern or issue?						

Is there anything else you would like to tell us? Please use back of form.

Optional Information

Name _____

Phone Number _____

Thank You From The Staff

Figure 6-1 Mammography survey form with patient complaint mechanism built in.

control policy. The form of documentation used is currently left to the discretion of individual facilities. The simplest type of documentation is a checklist posted in each imaging suite. The checklist must contain an area for the date, time, and who performed the task. Another method of documentation is a daily log.

When the infection control policy is written, it must comply with all federal, state, and local regulations. While writing the policy, it would be in the best interest of the facility to contact a qualified infection control person for assistance.

Radiologist Quality Assurance

QA for the mammography radiologist can occur in a variety of ways—double reading of films, correlation of radiology and ultrasound reports, correlation of radiology and pathology reports, a monthly radiology morbidity and mortality conference, and the medical outcomes audit. All of these mechanisms are a form of peer review and are intended to assist each radiologist in his growth process.

The ACR strongly recommends that mammograms be double read by radiologists. Double reading is a process by which a second radiologist reviews the same set of films that was previously read by another radiologist. This process was implemented to increase diagnostic sensitivity for breast cancer and studies, in general, have not demonstrated a significant increase in call back rate.

Suboptimal Image Tracking

The mammography radiologist has the responsibility to ensure that there is a mechanism for ensuring frequent positive and negative feedback for the technologist. This can be achieved by implementing a system for tracking suboptimal mammographic films, a mechanism for identifying and assisting radiographers who are having problems with primarily positioning and technique.

When monitoring suboptimal images, it is important to statistically track the suboptimal films by area, technologist, facility, and cause. Once this has been completed, a plan of action and a documentation process must be developed. This method is not designed to instill fear into the technologists but to enhance awareness of a problem that should be addressed. The way to address the problem is through education and a better understanding of what the problem is. Figure 6-2A and B provides an example of a documentation form for identifying suboptimal mammographic images. This particular style of documentation provides the radiologist a place for comments (i.e., feedback). The technologist and supervisor have sections for their comments, plus a section for a plan of action if needed.

Mammography Quality Assurance

Mammography QA focuses on the improvement of image quality through a systematic program of record keeping, equipment selection, and acceptance testing. An integral part of mammographic QA is the ability to track the performance and maintenance of equipment. This can be achieved by maintain-

Mammography Image Quality Action

Technologist: _____   Date: _____

Facility: _____   Radiologist: _____

Comments: _____

_____

_____

Patient Name: _____   Medical Record #: _____

<u>Repeat/Suboptimal Reason:</u>   (Circle Breast)   (Circle Projection)

Positioning	R	L	MLO	CC	Other _____
Patient motion	R	L	MLO	CC	Other _____
Blur	R	L	MLO	CC	Other _____
Light films	R	L	MLO	CC	Other _____
Dark films	R	L	MLO	CC	Other _____
Static	R	L	MLO	CC	Other _____
Artifact	R	L	MLO	CC	Other _____
Processor marks	R	L	MLO	CC	Other _____
Fog	R	L	MLO	CC	Other _____
Incorrect patient identification	R	L	MLO	CC	Other _____
Double exposure	R	L	MLO	CC	Other _____
Date of film missing	R	L	MLO	CC	Other _____
Missing films	R	L	MLO	CC	Other _____
Improper marking of lesions	R	L	MLO	CC	Other _____

<u>Place an "X" in the box:</u>

Mammo folder not written up   [ ]   Missing paperwork   [ ]

Incomplete history form   [ ]   Old/previous films not included   [ ]

Other: _____

Please place technologist and supervisor response on back

Figure 6-2 *A.* Obverse side of the mammography image quality action form.

Technologist response: _____

_____

_____

_____

_____

Technologist signature: _____ **Date:** _____

Supervisor's response: _____

_____

_____

_____

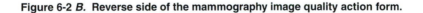

_____

Supervisor's signature: _____ **Date:** _____

Plan of action: _____

_____

_____

_____

_____

_____

_____

Figure 6-2 *B*. Reverse side of the mammography image quality action form.

ing a record on each piece of mammography equipment in the mammography imaging facility. There are a variety of ways that this could be done. The most common way is to keep a separate logbook on each piece of equipment from installation to removal. It is advisable that the record logs be kept in a central location as opposed to having the log in the room where the equipment is installed. Centralized record keeping ensures that maintenance and repair records can be readily found and reduces the chance of them being misplaced.

The selection of mammography imaging equipment should be made from the perspective of what is best for the patient and what will provide the most accurate clinical image for the patient. When selecting a new piece of imaging equipment the cost of the equipment should have little bearing on the decision if it is going to provide the images that may save a woman's life.

Once a piece of equipment has been selected, purchased, and installed, it should undergo a formal acceptance testing process. This may be done by the company or an independent consultant. Once the equipment has been certified as meeting the stated performance standards, it can be turned over to the facility.

Mammographic Quality Control

Mammographic quality control (MQC) focuses on the testing and monitoring of equipment in all areas of the mammography imaging facility. MQSA has established the type of equipment testing and monitoring required to be done in facilities that perform mammograms. The routine QC tests performed in a mammography imaging facility are listed in Fig. 6-3. The tests, which should be performed by the designated QC technologist and medical physicist, are listed in Table 6-7. The tests and protocols for performing them will be described later in this chapter. Record keeping is an essential part of MQC and the ACR is striving to have a uniform record keeping system. This author finds that the forms in the back of the ACR *Quality Control Manual* are quite satisfactory, except one. The processor QC form in the ACR manual, in my opinion, is not the best form to use because its structure leaves the possibility of inputting data incorrectly. I would strongly recommend using one of the processor monitoring forms developed by the film manufacturers. The forms to use are not included in this chapter because they are readily obtainable in the ACR's manual.

The primary cost for the QC program is in the test equipment. Figure 6-4 lists the type of QC equipment that a mammography QC program needs. The minimum cost to operate a mammography QC program is approximately $3000. The actual equipment costs for the QC program will vary depending on the type of equipment purchased.

TOOLS FOR QUALITY MANAGEMENT

MQM is a process that involves the analysis of tremendous amounts of data. To make sense of the raw data, individuals involved in the MQM process need to transform it into usable information. This can be achieved by utilizing tools that are specifically designed for the QM process. The tools used in this process are primarily the computer and the tools of statistical analysis.

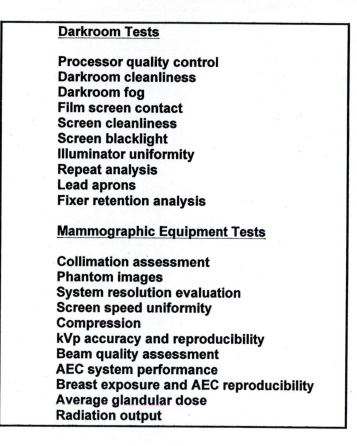

Darkroom Tests

Processor quality control
Darkroom cleanliness
Darkroom fog
Film screen contact
Screen cleanliness
Screen blacklight
Illuminator uniformity
Repeat analysis
Lead aprons
Fixer retention analysis

Mammographic Equipment Tests

Collimation assessment
Phantom images
System resolution evaluation
Screen speed uniformity
Compression
kVp accuracy and reproducibility
Beam quality assessment
AEC system performance
Breast exposure and AEC reproducibility
Average glandular dose
Radiation output

Figure 6-3 Mammography quality control tests.

The Computer

All the tools discussed in this chapter are critical to the MQM process; however, the most important tool is the computer. The computer is essential because it allows the individual to store and analyze a tremendous amount of data. The critical components of the computer are the storage capacity, speed, and type of software that is used.

The computer should have storage capacity of at least 1 gigabyte or higher. This amount of storage permits the storing of raw and computed data with ease. In addition, it is important to have sufficient random access memory (RAM) to ensure that the computer runs efficiently when handling multiple programs or tasks.

Select and install software that will provide you with the tools that are needed to adequately perform your QA and QC duties. The type of software to be installed should include a word processing, data base, and spreadsheet program.

Table 6-7
Mammography Quality Control Tests

Technologist Duties	Frequency of Test	Acceptance Parameters	Action to Be Taken
Darkroom cleanliness	Daily	0	—
Processor cleaning: crossover racks	Daily	0	—
Processor: developer temp	Daily	±0.5°F	Immediate
Processor: speed index	Daily	±0.15	Immediate
Processor: contrast index	Daily	±0.15	Immediate
Processor: base plus fog	Daily	±0.03 of total b + f	Immediate
Screen cleanliness	Weekly	0	—
Phantom images	Weekly	1.2 ± 0.20	Immediate
Visual checklist	Monthly	Pass/fail	—
Repeat analysis	Quarterly	<5%; preferred 2%	Within 30 days of test date
Fixer retention analysis	Quarterly	5 micrograms/cm^2 or a 3 on the hypo retention scale	Within 30 days of test date
Darkroom fog	Semiannual	Should not exceed a density of 0.05 in the fogged area	Immediate
Film-screen contact	Semiannual	Areas > 1 cm are not acceptable	Immediate
Compression force	Semiannual	Both Modes: 25–45 lb	Immediate
Compression deflection	Annual	<1 cm	Immediate
Light field luminance	Annual	160 lux	Within 30 days of test date
Lead aprons	Annual	0	Immediate

Medical Physicist Tests

Collimation	Annual	±2% of the SID	Within 30 days of test date
AEC system performance	Annual	±0.30 of the average	Within 30 days of test date
kVp accuracy and reproducibility	Annual	±5% of set kVp; a COV of ≤0.02 for reproducibility	Within 30 days of test date
Beam quality assessment	Annual	0.3 mm Al at 30 kVp	Within 30 days of test date
Breast exposure and AEC reproducibility	Annual	COV <0.05	Within 30 days of test date
Average glandular dose	Annual	3 mGy/exposure (0.3 rad/exposure)	Immediate
Radiation output	Annual	≥ 7.0 mGy/sec (800 mR/sec)	Within 30 days of test date
Film illuminator luminance	Annual	3000 cd/m^2	Within 30 days of test date
Reading room illuminance	Annual	50 lux	Within 30 days of test date
Evaluation of system resolution	Annual	A-C axis: parallel ≥13 lp/mm A-C axis: perpendicular ≥11 lp/mm	Within 30 days of test date
Uniformity of screen speed	Annual	Difference between the maximum and minimum OD <0.30	Within 30 days of test date
Image quality evaluation	Annual	See ACR QC Manual	Immediate
Artifact evaluation	Annual	See ACR QC Manual	Within 30 days of test date
Grids	Annual	Optical density of 1.20 ± 10	None Set
Focal spot size	Annual	NEMA Standards	None Set

Test Equipment	Approximate Cost
Sensitometer	$800
Densitometer	$800
Digital thermometer	$200
Screen contact wire mesh	$130
Digital light meter	$350
Mammographic phantom	$700
Bathroom scales	$ 50
Total	$3030

Figure 6-4 Mammography quality control equipment.

Statistical Tools

The statistical analysis tools that are discussed in MQM are referred to as descriptive statistics because they are used to describe an event. The intent of this section is to provide the reader with a basic overview of descriptive statistics and examples of where they may be applied in the MQM process. The reader should keep in mind that the descriptive statistics discussed here could be calculated by using a personal computer that has a commercially available statistical package or spreadsheet, which is the most efficient way to calculate any of the descriptive statistics discussed in this chapter. Descriptive statistics that are used in MQM include measures of central tendency, measures of dispersion, frequency distributions, and sample size.

Measures of Central Tendency

A number that is used to describe or characterize a distribution of numbers is called a measure of central tendency. The mean, median, and mode are measures of central tendency.

- *Mean:* The **mean** is the average of a group of numbers. The mean is the most commonly used measure of central tendency because of its stability. The mean is determined by adding the values and dividing by the number of values (Fig. 6-5). From a mammography imaging perspective, the mean may be used when describing the average turn around times for procedures done in the imaging facility, the average number of films repeated per technologist, the average cost of a procedure, or the average number of films per examination.
- *Median:* When the values of a group of numbers are very large or very small, the mean may not be representative of that group and the median should be used. Before determining the median, it is important to arrange

What is the mean of the following groups of numbers?

20
58
13
128
75
6
$\Sigma X = 300$

$$\overline{X} = \frac{\Sigma X}{n}$$

ΣX is the sum of the numbers
n is the total number of numbers

$\overline{X}$ is the mean

$$\overline{X} = \frac{300}{6} = 50$$

Figure 6-5 Determining the mean of a group of numbers.

the values either from the highest to lowest or the lowest to the highest value. The **median** is the midpoint of the values after they been arranged. Figure 6-6 illustrates how the median is determined. In MQM imaging the median is rarely used because of its instability.

- *Mode:* The **mode** is the most frequently observed number in a set of numbers. The mode does not require any calculation. From the medical imaging perspective, the mode has little or no application in the handling of raw data. Figure 6-7 demonstrates the determination of mode.

Measures of Spread (Dispersion)

Numbers that describe the spread around the mean are called measures of spread or dispersion. Typically these are range, percentile, standard deviation, and coefficient of variation.

What is the median?

125
100
75 ⇐ Median
50
25

Figure 6-6 Determining the median.

> **The repeat/reject rate for a twelve month period is 10%, 5.5%, 15%, 10%, 4.5%, 6%, 7%, 5%, 10%, 9%, 6.5%, and 11%. What is the modal repeat/reject rate?**
>
> **The mode is 10% because it appears the most often.**

Figure 6-7 Determining the mode.

- *Range:* The range is the lowest and highest number in a group of numbers. The easiest way to determine the range of a set of number is to rank order them from lowest to highest or vice versa (Fig. 6-8). Range has very little real application in mammography imaging.
- *Percentile:* The percentile is a number or score that falls at or below a given percentage. The percentile scale is used to describe percentiles. The most commonly used percentiles are the 25th, 50th, and 75th percentiles. Percentiles are frequently used in health care to compare some specific procedure or operation of the institution with the same procedure or operation at other institutions in the same area or nationally. Percentiles can be readily used in mammography imaging to compare turn around times of various procedures (i.e., screening examinations, diagnostic examinations, etc.), repeat rates, radiologist QA, and potentially many other items that are done as performance improvement opportunities. The most efficient way to calculate percentile is to use the statistical analysis package that comes with the majority of spreadsheet programs that are on the market today.
- *Standard deviation:* The range of variation around the mean is called **standard deviation.** This is the most commonly used dispersion measure in health care. In mammography it is used as a calculation in many of the physicist tests discussed later in the chapter. It is a powerful tool that can be used in medical

> **What is the range of the following 4.5, 10, 8, 23, 6, and 15?**
>
> **23**⇐ **Highest number**
> **15**
> **20**   **The range is 4.5 and 23.**
> **8**
> **6**
> **4.5**⇐ **Lowest number**

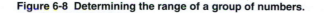

Figure 6-8 Determining the range of a group of numbers.

outcomes audit. Standard deviation is typically shown as *SD* or the small Greek letter sigma (σ). Standard deviation is calculated by using the following formula:

$$SD\ (\sigma) = \sqrt{\frac{\Sigma\,(X - \overline{X})^2}{N}}$$

Where *X* is the raw score or number, $\overline{X}$ is the mean, and *N* is the number of scores. Figure 6-9 illustrates how standard deviation is calculated.

What is the standard deviation of the following group of numbers?

    3, 5, 7, 9, and 11

Step 1: Determine the mean ($\overline{X}$).

    The mean is 7.

Step 2: Calculate the standard deviation.

$$SD\ (\sigma) = \sqrt{\frac{(3-7)^2 + (5-7)^2 + (7-7)^2 + (9-7)^2 + (11-7)^2}{5}}$$

$$SD\ (\sigma) = \sqrt{\frac{16 + 4 + 0 + 4 + 16}{5}}$$

$$SD\ (\sigma) = \sqrt{\frac{40}{5}}$$

$$SD\ (\sigma) = \sqrt{8}$$

The standard deviation is 2.83.

Figure 6-9 Calculating the standard deviation.

- *Coefficient of variation:* There are times that it will be necessary to compare two or more measures of dispersion. When that time comes, a direct comparison may lead to a false conclusion. The best way to avoid this is to use the coefficient of variation. The **coefficient of variation (CV)** is a useful statistic because it is a relative measure of dispersion. The CV is the standard deviation (σ) divided by the mean ($\bar{X}$). The number that expresses CV is always stated as a fraction (i.e., 0.01). The coefficient of variation is expressed as the following formula:

$$CV = \frac{\sigma}{\bar{X}}$$

In mammography the medical physicist uses the CV in conjunction with the mean and standard deviation when measuring reproducibility of x-ray generators. Figure 6-10 illustrates the application of the formula in medical imaging.

Frequency Distributions

A frequency distribution is used to describe data by how often an event or a situation occurs. The simplest way to use a frequency distribution is to group the data into categories. Frequency distributions could be used in mammography to determine how often a particular situation or event is occurring (i.e., suboptimal film tracking, repeat analysis, causal repeat rates, etc.). Figure 6-11 shows how a frequency distribution might be used in mammography.

Sample Size

Sample size is determined by what you are attempting to study. It should be adequate to obtain the required data for the problem that is being studied. When the sample size is too small, the tabulated results will not be accurate. When the sample size is too large, the amount of data will be too ponderous to calculate. It is important to select a sample size that will meet the current need. In medical imaging there are no clear-cut guidelines for selecting the size of the sample. To obtain reliable data, it is critical that the sample be selected in a random fashion (i.e., one out of five, etc.). Randomization reduces the possibility of skewing. The ideal sample size should be no less than 30 and no greater than 100. This range provides an adequate sampling base for almost any study that would occur in the mammography facility.

THE DARKROOM

There are no strict guidelines on the size of a darkroom. Over the span of my career, I have seen darkrooms from the size of two offices to the size of small closets. Darkrooms should have ample room to allow unimpeded movement and adequate storage space. All darkrooms must share some commonalties, such as ventilation, lighting (ambient and safe), temperature control, humidity control, storage, loading benches, and easy access.

What is the coefficient of variation for four exposures using a technique of 200 mA 0.5 sec and 80 kVp? The four exposures yielded mR readings of 425, 420, 423, 426.

$$CV = \frac{\sigma}{\overline{X}}$$

Step 1: Determine the mean and standard deviation.

$$\overline{X} = 423.5 \qquad SD\ (\sigma) = 2.29$$

Step 2: Calculate the coefficient of variation.

$$CV = \frac{2.29}{423.5}$$

$$CV = 0.005$$

The estimated coefficient of variation of radiation exposures shall be no greater than 0.05. The CV for this exposure is within the accepted limits.

Figure 6-10 Calculating the coefficient of variation.

Tech	# of repeats/week	Tech	# of repeats/week
A	0	K	5
B	2	L	2
C	1	M	3
D	2	N	4
E	4	O	1
F	3	P	1
G	2	Q	3
H	2	R	2
I	3	S	3
J	4	T	4

Figure 6-11 Frequency distribution showing the number of repeat films per week for a selected group of technologists.

One problem being encountered in darkrooms today is the control of dust and dirt when a dropped ceiling is used. There are several ways to control this problem. The least expensive method involves covering the ceiling tiles with shrink wrap plastic. This will prevent dust and dirt from falling onto work surfaces and into cassettes.

The temperature and relative humidity of the darkroom room and film storage area should be checked on a daily or weekly basis, whichever is deemed appropriate by the administration of the Medical Imaging Department. Air circulation of the darkroom must be checked by plant operations of the institution semiannually or annually. The people who are actually doing the checks will determine the frequency of air circulation checks (Fig. 6-12).

Film Storage

Proper storage of x-ray film in the Mammography Imaging Facility is a crucial part of any radiographic quality assurance program. Failure to properly store film will result in film artifacts, loss of image quality, repeat films, missed diagnoses, and increased cost to the department and the consumer.

Film should be stored in an area free of temperature and humidity extremes and any potential exposure to x-radiation. The storage room should be environmentally controlled with the relative humidity between 30% to 50% and the room temperature maintained between 50° and 70°F. These environmental conditions also apply to the darkroom.

Film should be stored vertically either on end or on the side. Boxes of film should never be stored flat or stacked on top of each other. Always rotate the stock and use the oldest stock first. The easiest way to do this is to store the film by expiration date. X-ray film will start aging (base + fog increases) approximately 6 months after the expiration date. Base plus fog (b + f) is the inherent density in a sheet of x-ray film prior to exposure to x-rays. Some departments use a color coding system for rotating film stock. Poor or improper film storage can result in poor image quality and film artifacts such as static.

Film Artifacts

Film artifacts originate from the automatic processor or are due to improper film handling by department personnel in the darkroom. Common automatic

---

◆ **Air Circulation: 10 complete air exchanges per hour**

◆ **Temperature: 50° to 70°F**

◆ **Relative Humidity: 30% to 50%**

Figure 6-12 Darkroom and film storage environment guide.

Table 6-8
Common Parallel Processing Artifacts: Guide Shoe Marks

Artifact Appearance	Cause
Lines that are parallel to the direction of film travel	Guide shoe set too close to the adjacent roller
Plus density, minus density, or minus density with surface damage	Crossover guide shoes on single-emulsion film processed emulsion side up
Evenly spaced intervals (1 inch, 1/8 inch)	Turnaround guide shoes on single emulsion film processed emulsion side down
Continuous or short length	Appear as plus density when pressure is exerted on the emulsion side of the film, usually from guide shoes in the developer section of the processor
Usually found on the leading edge and/or the trailing edge of the film, but can be found anywhere	Appear as minus density without surface damage when pressure is exerted on the emulsion side of the film, usually from guide shoes in the fixer-to-wash crossover
	Appear as minus density with surface damage when emulsion is gouged off the film base anywhere in the film path

Courtesy of Eastman Kodak, used with permission.

processor artifacts are described in Tables 6-8 through 6-24. Common film handling artifacts are described in Tables 6-25 and 6-26.

Artifacts that originate in the automatic processor may be reduced or even eliminated by instituting a careful preventative maintenance program. Whenever the processor chemistry is changed and the processor is cleaned, deep racks and crossover assemblies should be checked for rollers that are bad (worn, pitted, etc.), gears that are worn or missing teeth, and chains that are

Table 6-9
Common Parallel Processing Artifacts: Delay Streaks

Artifact Appearance	Cause
Randomly spaced narrow bands of varying widths	Build up of oxidized developer on the developer-to-fixer crossover assembly (build-up prevents uniform development of the film(s) leading edge)
Parallel to the direction of film travel	Low solution levels can cause delay streaks when rollers are not kept wet
Usually plus density	
Usually seen starting at the leading edge of the first film fed into the processor after it has been unused for an extended period of time	

Courtesy of Eastman Kodak, used with permission.

Table 6-10
Common Parallel Processing Artifacts: Entrance Roller Marks

Artifact Appearance	Cause
Plus density bands 1/8 inch wide	Excessive pressure on the emulsion of the film from the entrance rollers
Parallel to the direction of film travel	Moisture on the entrance rollers

Courtesy of Eastman Kodak, used with permission.

Table 6-11
Common Perpendicular Processing Artifacts: Film Hesitation Marks and Stub Lines

Artifact Appearance	Cause
Plus density located 1⅝ inches from the leading edge of the film	Improper guide shoe positioning in the developer turnaround assembly
Perpendicular to the direction of film travel	Nonuniform film speed resulting from malfunctioning rack or drive component (warped or rough rollers, rack drive chain too loose or too tight, malfunctioning gears)
	Poor quality, exhausted, or contaminated chemicals
	Build-up of chemicals on the rollers
	Processor or film emulsion design

Courtesy of Eastman Kodak, used with permission.

Table 6-12
Common Perpendicular Processing Artifacts: Chatter

Artifact Appearance	Cause
Plus-density lines consistently spaced	Too loose or too tight developer rack drive chain, gears, or developer-to-fixer crossover assembly drive mechanism
Perpendicular to the direction of film travel	

Courtesy of Eastman Kodak, used with permission.

Table 6-13
Common Perpendicular Artifacts: Slap Lines

Artifact Appearance	Cause
Broad, plus density line located 2⅛–2¼ inches in from the trailing edge of the film	Occurs when the trailing edge of a film releases abruptly from the developer-to-fixer crossover and slaps the top center roller of the fix rack
Perpendicular to the direction of film travel	

Courtesy of Eastman Kodak, used with permission.

Table 6-14
Common Perpendicular Processing Artifacts: Pi Lines

Artifact Appearance	Cause
Plus-density line just short of film edge with stub lines that go almost to the film edge 3.14 inches from leading edge	Emulsion on the roller A problem with the air/solution interface rollers Dirty rollers Newly cleaned rollers

Courtesy of Eastman Kodak, used with permission.

Table 6-15
Common Random Processing Artifacts: Drying Patterns/Water Spots

Artifact Appearance	Cause
Narrow wavering bands or spots with a mottled, washed out, or shiny appearance	Depleted photochemicals Under-replenished photochemicals
Readily seen by reflected light	Poor squeegee action at wash rack exit
Can be seen by transmitted light when severe	Air tube missing or clogged
Occur at random intervals parallel or perpendicular to the direction of film travel	Dirty or inoperative dryer rollers Excessive dryer temperature

Courtesy of Eastman Kodak, used with permission.

Table 6-16
Common Random Processing Artifacts: Wet Pressure

Artifact Appearance	Cause
Random plus-density fluctuations that may look like noise or quantum mottle on film	Rough, blistered, or warped rollers in the developer rack or developer-to-fix crossover, exerting excessive pressure on the film emulsion Exhausted developer

Courtesy of Eastman Kodak, used with permission.

Table 6-17
Common Random Processing Artifacts: Surface Scratches

Artifact Appearance	Cause
Random, plus-density marks indicating pressure on the film emulsion	Processor components especially dryer rollers and air tubes, improperly maintained, or out of position after maintenance
Random, minus-density marks indicating the emulsion was scraped off the film base	

Courtesy of Eastman Kodak, used with permission.

Table 6-18
Common Random Processing Artifacts: Flame Patterns

Artifact Appearance	Cause
Variations in film density resembling a flame	Low recirculation rates Less likely to occur with seasoned chemicals

Courtesy of Eastman Kodak, used with permission.

Table 6-19
Common Random Processing Artifacts: Run Back

Artifact Appearance	Cause
Random, plus-density "dribble" or "scallop" on the trailing edge of the film	Developer solution runs back down the trailing edge of the film as the film enters the fixer, causing increased and uncontrolled development

Courtesy of Eastman Kodak, used with permission.

Table 6-20
Common Random Processing Artifacts: Bent Corners

Artifact Appearance	Cause
A corner of the film is bent	Excessive recirculation of changes in the path of the film as it is transported through the processor

Courtesy of Eastman Kodak, used with permission.

Table 6-21
Common Random Processing Artifacts: Pick-Off

Artifact Appearance	Cause
Random, small minus-density spots	Rough and dirty rollers in poorly maintained processors
Readily detectable on single-emulsion film	Nonuniform or inconsistent transport speed
Emulsion has been removed down to the film base	Poor quality chemicals

Courtesy of Eastman Kodak, used with permission.

Table 6-22
Common Random Processing Artifacts: Dye Stain

Artifact Appearance	Cause
A pink color seen in the clear area of the film	Incomplete removal of sensitizing dye during processing due to incomplete or inadequate fixing or washing

Courtesy of Eastman Kodak, used with permission.

Table 6-23
Common Random Processing Artifacts: Brown Films

Artifact Appearance	Cause
Processed film has turned brown	Inadequate washing or fixing of the film

Courtesy of Eastman Kodak, used with permission.

Table 6-24
Common Random Processing Artifacts: Skivings

Artifact Appearance	Cause
Emulsion appears 3.14 inches distance from the leading edge of the film	Nonuniform film transport speed, poor processor film path design, film slitting, cutting, or finishing
	Film emulsion formulation or inadequate or hardener-depleted developer solution

Courtesy of Eastman Kodak, used with permission.

Table 6-25
Common Random Processing Artifacts: Static

Artifact Appearance	Cause
Random, plus-density marks that resemble tree branches, smudges, or dots and dashes	Static infrequently occurs as a result of processing; it is usually caused by low relative humidity in the darkroom, synthetic clothing worn by operators, etc.

Courtesy of Eastman Kodak, used with permission.

Table 6-26
Film Handling Artifacts

Artifact Appearance	Cause
Shadow images (minus density)	Dirt and dust in darkroom and image receptors
	Screens and image receptors must be thoroughly cleaned to eliminate shadow images
	The darkroom must be as clean as possible
	Use an ultraviolet light device to help detect areas where dust and dirt accumulate
Scratches (minus and plus density)	More likely to occur from handling, not processing
	Carelessly placing film in the film bin
	Routinely slamming the film bin
	Carelessly removing film from the film bin and loading image receptor
	Sliding film across dirty film feed tray
Static (plus density)	Usually caused by handling film in a darkroom with low relative humidity
	Use a humidifier to raise relative humidity to 30–50%
	Personnel should wear natural fibers and use antistatic laundry products
Fingerprints (minus and plus density)	Minus density fingerprints result from moisture on the film prior to exposure
	Plus density fingerprints result from moisture on the film after exposure and prior to processing
	Keep hands clean and dry
Pressure marks (plus density)	Stacked cases of film
	Exposed film carelessly loaded
Stress marks	Holding film incorrectly
Kink marks (minus and plus density)	Pressure from fingernails
Film feeding errors	May cause many different types of artifacts

Courtesy of Eastman Kodak, used with permission.

loose. A quick visual inspection should be performed daily when the crossover rollers and the exposed rollers of the deep racks are wiped off. Any damage or anomaly should be reported to the appropriate person.

Film handling artifacts will never be eliminated in a Medical Imaging Department. This type of artifact can be reduced with proper inservice training of all personnel. It is important that environmental conditions and film storage practices be monitored to help in reducing film artifacts.

REPEAT ANALYSIS

The repeat analysis program is a critical element of the MQM program. The repeat analysis process is a well-defined method that determines whether problems exist and the causes of these problems. An analysis of repeats consists of looking at the number of repeat films, the number of rejected films, and the number of waste films. Repeat films are those films that are repeated for a reason (i.e., positioning, technique, motion, etc.). Waste films are films that are thrown away because they are black, green (unexposed), clear, or sensitometric. Rejected films are a reflection of the total number of films that are being discarded by the Mammography Imaging Facility. Adding the total number of repeat films and the total number of wasted films arrives at the number of rejected films.

There are two types of repeat analysis tools that may be used by the imaging department. They are repeat analysis by projection and the causal repeat analysis for specific cause. One must perform the actual repeat analysis prior to doing a causal repeat analysis.

Unlike the radiographic repeat analysis discussed in Chap. 3, there are specific guidelines established for the mammography repeat analysis. It is done quarterly, and for it to be meaningful there must be a patient volume of at least 250 patients. Individual facilities may wish to collect and tabulate the data more frequently, but the data should be reported quarterly.

Repeat Analysis

Rationale
This procedure is designed to provide the Mammography Imaging Facility with a means for analyzing the cause of mammographic repeat and reject films.

Testing Frequency
The reject analysis should be performed quarterly.

Equipment
- Pencil

- Calculator
- Repeat analysis form
- Illuminator
- Reject films

Procedure

A. At the end of the repeat analysis phase calculate the total number of films used during the this time. This number may be obtained by using the inventory method or the film estimation method. The film inventory method is more accurate and takes a little more time than the estimation method

B. Methods for calculating total films used.
  - Film inventory method

    At the beginning of the repeat analysis phase take an initial inventory (II) of all film in the department and record this number on the film inventory log (see Fig. 3-2).

    At the end of repeat analysis phase, take a final film inventory (FFI) of all film in the department and record this number on the film inventory log.

    At this time, determine if any new film shipments (NFS) have been received and record this number on the film inventory log.

    Determine the total films used with the formula

    $$TFU = (II + NFS) - FFI$$

  - Film estimation method

    $TFU = 3.5 \times$ the number of examinations performed

    3.5 is a constant that reflects the average number of films used per examination.

    The number of examinations performed reflects the number of examinations done during the analysis period.

C. Obtain rejected/repeated films from mammographic areas.

D. Determine the cause of each repeat, reject, and waste film; record the films in the appropriate area of the repeat analysis form.

E. Perform the following tasks.
  - Calculate the number of repeat films, reject films, and waste films.
  - Calculate the repeat percentage.

$$\text{Repeat \%} = \frac{\text{\# Repeat Films}}{\text{TFU}} \times 100\%$$

  - Calculate the reject percentage.

$$\text{Reject \%} = \frac{\text{\# Repeat Films plus Waste Films}}{\text{TFU}} \times 100\%$$

• Calculate the waste percentage.

$$\text{Waste \%} = \frac{\text{\# Waste Films}}{\text{TFU}} \times 100\%$$

F. Record the films in the appropriate area of the repeat analysis form.

Acceptance Parameters

• The ACR states that the repeat should be less than 2%, but a 5% repeat rate is probably adequate.
• MQSA states that if the total repeat or reject rate changes from the previous determined rate by more than 2% of the total films included in the analysis, the reason(s) for the change shall be noted.

Record Keeping

A record should be kept that documents the date of the test, who performed the test, the results of the test, and the corrective action taken.

Potential Problems

The most often encountered problem is the failure to account for all repeat films. This will result in an inaccurate repeat rate.

Causal Repeat Analysis

The implementation of a casual repeat analysis as part of a MQM program is strongly recommended. Causal repeat analysis is an additional tool that will enhance the overall repeat analysis program of the mammography imaging department. The causal repeat analysis can determine what portion of the overall repeat rate is the result of a specific cause (i.e., positioning). All that one needs to calculate the causal repeat rate is the repeat analysis form, a calculator, and following formula:

$$\text{Causal Repeat Rate (\%)} = \frac{\text{Number of Repeats for a Specific Cause}}{\text{Number of Total Repeats}} \times 100$$

Examples for calculating causal repeat rate can be found in Chap. 3.

Ultraviolet Light Test for Darkroom Cleanliness

Rationale

This test is designed to confirm that the darkroom is free of dirt, dust, and any foreign material.

Testing Frequency

This test should be performed weekly, preferably at the beginning of the work-week.

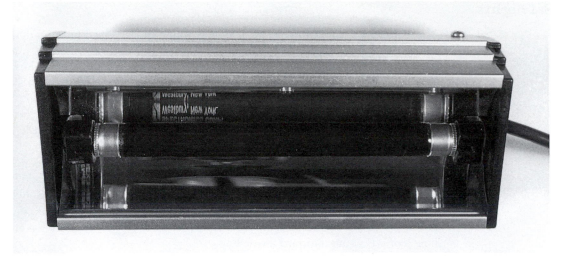

Figure 6-13 Ultraviolet light used for darkroom cleanliness checks and image receptor checks.

Equipment
• Ultraviolet light (UV) (5 to 10 V) (Fig. 6-13)

Procedure
A. Plug in the UV light at a convenient outlet in the darkroom.
B. If applicable, close all doors leading into the darkroom.
C. Turn on the UV light.
D. Turn off all safelights and overhead lights.
E. Carefully examine all work surfaces with the UV light. Dirt, dust, and particulate matter will glow under the UV light.
F. Carefully examine all walls, corners, ceilings, and other areas where dirt and dust might accumulate with the UV light.
G. Record the results.

Acceptance Parameters
Acceptance parameters are determined by the ACR and are based on the MQSA. MQSA requires that the darkroom be totally free of dust and dirt.

Record Keeping
A record should be kept that documents the date of the test, who performed the test, the results of the test, and the corrective action taken.

Potential Problems
• Suspended or dropped ceilings pose a problem because they trap dust and dirt.
• Every time the darkroom door is slammed, a dropped ceiling generally vibrates and dust, dirt, and particulate matter come free, contaminating the work surfaces of the darkroom and image receptors.

Safelights

There are essentially two types of safelights found in a medical imaging darkroom, the safelight used with calcium tungstate films and the safelight used with rare earth films. The safelight used with calcium tungstate films has a Wratten 6-B filter and the safelight for rare earth films has a GBX-2 filter. The most commonly used safelight is the GBX-2.

When installing or servicing a safelight, it is important that a visual check be done to ensure that the filter is intact and that there are no apparent light leaks in the filter housing. It is just as important to check the wattage of the light bulb being used and the distance the safelight is from the loading bench. The light bulb used for a safelight should be 7½ Watts. The safelight should be mounted no less than 36 inches from the loading bench. Mounting a safelight less than 36 inches away will result in fogging of the film. A 15-Watt bulb may be used with the GBX-2 safelight filter if it is 4 feet or higher from the loading bench or it is pointed toward the ceiling.

Safelight Test

Rationale

This test is designed to confirm that the safelights and other unsafe light will not fog the film(s) being handled in the darkroom.

Testing Frequency

Safelights should be tested semiannually or when films exit the processor fogged.

Equipment

- 8 × 10 mammography image receptor and film
- Mammographic phantom (Fig. 6-14)
- Lead mat
- Timer or a clock with a secondhand or a stopwatch
- Densitometer
- One piece of 8- × 10-inch cardboard
- One piece of 4- × 10-inch cardboard

Procedure

A. Turn off all lights in the darkroom and check for any light leaks. If any light leaks are detected repair them.

B. Turn off the safelights in the darkroom and load the 8 × 10 image receptor with the mammography film.

C. Place the image receptor in the image receptor holder of the mammographic unit.

D. Place mammographic phantom on top of the image receptor holder and position the edge of the phantom with the chest wall side of the image receptor.

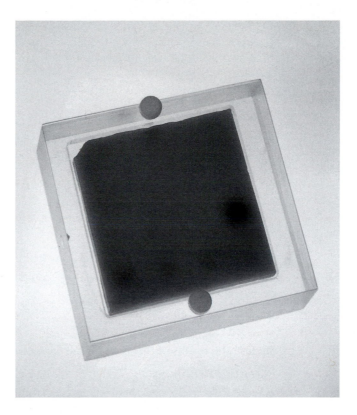

Figure 6-14 Mammographic phantom used for the darkroom fog test and phantom images test. *(Courtesy of Nuclear Associates, used with permission.)*

E. Place the compression device of the mammographic unit in contact with the phantom.
F. One of the following should be done:
- If automatic exposure control (AEC) is to be used, the AEC sensor should be in the same location as previous phantom images.
- If a manual exposure is to be used, then select an appropriate mA and exposure time.
G. Make an exposure that would be appropriate for a 4.0 to 4.5 centimeter compressed breast.
- The exposure should produce an optical density between 1.2 and 1.5.
H. Remove the image receptor from the image receptor tray.
I. Turn off all lights in the darkroom.
J. Place the film on the loading bench emulsion side up under the safelight to be tested.
K. Cover the half of the phantom image with cardboard or opaque paper. The cardboard or opaque paper should be perpendicular to the chest wall edge of the film.

L. Turn on the safelight to be tested and expose the film for 2 minutes.
M. Immediately turn off the safelight and process the film.
N. Using the densitometer measure the density of the unfogged and fogged images.
   • Both density measurements should be made directly adjacent from each other.
   • The measurements should be obtained as close to the line separating the fogged and unfogged areas of the film as possible.
   • The density measurements should not be obtained in areas where there are test objects.
O. The amount of fog is determined by subtracting the unfogged portion of the film from the fogged portion.
P. Record the densities and the amount of fog in the QC log (Fig. 6-15A and B).

Acceptance Parameters

The ACR and MQSA specify that fog should not be greater than an optical density of 0.05.

Record Keeping

A record should be kept that documents the date of the test, who performed the test, the results of the test, and the corrective action taken.

Potential Problems

• Light leaks in the darkroom will cause erroneous results.
• Leaving the safelight on while loading or unloading the image receptor may result in error.
• Exposing sections of film for longer than 2 minutes may result in increased density readings.
• Having the wrong wattage of bulb in the safelight may result in increased density readings.
• Using the wrong type of film will result in inaccurate density readings.
• Having safelights at less than the prescribed distance will result in increased fog and increased density readings.

AUTOMATIC PROCESSORS

Automatic processors may be purchased with a variety of processing times. The available processing times range from 45 seconds to 3½ minutes. Processors that have a 45-second processing time are called rapid action processors, while processors that have a processing time greater than 90 seconds are referred to as extended time processors. The standard processor in most Medical Imaging Departments is the 90-second processor, which serves a variety of imaging demands. There are two QC tests that should routinely be performed

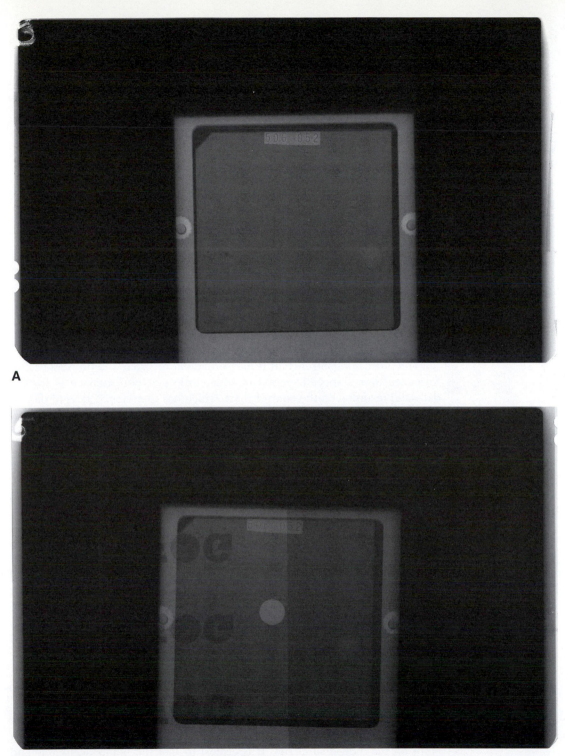

A

B

Figure 6-15 *A.* Normal darkroom test film. *B.* Darkroom test film with increased fog that resulted from the use of the wrong wattage of light bulb.

on automatic processors. They are sensitometry or processing monitoring and immersion time. Of these tests, processor monitoring and immersion are the most critical tests to perform.

Establishing and Maintaining a Processor Monitoring Program

Processor monitoring is a fairly routine task that is done daily at approximately the same time and on all processors in the Mammography Imaging Facility. The standard for processor monitoring has been established by the MQSA guidelines and should be used for both mammography film processors and diagnostic film processors. All that is needed to perform processor monitoring is the film, processor control chart, sensitometer, densitometer, and thermometer.

The type of film used for processor monitoring will be mammography film. If a processor is serving double duty running both mammography films and diagnostic films, then mammography film should be used for the processor monitoring.

The processor control chart is the permanent record of the processor's performance over a specific period of time. Processor performance is tracked daily and recorded on the control chart, which has room for 31 days of data. A new control chart should be started at the beginning of each month. Processor control charts should be kept on file for at least 24 months to provide a performance history of the processor. The processor control chart is divided into six specific sections for the recording of information. The upper section is for documenting the processor, type of film, emulsion number, year, date the crossover is performed, and crossover emulsion number. The next section is the area for the month, date, and initials of who performed the test. The third, fourth, fifth, and sixth sections of the control chart are for recording the medium density (speed index), density difference (contrast index), b + f, and developer temperature. On the reverse side of the control chart is an area for making comments about processor performance. The medium density and density difference portions of the processor control chart have upper and lower limits established. These limits are ±0.15 of the midpoint of the graph. If either speed or contrast exceed or fall below this number, it is important to stop running films and find the cause of the problem. If processor values either exceed or fall below ±0.10 of the midpoint, one should be on the alert for potential problems with the processor chemistry. When this occurs, it will be necessary to run several filmstrips to monitor the performance of the processor and make the determination if the service engineer should be called. Table 6-27 is a trouble shooting guide for processor control charts. Once the data have been plotted on the control chart, it will be necessary to connect each point on the individual charts. It is critical to plot the points accurately and evaluate the chart for trends and points out of control. A trend is a series of three to five consecutive data points that present either as an upward or down-

Table 6-27
Troubleshooting Guide for Processor Control Charts

Control Parameter	Film Appearance	Probable Causes	Corrective Action
↑ Speed index	Film density too high	Developer temperature too high	Check developer thermostat setting; check incoming water temperature
↑ Contrast index		Developer replenisher improperly mixed	Drain and remix developer
↑ Base + fog		Developer contaminated with fixer	Drain and rinse tanks and mix fresh chemistry
			Use splash guard when removing fixer rack to avoid contamination
↓ Speed index	Film density too low	Developer temperature too low	Adjust developer thermostat to correct setting
↓ Contrast index		Developer exhausted	Check replenishment rates and/or mix fresh chemistry
↓ Base + fog			Change chemistry; follow mixing instructions included with chemistry
		Developer improperly mixed	Check processor overflow drain
		Developer diluted	Check tanks for possible leaks
↑ Speed index	↑ Fog level	Developer contaminated with fixer	Drain and rinse tanks; mix fresh chemistry and replace filter
↓ Contrast index	↓ in overall film density	Fixer replenishment rate inadequate	Drain tank and reset fixer replenishment rate to correct level
↓ Base + fog			
↑ Speed index	↓ Fog level	Fixer contaminated with developer	Drain and rinse tanks; mix fresh chemistry
↑ Contrast index	↓ in overall film density	Developer improperly mixed	Change chemistry; follow mixing instructions included with chemistry
↓ Base + fog		Developer starter inadequate	Drain and rinse tanks; mix fresh chemistry, add correct amount of starter
		Excessive developer replenishment	Drain developer tank and refill with fresh developer; add correct amount of starter
		Developer completely oxidized	Adjust developer replenishment rates
			Check replenishment rates and/or mix fresh chemistry
↑ Speed index	Loss of image contrast	Developer improperly mixed, overdiluted, or oxidized	Mix fresh chemistry
↓ Contrast index			Consider making a limited amount of chemistry
↓ Base + fog		Developer replenishment rate inadequate	Drain developer tank and refill with fresh developer; add correct amount of starter

ward pattern on the graph. When a trend falls within the acceptable processor limits, it is still okay to perform clinical images. However, if the trend falls above or below the acceptable limits, the technologist will need to stop running clinical images and determine what is causing the problem. A point out of control is a data point that is outside of the established control limits. When this occurs, the point must be circled and another strip run within 30 minutes of the first strip. Trends and points out of control must be documented in the remarks section of the processor control chart. Figures 6-16A and B illustrate a trend and point out of control.

A device called a sensitometer (see Fig. 3-8) produces the filmstrip that is used for processor monitoring. The sensitometer is a battery operated electromechanical device that imprints a 21-step wedge on a piece of film (see Fig. 3-9). Sensitometers used in medical imaging have two exposure settings identified as blue and green. The exposure switch is located on the front corner of the sensitometer. The purpose of this switch is to allow for the use of film that is sensitive to either blue or green light. It is important to check that the proper switch position is used for the type of film used. When exposing a film with the sensitometer, a tonal sound is emitted to denote that the film has been exposed. The quality of the sound and the duration of the exposure are different for the blue and the green settings. The blue exposure setting emits a lower and quicker sound than the green exposure setting. When exposing a film with the sensitometer, it is important to wait approximately 15 to 20 seconds between exposures. This should be done to allow the sensitometer to stabilize. The sensitometer should be sent back to the manufacturer for calibration every 12 to 18 months. The ACR requires that sensitometers be recalibrated every 18 months.

It is important that all sources of potential error be controlled as much as possible. A potential source of error that can occur with the sensitometer is how frequently the battery is changed. The battery in the sensitometer should be changed either quarterly or semiannually. When the decision is made to replace the battery it is also very important to run film strips pre- and post-battery change. This is the only method that will confirm that speed and contrast values have not changed between battery changes. Failure to change the battery of the sensitometer either quarterly or semiannually may result in erroneous data being plotted on the processor control chart.

The densitometer (see Fig. 3-13A, B, and C) is an electromechanical device that is used to read the optical density of a film or the preselected density steps from a film that has been exposed. When a densitometer is purchased, there is a pre-exposed calibration strip (see Fig. 3-14) that may be used to periodically check the calibration of the unit. It is important to remember that the calibration strip has an expiration date and should be replaced every 18 to 24 months; it is an organic material and degrades when exposed to any light source. When using the densitometer, it is important to turn the unit on and let it warm up. Once it has warmed up, it will be necessary to zero the unit prior to use. Each time a density reading is taken, the unit should be zeroed

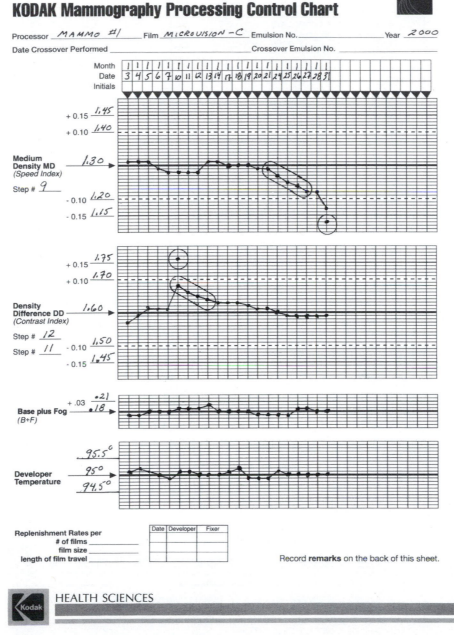

Figure 6-16 A. Control chart illustrating points out of control and trends in both the contrast index and speed index.

Remarks

Date	Action
1-10	CONTRAST INDEX VALUES beyond ACCEPTED AIMS. NO MAMMOGRAMS RAN; 2nd strip RAN AT 9 a.m. VALUES WITHIN AIMS.
1-31	Speed index VALUES below ACCEPTED AIMS. 2 ND strip RAN AT 9 a.m. VALUES STILL low. NO MAMMOGRAMS RAN; SERVICE CALLED.

Remarks

Date	Action

More than quality imaging

Kodak

M7-173   Printed in U.S.A.   © Eastman Kodak Company, 1995   Kodak is a trademark.

Figure 6-16 *B.* **Reverse side of control chart with remarks.**

again to ensure that the next reading is accurate. Like the sensitometer, the densitometer has to be periodically recalibrated. It should be sent back to the manufacturer for calibration every 12 to 18 months. The ACR requires that densitometers be recalibrated every 18 months.

The temperature of the developer should be checked daily and recorded on the processor control chart. The temperature should be measured with either a digital thermometer (Fig. 6-17) or a nonmercury analog thermometer. Do not use a mercury-filled glass thermometer to measure the temperature of the developer because there is always the possibility of the thermometer breaking and contaminating the developer. The temperature for the developer should be within ±0.5 degrees of the aim temperature, which is generally 35°C (95°F).

When starting a processor monitoring program from scratch, the processor or processors being monitored should be thoroughly cleaned, new chemistry

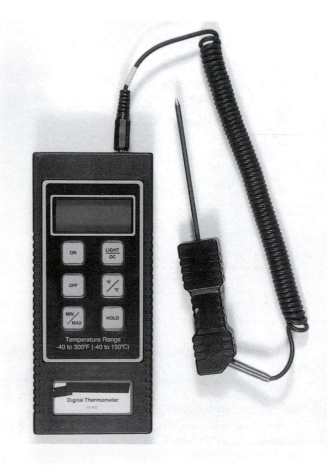

Figure 6-17 Digital thermometer used to monitor processor temperatures.

mixed, solution temperatures checked, and the replenishment rates checked and adjusted if necessary. Once this has been accomplished, aim values should be established for the processors being monitored. The simplest way to do this is with a 5-day average of the b + f, the mid-density step (speed index), and the density difference between high and low density steps (contrast index). The new aim values are the average b + f, speed index, and contrast index. The steps and values associated with these terms are described in the automatic processor monitoring protocol.

Processor Preventive Maintenance

Processor preventive maintenance is a critical and integral component of the processor monitoring program. Failure to have a preventive maintenance schedule can lead to needless downtime and loss of revenue. Preventive maintenance is an ongoing task that has daily and monthly components (Table 6-28). A qualified processor service engineer should perform the monthly component of the preventive maintenance program. It is important that, when the monthly preventive maintenance is done, all worn or damaged parts be replaced at that time.

Automatic Processor Monitoring Protocol

Rationale
- This test is designed to confirm that there is consistency in density from image to image.
- This test is designed to confirm that uniformity exists between processors when more than one processor is found in the Mammography Imaging Facility and adjacent areas.

Table 6-28
Preventive Maintenance Chart

Daily	Monthly
Wash evaporation covers with warm water.	Check replenishment rates.
Clean crossover racks with warm water; rotate and clean rollers.	Check feed tray alignment.
	Clean and check deep racks for any needed repairs.
Check for deposits above solution level and clean if necessary.	Clean and check crossover racks for any needed repairs.
Check dryer area for deposits and clean if necessary.	Drain and clean processor tanks.
	Follow manufacturer's recommendation for lubrication of gears.
Keep top of processor open overnight to vent trapped fumes and reduce chemical buildup.	Check all tubing and connections for leaks.
Run and check clearing films.	Check entrance roller detector switches for proper engaging and disengaging.

Testing Frequency
Monitoring of the processor is done daily.

Equipment
- Sensitometer
- Densitometer
- 18- × 24-centimeter QC film
- Thermometer (nonmercury); may be either digital or analog
- Processor control chart
- Felt tip marker
- Pencil

Procedure
A. Warm up the processor for a minimum of 30 minutes.
B. Check the developer temperature.
C. Record the developer temperature on the processor control chart.
D. Expose the emulsion side of the film with the sensitometer. The film is generally exposed on the right and left sides.
E. Process the film by feeding the long axis of the film emulsion side up into the processor.
F. Use the densitometer to measure b + f, which may be any clear area on the film or the first step of the stepwedge. Base plus fog is generally around 0.18.
G. Use the densitometer to measure the following data points on each side of the film strip:
   - The speed index, which is a midrange density (usually Step 11). The midrange density should be near but not less than 1.2 (1.0 above b + f).
   - The high-density step (usually Step 13), which should have a density near 2.2 (2.0 above b + f).
   - The low-density step (usually Step 9), which should have a density near but not less then 0.45 (0.25 above b + f).
   - Average the data points for the low-, mid-, and high-density steps.
H. Calculate the contrast index, which is determined by subtracting the high minus low densities.
I. Record the b + f, the speed index, contrast index on the processor control chart.
J. Developer temperature, b + f, speed, and contrast are recorded daily. It is important for the technologist to observe any trends that occur and report them.
K. If the numbers obtained for speed and contrast exceed the upper dotted line of the graph or go below the lower dotted line of the graph it will be necessary to run another strip to verify the accuracy of the original reading.

Acceptance Parameters
- The b + f should be within ±0.03 of the total b + f.
- The speed index should be within ±0.15.

- The contrast index should be within ±0.15.
- The developer temperature should be within ±0.5°F.

Record Keeping

- A record should be kept that documents the date of the test, who performed the test, the results of the test, and the corrective action taken.
- Processor strips should be maintained for at least 12 months.

IMPORTANT REMINDER

- Processor control strips should be kept for at least 1 year, and preferably 18 months.
- The temperature, density values, date, and time should recorded daily on the processor strips with a felt tip marker.

Potential Problems

- Over- or under-replenishment of the chemistry will have an impact on the speed and contrast indices.
- Increased or decreased developer temperature will impact the speed and contrast indices and b + f.

IMPORTANT REMINDER

- Processor monitoring should be done at the same time every day.
- A trend is a series of points in either a downward or upward pattern on the processor control chart. If the points fall out of established limits corrective action must be taken.

Processor Monitoring: Alternative Method

Rationale

This test is designed to confirm that the automatic processor is within acceptance criteria when the sensitometer is not available.

Testing Frequency

This procedure is done daily for a maximum period of 2 weeks.

Equipment

- 8 × 10 image receptor
- Lead mat
- Mammographic phantom
- Desitometer

Procedure

A. Perform the following tasks, prior to performing the procedure.

- Turn on the mammographic unit.
- Place the image receptor in the image receptor holder of the unit.
- Place the mammographic phantom on top of the image receptor holder.
- Center the phantom to the center of the image receptor, with the contrast object in place.
    Verify that the AEC detector is under the center of the wax insert and in the same location for all phantom images.
- Place a lead mat on one side of the phantom. The lead mat is used to create a clear area on the film for the measurement of b + f.

B. Expose and process the film.
- The selected technical factors should be sufficient to achieve proper background density.

C. Use the densitometer to measure the optical density
- at the center of phantom image.
- of the phantom image background.
- of the image contrast object.
- of the b + f density.

D. Record the density readings in the QC log.

Acceptance Parameters

- The optical density at the center of the phantom image is at least 1.20.
- The optical density at the center of the phantom image should not vary more than ±0.20 from established operating level.
- The density difference between the background of the phantom and that of the added test object, used to assess image contrast, is measured and must not vary more than ±0.05 from the established operating level.
- The b + f density must be within ±0.03 of the established operating level.

Record Keeping

A record should be kept that documents the date of the test, who performed the test, the results of the test, and the corrective action taken.

Potential Problems

Failure to follow the protocol may lead to erroneous results.

IMPORTANT REMINDER

- This protocol is to be used only when the sensitometer is unavailable.

Immersion Time: Time-in-Solution Test

Rationale

This test is performed to confirm that the immersion time of a film is within the manufacturer's specifications.

Testing Frequency

This test should be performed annually or when there is a suspected problem with development time.

Equipment

- Time in solution (TIS) tool (Fig. 6-18)
- Stopwatch
- Magnet
- Calculator

Procedure

A. Remove the lid of the processor.
  - For newer processors, once the lid has been removed, a magnet should be placed near the microswitch to keep the processor running. This is not necessary for older processors.
B. Locate the following mechanisms in the processor.
  - The 1/4-inch gap between the entrance roller assembly and the guide shoe.
  - The gap between the developer to fixer crossover and the guide shoe.
C. Place the test tool against the feed tray guide on the right side and feed the leading edge of the test tool into the processor.
  - The leading edge of the test tool will be the "T."
D. Prepare to begin timing when the black line on the test tool crosses the gap in the entrance roller assembly. The stopwatch should be in your hand.
E. Start timing when the top of the "T" reaches the gap of the entrance roller.
F. Stop timing when the top of the "T" reaches the gap in the developer to fixer crossover rack.

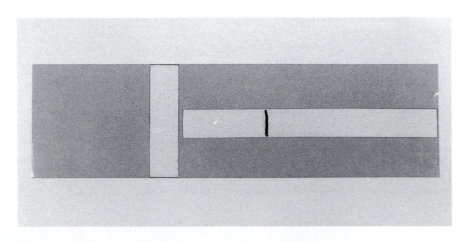

Figure 6-18 Time-in-solution (TIS) test tool.

G. The timing sequences should be done a minimum of five times, and then take an average to determine the developer time.

Acceptance Parameters

Check with the manufacturer to see what the acceptance parameters for immersion time are.

Record Keeping

A record should be kept that documents the date of the test, who performed the test, the results of the test, and the corrective action taken.

Potential Problems

Failure to start the stopwatch at the correct time will lead to misinterpretation of test results.

CROSSOVER PROCEDURES

Crossover procedures are done to ensure that there is consistency between the film emulsions that are being used for processor sensitometry. A crossover procedure should be performed about every 4 to 6 weeks or sooner, depending on the number of processors being monitored. It is important that crossover procedures be done for all processors that are used to process mammography images. When monitoring multiple processors using the same emulsion, it will become necessary to perform a crossover procedure more frequently. When doing crossover procedures it is important to remember that the crossover should be done when the processor chemistry is stable and not immediately after a preventive maintenance procedure has been done.

Crossover Procedure for Processor Monitoring Film

Rationale

This procedure is designed to reference the speed index, contrast index, and b + f of a new box of film to the old box of film currently used for processor monitoring.

Frequency

A crossover procedure should be done approximately every 4 to 6 weeks.

Equipment

- Crossover film (old and new emulsions)
- Sensitometer
- Densitometer
- Calculator
- Pencil
- Processor control chart

- Felt tip marker
- Red pen
- Crossover worksheet

Procedure

A. When a new box of film is used for processor monitoring, cardboard should be placed in front of the last 5 or 10 sheets of film in the box.
B. The crossover procedure should be performed when there are five sheets of film left in the old box.
C. The crossover procedure should be performed in total darkness to eliminate any possibility of unwanted fog from the safelight.
D. When the cardboard is reached, expose the emulsion sides of last five sheets of film with the sensitometer.
E. Take the first five of the new box of film and repeat Step D.
F. Identify the new film from the old film by marking the emulsion side of the film with a lead pencil. Some sources recommend that this be done in the area of the film notches.
G. In total darkness alternately process the old and new films. Feed the film lengthwise into the processor.
H. With a densitometer read the densities normally used for determining b + f, low density, mid-density, and high density.
I. Calculate the contrast index for each film.
J. For the five old and new films, determine the average b + f, speed index, and contrast index. Record these values on the crossover calculation form (see Fig. 3-17).
K. Subtract the old film values from the new film values.

   (New b + f) − (Old b + f) = Difference (+ or − or no change)

   New Speed Index − Old Speed Index = Difference (+ or − or no change)
   New Contrast Index − Old Contrast Index = Difference
   (+ or − or no change)
L. If there is a negative difference between the new and old values, the original processor control parameters should be reduced and a new processor control chart started.
M. If there is a positive difference between the new and old values, the original processor control parameters should be increased and a new processor control chart started.
   - Instead of starting a new control chart, it is acceptable to take a red pen and draw a line on the old chart between the previous day and the day of the crossover. The new aim values for the processor should be written in red in the right hand margin of the control chart and identified as "New Aim Values." On the back of the control chart there should be a notation that the crossover was performed.
N. If there is no difference, the original processor control parameters will stay the same.

O. The new processor control parameters should be put in statement form and included in the processor QC log.

Record Keeping

- All control strips should be kept in a notebook or file for at least 12 months, preferably 18.
- The temperature, density values, date, and time should be recorded daily on the processor strips with a felt tip marker.
- The crossover procedure worksheet should be kept as a reference in the processor QC notebook.

Potential Problems

- Failure to do the crossover procedure in total darkness may lead to inaccurate results.
- Failure to follow the described procedure may cause erroneous results.

IMPORTANT REMINDER

- If, for some reason, the box of film set aside for processor monitoring is used up before a crossover procedure can be done an alternate method for establishing new aims will need to be used. The following may be done to establish new aims for the b + f, speed index, and contrast index:
  - An average of the previous 30 days may be done.
  - Using the new film emulsion, a 5-day average may be done.

Hypo Retention Test

Rationale

This test is designed to confirm that the films exiting the automatic processor have been properly fixed and washed.

Testing Frequency

This test is performed quarterly or when a processing or archival problem is suspected.

Equipment

- A commercially available hypo estimator kit
- One sheet of unexposed mammography film

Procedure

A. Process one unexposed mammography film.
B. Follow the manufacturer's directions for the hypo estimator. Generally this entails placing drop of the test solution on the emulsion side of the film.
C. The test drop should be allowed to stand for approximately 2 minutes. The standing time may vary from manufacturer to manufacturer.
D. With a paper towel, tissue, or lint-free cloth blot off the excess solution.

E. Place the film on a white sheet of paper and compare it with the fixer retention estimator.
  • To reduce potential error the estimator should be placed over the film.

Acceptance Parameters

The estimated amount of residual fixer (hypo) should be less than 0.05 grams per square meter or 5 micrograms per square centimeter.

Record Keeping

A record should be kept that documents the date of the test, who performed the test, the results of the test, and the corrective action taken.

Potential Problems

• Test solution that is used past its expiration date will provide erroneous results.
• Failure to read the film immediately after the excess solution has been removed may cause erroneous results.

ACCESSORY DEVICES

Accessory devices include image receptors, illuminators, lead protective devices, and grids.

Image Receptor

The image receptor deals with the total film-screen imaging system used in medical imaging and mammography (Thompson et al., 1994; MQSA, 1999). The intensifying screens of the image receptor are constructed in such a way that they are durable and can last for many years. However, the longevity of intensifying screens is in direct proportion to the care provided by the user. Failure to take proper care of intensifying screens will lead to decreased imaging capabilities and a loss of imaging quality. MQSA requires that mammographic screens be cleaned weekly.

With everyday use, intensifying screens receive scratches, nicks, and stains to the phosphor layer, which can result in the appearance of artifacts on the radiographic image. It is critical that care be exercised when unloading the image receptors. At the time of cleaning, it is also important to carefully inspect the screens for any type of defect. It is possible that there are stains and scratches that are not readily visible to the naked eye. To ensure that there are no invisible defects, a blacklight (see Fig. 6-13) should be used to examine the image receptor for defects

Another aspect of intensifying screen care is the routine checks that should be performed to assure that there is proper film-screen contact in all of the image receptors of the Mammography Imaging Facility. The easiest way to achieve this is to perform the screen contact test and the blacklight test at the same time that the intensifying screens are cleaned.

Image Receptor: Film-Screen Contact Test

Rationale
This test is designed to confirm that all image receptors in the Mammography Imaging Facility have perfect film-screen contact.

Testing Frequency
Image receptor film-screen contact should be checked semiannually or when there is a suspicion or indication that imaging resolution is being lost due to poor film-screen contact.

Equipment
- Mammographic room
- Wire mesh test tool (Fig. 6-19)
- All image receptors in the mammography area
- Acrylic sheets
- Densitometer

Procedure
A. Place the image receptor on top of the image receptor holder and place the wire mesh test tool on top of the image receptor.
B. If needed place the acrylic sheets on top of the compression paddle and move the compression paddle as close to the x-ray tube as possible.

Figure 6-19 Mammography screen contract tool. *(Courtesy of Nuclear Associates, used with permission.)*

C. Set a manual technique that will provide an optical density of 0.70 to 0.80 in the image near chest wall edge. The kVp used will be between 25 and 28.
D. Expose the image receptor.
E. Process the film.
F. Use the densitometer to measure the density of the film.
G. Repeat Steps A through F for all remaining image receptors.
H. All radiographs of the image receptors should be viewed at a distance of at least 3 feet on a single illuminator in a dimly lit room (Fig. 6-20A and B).

Acceptance Parameters

- Poor film-screen contact results in a degraded image because the image resolution has been lost.
- MQSA currently does not have established acceptance parameters for this test.

Figure 6-20 *A.* Radiograph demonstrating satisfactory film-screen contact.

Figure 6-20 *B.* **Radiograph demonstrating the loss of detail from poor film-screen contact.**

- The ACR recommends
  - that areas of greater than 1 centimeter in diameter of poor contact should not be tolerated and the image receptors be removed from service.
  - that multiple areas of less than 1 centimeter in diameter should not be tolerated and the image receptors be removed from service.

IMPORTANT REMINDER

- Areas of poor contact will appear darker than areas of good contact.
- Areas of poor contact will demonstrate loss of detail or blurring of the wire mesh.

Record Keeping

A record should be kept that documents the date of the test, who performed the test, the results of the test, and the corrective action taken.

Potential Problems

Films that are over- or underexposed cannot be easily analyzed for film-screen contact.

Image Receptors: Ultraviolet Light Test

Rationale

This test is designed to confirm that the image receptors in the Mammography Imaging Facility are free of dirt, dust, foreign material, and invisible flaws or impurities in the intensifying screens.

Testing Frequency

This test should be performed semiannually, when image quality appears to be degraded, when an image receptor appears damaged, or when the screens of the image receptor are cleaned.

Equipment

- Ultraviolet light/blacklight (5 to 10 V)
- All image receptors in the mammography area

Procedure

A. After the screens of the image receptor have been cleaned, take them into the darkroom and place them open on the loading bench.
B. Plug in the UV light at a convenient outlet in the darkroom.
C. If applicable, close all doors leading into the darkroom.
D. Turn on the UV light.
E. Turn off all safelights and overhead lights.
F. Carefully examine the open image receptors with the UV light. Dirt, dust, and invisible and visible defects in the screens will glow under the UV light.
G. If there is dust or dirt still on the image receptors, they should be cleaned again.
H. Image receptors that have either visible or invisible defects in their intensifying screens should be taken out of circulation and replaced when possible.

Acceptance Parameters

Currently there are no stated parameters for image receptors.

Record Keeping

A record should be kept that documents the date of the test, who performed the test, the results of the test, and the corrective action taken.

Potential Problems

Suspended or dropped ceilings pose a problem because they trap dust and dirt. Every time the darkroom door is slammed, this type of ceiling generally vibrates and dust, dirt, and particulate matter come free, contaminating the work surfaces of the darkroom and image receptors.

Illuminators

Film illuminators (viewboxes) are commercially available in a variety of formats. They may be purchased as a single unit or in multiple units. Film illuminators over the last 25 years have evolved into sophisticated motorized devices with the capability of displaying films on as many as 50 different patients. Illuminators, whether or not they are motorized or nonmotorized, have a variety of commonalties but the two most important are they must have a light and power source for the physician to view radiographs. There are film illuminators used for viewing diagnostic radiographic images and illuminators for viewing mammographic images. The film illuminators used for reading mammographic images are governed by MQSA regulations.

The ability of the radiologist to accurately interpret mammogram images depends on the viewing conditions that are present in the reading room environment. The primary nontechnical factors are the brightness of the illuminator and the ambient light levels in the viewing room. It is important that the light bulbs of the illuminator are spectrally matched and have the same intensity. Therefore, it is necessary to replace all light bulbs in the illuminator when one goes bad. This will provide a uniform viewing environment. It is critical that the ambient lighting of the viewing room be kept at a standard level to help ensure the accuracy of film reading. The ambient lighting in the mammography viewing area should not exceed 50 lux.

When discussing illuminators, two characteristics that should be mentioned are illuminance and luminance. The basic unit for illuminance is the lux; 1 lux is equal to 1 lumen per square meter. **Illuminance** is generally defined as the quantity of light that falls on a surface. The basic unit for luminance is the candela per square meter (cd/m^2); 1 cd/m^2 is equal to 1 nit. **Luminance** is the amount of light being emitted from the surface of the light source. It is the brightness of the illuminator. In medical imaging, luminance is the standard used when monitoring the brightness level of film illuminators. Film illuminators that are used to view mammograms should have a brightness level of 3000 cd/m^2. The maximum density that can be visualized at 3000 cd/m^2 is an optical density of 3.10. Determining the brightness output of an illuminator can be achieved by using a photometer (Fig. 6-21). The photometer is the more accurate than the light meter. Table 6-29 is a simple conversion table for light units. Table 6-30 is a table of light units commonly used in medical imaging.

Illuminator Uniformity: Luminance

Rationale

This test is designed to confirm that all illuminators used for interpreting or quality control of mammography images meet or exceed minimum levels.

Testing Frequency

All illuminators used for viewing and interpreting mammography should be checked annually or when light bulbs are replaced.

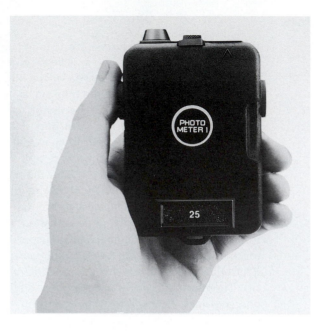

Figure 6-21 Photometer used to measure the luminance level of a film illuminator room illuminance. *(Courtesy of Nuclear Associates, used with permission.)*

Equipment

- Photometer
- Illuminators
- Calculator
- Record form

Procedure

A. Reduce the ambient light to normal viewing levels.
B. The illuminator should be turned on 30 minutes prior to the measurement.
C. Place the photometer parallel to and facing the illuminator surface; set the photometer to read cd/m^2.

Table 6-29
Conversion Table for Luminance

To Convert From	To	Multiply By
Lux	Footcandles	10.8
Footcandles	Lux	0.093
Nit (candela/m² [cd/m²])	Footlamberts	3.43
Footlamberts	Nit	0.292

Table 6-30
Light Units Used in Medical Imaging

Unit	Equivalent Unit
1 nit	1 cd/m²
1 footlambert	3.426 nits
1 lux	1 lumen/m²
1 footcandle	10.764 lux

D. Take the readings and record the data.

E. Repeat Steps A through D for the remaining illuminators in the mammography viewing area.

Acceptance Parameters

• MQSA does not have requirements for illuminator luminance levels.

• Luminance levels for interpreting mammograms should be at least 3000 cd/m².

Record Keeping

A record should be kept that documents the date of the test, who performed the test, the results of the test, and the corrective action taken.

Potential Problems

Illuminators that have different bulb wattages and colors will lead to reading errors.

IMPORTANT REMINDER

• It is critical that all illuminator readings be conducted in the same lighting conditions that a radiologist would read films. Ambient light should be strictly controlled.

• The viewing surface of the illuminator should be cleaned regularly.

• When one light bulb in illuminator is replaced, the other light bulbs in the bank of illuminators should be replaced to ensure that uniformity is maintained.

Room Illuminance

Rationale

This test is designed to confirm that the illumination levels of the mammography viewing areas are within the recommended levels and that viewing conditions are optimized.

Testing Frequency

Room illumination levels should be checked on a semiannual basis.

Equipment
- Photometer
- Calculator

Procedure
A. Reduce the ambient light to normal viewing levels.
B. Set the photometer to read lux. Follow the manufacturer's guidelines.
C. With the photometer in hand, take readings from different areas of the viewing room. The author suggests that readings be taken from the center of the viewing room and if possible three other areas of the room.
D. Once the readings have been obtained they should be averaged and the final value recorded.

Acceptance Parameters
- MQSA does not have requirements for room illumination levels.
- Room illumination levels for mammographic reading rooms should be no higher than 50 lux.

Record Keeping
A record should be kept that documents the date of the test, who performed the test, the results of the test, and the corrective action taken.

Potential Problems
Failure to follow the described procedure may lead to erroneous results.

LEAD PROTECTIVE DEVICES

There are a variety of lead protective devices found in the majority of all Mammography Imaging Facilities. They include aprons, gloves, thyroid shields, and gonad shields. The lead protective devices used in general diagnostic imaging are constructed from lead-impregnated vinyl-like materials and have a thickness of between 0.25 and 1.0 millimeter. Typically the standard is 0.5 millimeter. Lead protective devices may be evaluated either radiographically or fluoroscopically. The most expedient and cost-effective method is to use fluoroscopy for the evaluation. Although there is no Federal law mandating the frequency that lead protective devices be checked for cracks and tears, it should be done regularly. The frequency of surveying lead protective devices should be done upon receipt and at least annually (Lin et al., May 1988). The permanent record can also serve as an inventory for the department.

Lead Protective Devices

Rationale
This test is designed to confirm that all lead protective devices are free of cracks and other defects.

Testing Frequency
All lead protective devices should be checked annually.

Equipment
- All lead protective devices
- Fluoroscopic room

Procedure
A. Set the generator for fluoroscopic mode.
B. Place the lead protective devices individually on the tabletop.
C. Each protective device is carefully examined under fluoroscopy for any flaws or defects.
D. When a protective device is found to be flawed, it should be removed from circulation and identified in some fashion.

Acceptance Parameters
There is a zero percent tolerance for lead protective devices.

Record Keeping
A record should be kept that documents the date of the test, who performed the test, the results of the test, and the corrective action taken.

Potential Problems
There are no potential problems that are encountered with this test.

IMPORTANT REMINDER

- Lead aprons, gloves, and lead mats used for shielding *should never* be folded. Lead aprons and half aprons should be hung correctly on the apron racks. Lead gloves should be placed on the glove stand on the apron rack. Lead mats should be placed in their designated areas. Lead protective devices should be properly cared for.

GRIDS

The primary purpose of a grid is to improve radiographic contrast by absorbing the scatter radiation produced during an exposure before it reaches the film. Grids in mammography are reciprocating and move at the same rate throughout the exposure. The majority of mammography grids are linear and all mammography grids are focused for the SID of the unit. Carbon fiber interspacing is used in mammography grids to allow for minimal attenuation of the primary photons. Mammography grids have a grid ratio from 3.5:1 to 5:1, with 30 to 50 lines per centimeter. After a grid is manufactured, test radiographs are made of the grid to ensure that it is functioning properly. When a mammography unit is installed, the grid should be checked to ensure that the grid has not been damaged during shipment. This is also a quick test that can be performed when one suspects that a grid has been damaged. The technique selected for the initial check will depend on the speed of the mammographic imaging system. Once the grid has been checked, grid uniformity should be checked on regular basis. Grid uniformity tests are not currently mandated by MQSA.

Grid Uniformity Test

Rationale

This procedure is designed to confirm that the interspacers of the grid are uniform and not producing any type of artifact in the image.

Testing Frequency

This test should be conducted annually on all grids in the mammography area.

Equipment

- Homogenous mammography phantom (aluminum or Lucite)
- Image receptor (will be determined by the size of the grid being checked)
- Grid
- Densitometer

Procedure

A. Place the image receptor in the Bucky tray.
B. Place the homogenous phantom on top of the grid being tested.
C. Select a technique that is appropriate for the grid ratio and that would produce a density of 1.5.
D. Expose and process the film.
E. After processing the film, use the densitometer to take readings from the center of the film and all four quadrants. Compare the density readings.
F. Record the results.

Acceptance Parameters

- The ACR and MQSA do not have requirements or guidelines for ensuring the integrity of mammography grids.
- NCRP Report #99 makes the following recommendations.
  - Films should be uniform with an optical density of ±0.10.

Record Keeping

A record should be kept that documents the date of the test, who performed the test, the results of the test, and the corrective action taken.

Potential Problems

- Failure to have the proper technique set could cause inaccurate results.
- Failure to have the x-ray tube perpendicular could provide the radiographer with inaccurate readings.
- If the grid movement mechanism is not functioning properly, inaccurate results could occur.

> **Points to Ponder**
> - If there is a lack of uniform density in the films produced using the Bucky, the grid alignment test should be performed immediately.

THE TUBE AND COLLIMATOR

When discussing the x-ray tube and collimator, it will be necessary to briefly discuss how x-rays are produced, the formation of the focal spot, and the basic construction of the collimator. The production of x-rays requires a source of electrons, a means of accelerating the electrons, and some way to suddenly stop the electrons. This is achieved by having an anode and cathode enclosed in a glass tube that has had all of the air removed. The source of the electrons is the cathode, which generally has two filaments. The electrons are boiled off the filament when a current heats the filament. When a voltage is applied to the cathode the speed of the electrons is increased and they are accelerated at or near the speed of light across a very short distance (less than 1 inch) toward the anode. Upon reaching the anode, the high-speed electrons are suddenly stopped and x-rays are produced. The electron to x-ray energy conversion is an inefficient process; less than 1% of the resulting energy is in the form of x-rays. The remaining energy conversion is in the form of heat (>99%).

The x-rays that are produced are Bremsstrahlung and characteristic. **Bremsstrahlung x-rays** are the result of the incident electrons interacting with the nuclei of the target atoms. **Characteristic x-rays** are produced when incident electrons interact with the inner shell (K shell) electrons of the atom. The x-rays produced by this interaction will be characteristic of the target material. The type of target material used influences both the discrete (characteristic) and the continuous (Bremsstrahlung) portions of the x-ray emission spectrum. As the atomic number of the target material increases, there is a shift in the discrete portion of the x-ray emission spectrum to the right. Therefore more x-rays will be produced per unit of energy and the energy of the characteristic x-rays will be higher. The continuous portion of the x-ray emission spectrum will increase in quantity but there is only a slight change in quality (energy). In mammography the most commonly used anode material is molybdenum (Mo). The use of molybdenum as target material provides a wide range of kilovoltage selections (24 to 30) for imaging breast tissue and as a result of this there is less loss of contrast when compared to other anode materials. Other anode materials used in mammography are rhodium (Rh) and tungsten (W). Rhodium is used in the 26 to 32 kV ranges and tungsten is used in the 22 to 26 kV ranges. Rhodium and tungsten produce a higher energy spectrum but as a result there is a loss of contrast in the image. Using different filters for a specific anode can offset the imaging difficulties encountered with molybdenum, rhodium, and tungsten. It has generally been accepted that when using a molybdenum target one had to use a 0.03 millimeter-Mo filter. The purpose of the filter is to remove the low-energy x-rays that normally would have been absorbed by the breast tissue. However, using a different anode/filter combination provides the technologist with imaging options for large patients and glandular breasts.

Focal spot size is determined by several factors (Fig. 6-22), but it is important to remember that x-rays originate from a point source on the anode. When the focal spot is projected onto the image receptor, its actual shape is rectangular. All of the factors identified in Fig. 6-27 are of great importance in determining focal spot size, but the steepness of the anode angle plays an important role in determining the size. It is important to keep in mind that anode angle is measured from the perpendicular. The standard anode angle for mammographic applications is approximately 7°. A steep anode angle will result in a smaller focal spot size, which will produce greater resolution but will have a heat loading limitation. In other words, the x-ray tube will need to cool longer before additional exposures can be made and lower mA techniques should be used. An x-ray tube with a target angle that is less steep will have a larger apparent focal spot that can accept more of a heat load but has a decrease in resolution (Fig. 6-23). This trade off will allow more heat loading and, therefore, the use of higher mA techniques. In mammography, the typical focal spot sizes used are 0.4 millimeter or smaller for routine work and 0.15 millimeter or smaller for magnification work.

Collimators used in mammography are designed to provide the mammographer with the ability to cone to the size of the image receptor. At the chest wall the field should extend just slightly past the image receptor to prevent the exclusion of breast tissue (Kimme-Smith et al., 1997; Wentz, 1997).

There are a variety of quality control tests that should be performed on the tube and collimator to ensure that they are within acceptance parameters. When either the tube or collimator is not within acceptance parameters, service must be called immediately. The tests performed are focal spot size, collimator assessment, and light field illumination.

◆ **Filament size and shape**

◆ **Filament position within the focusing cup**

◆ **Physical dimensions of the focusing cup**

◆ **Distance between the anode and cathode**

◆ **Anode angle**

Figure 6-22 Factors that determine focal spot size.

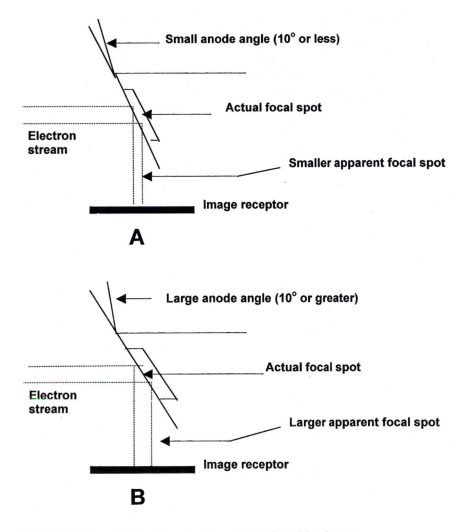

Figure 6-23 The relationship between anode angle and focal spot.

Focal Spot Size: Slit Camera

Rationale

This test is designed to confirm that the small and large focal spots are within the tube manufacturer's stated specifications.

Testing Frequency

Focal spot size should be checked annually, when the x-ray tube has been replaced, or as workload dictates.

Equipment

- Slit camera with a slit aperture of 0.01 millimeter (Fig. 6-24A and B)
- Mammographic image receptor and film
- Lead marker to designate anode-cathode direction
- Optical comparator with a built-in graticule of 0.1-millimeter divisions and a magnification capability of 10× to 50×

Procedure

A. Remove the compression paddle.
B. Place the slit camera test apparatus on top of the image receptor holder near the chest wall side of the holder.
C. Extend the legs of the test apparatus to provide maximum magnification.
D. The test apparatus alignment tool should be placed in the test stand. Use the collimator light to align the five lead beads. The test stand may extend beyond the image receptor holder a little bit.
E. A piece of intensifying screen is then placed on the base of the test stand.
F. Turn out the room lights and make a 1-second exposure using a low mAs at 28 kVp.
   - While the exposure is being made observe the image on the intensifying screen.
   - If necessary adjust the test device, so that the lead beads are aligned.
   - Repeat this step until alignment is achieved.
G. Remove the alignment device and replace it with the slit camera.
H. Place the load mammographic image receptor in the tunnel of the test stand.
I. Select the small focal, 30 kVp at the highest mA possible and an exposure time that will produce an optical density between 0.80 and 1.20.
J. Produce two images, one with the slit parallel to the anode-cathode axis and the second one perpendicular to the anode-cathode axis.
K. Process the exposed film (Fig. 6-24B).
L. If applicable, repeat Steps H through K for the large focal spot.
M. Calculate the focal spot sizes.
N. Calculate the magnification (*M*) using the following formula:

$$M = \frac{\text{Image Size}}{\text{Object Size}} - 1$$

O. Use the optical comparator to measure the parallel dimension (d_{parallel}) and the perpendicular dimension (d_{perp}).
P. Compute the focal spot sizes using the following formula:

$$\text{FSS}_{\text{parallel}} = \frac{d_{\text{parallel}} - s\,(M+1)}{M} \qquad \text{FSS}_{\text{perp}} = \frac{d_{\text{perp}} - s\,(M+1)}{M}$$

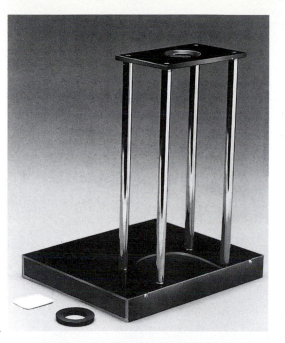

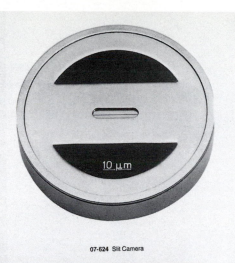

07-624 Slit Camera

NUCLEAR ASSOCIATES
A Division of VICTOREEN, INC.
100 VOICE ROAD
CARLE PLACE, NY 11514-1593
(516) 741-6360
VICTOREEN A Subsidiary of Sheller-Globe

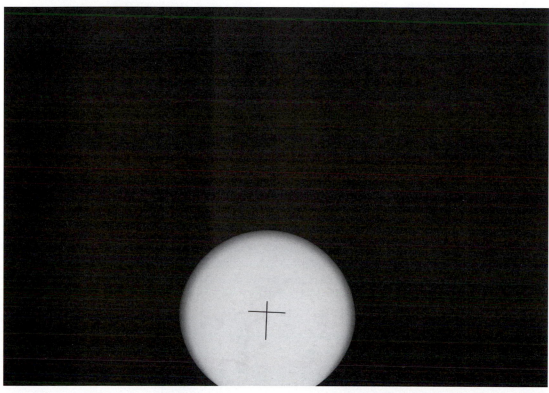

Figure 6-24 *A.* Slit camera and test stand for measuring focal spot size. *(Courtesy of Nuclear Associates, used with permission.) B.* Slit camera image. *(Courtesy of Michael Biddy, Phoenix Technology.)*

Acceptance Parameters

Focal spot sizes are based on specifications established by the National Electrical Manufacturers Association (NEMA).

Stated Focal Spot Size	Maximum Measured Dimension (Perpendicular)	Maximum Measured Dimension (Parallel)
0.10 mm	0.15 mm	0.15 mm
0.15 mm	0.23 mm	0.23 mm
0.20 mm	0.30 mm	0.30 mm
0.30 mm	0.45 mm	0.65 mm
0.40 mm	0.60 mm	0.85 mm
0.60 mm	0.90 mm	1.30 mm

Record Keeping

A record should be kept that documents the date of the test, who performed the test, the results of the test, and the corrective action taken.

Potential Problems

Failure to follow the test protocol may introduce error.

Collimation Assessment

Rationale

This test is designed to confirm that the collimator does not allow significant radiation beyond the edges of the image receptor.

Testing Frequency

The collimator should be checked annually or when the tube has been replaced.

Equipment

- Four pennies and one nickel
- Two 8- × 10-inch mammographic image receptors
- Two 10- × 12-inch mammographic image receptors
- A sheet of 1-inch thick acrylic

Procedure

A. Place the 8- × 10-inch image receptor in the Bucky tray of the mammographic unit.
B. Load the second 8- × 10-inch image receptor with film. It is important to have emulsion side of the film away from the intensifying screen.
C. Place the second image receptor face down on top of the image receptor holder.
   - The back of the image receptor should be toward the x-ray tube.

- The image receptor should extend approximately 1 centimeter beyond the chest wall side of the image receptor holder.
D. Remove the compression paddle.
E. Turn on the collimator light.
F. After turning on the collimator light place the four pennies inside the light field with one edge of each penny just touching the edge of the light field. The penny on the chest wall side should be moved approximately 2 inches to the right to avoid interfering with the AEC sensor.
G. Place the nickel on the chest wall side approximately 2 inches to the left of the AEC sensor.
H. Expose the film using AEC.
I. Process the film.
J. Measure the image and record the data (Fig. 6-25).
K. Repeat Steps A through J for the 10- × 12-inch image receptor.

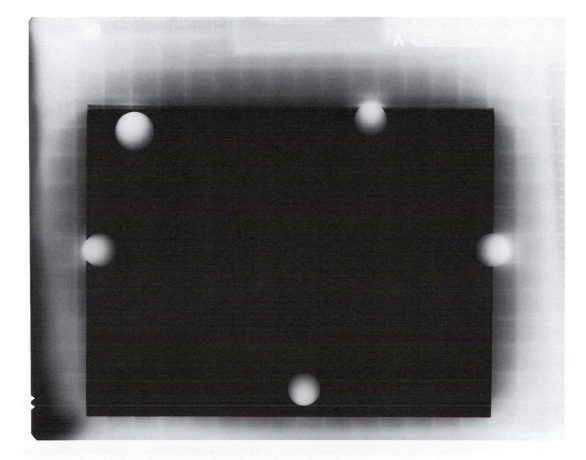

Figure 6-25 Mammography collimation assessment film.

Acceptance Parameters

- MQSA requires that the x-ray field does not extend beyond any edge of the image receptor by more than 2% of the SID.
- 21 CFR 1020.31 (d) (2) states that
  - The x-ray field should not extend beyond any of the four sides of the image receptor by more than +2% of the SID.
  - At the chest wall side, the radiation field must extend to the edge of the film to ensure that no breast tissue is missed adjacent to the chest wall.

Record Keeping

A record should be kept that documents the date of the test, who performed the test, the results of the test, and the corrective action taken.

Potential Problems

Failure to follow the test protocol could introduce error into the measurements.

Light Field Illumination Test

Rationale

This procedure is designed to confirm that the illumination level of the collimator light is visible in the lighting conditions that are routinely used during positioning.

Testing Frequency

- The illumination level of the collimator light field is checked when a piece of equipment is installed or removed and reinstalled in another location.
- The illumination level of the collimator light field should be checked annually or as often as the management of the Mammography Imaging Facility deems it necessary.

Equipment

- Photometer (see Fig. 6-21)

Procedure

- A. Adjust the ambient lighting to levels that would be used during a routine radiographic procedure.
- B. Set the tube at a distance of 40 inches (100 centimeters) or at the maximum SID, whichever is less.
- C. Adjust the collimator to an appropriate field size (i.e., 24 × 30 centimeters, etc.).
- D. Divide the light field at the image receptor into four equal quadrants.
- E. Turn the photometer on and take a reading in the center of each quadrant.
- F. Average the readings and record the results.

Acceptance Parameters

The Code of Federal Regulations 21 1020.31 (2) requires that the light field illuminance be no less than 160 lux or 15 footcandles at an SID of 40 inches.

Record Keeping

A record should be kept that documents the date of the test, who performed the test, the results of the test, and the corrective action taken.

Potential Problems

- Low batteries in the photometer may lead to readings that are not accurate.
- Failure to have the photometer set on the correct units will be a source of error.

THE GENERATOR

In the United States, for mammography equipment there are two types of x-ray generators available for producing x-rays—three phase and high frequency. As the power of an x-ray generator increases there is a corresponding affect on the x-ray emission spectra (Table 6-31). This effect can be readily seen in the quality of films produce in the mammography imaging facility. The advantages that are obtained from increasing generator power include more efficient x-ray production, reduction of radiation exposure to the patient, the selection of higher mA techniques, and the selection of faster exposure times.

Under MQSA, a qualified medical physicist is required to perform the majority of QC tests discussed in this section. The only test that a technologist can perform is the phantom image test. There is a variety of test equipment available on the market to perform the tests described in this chapter. This

Table 6-31
How the Generator and Tube Affect the X-Ray Emission Spectra (Quality and Quantity)

As Factor Increases	Affect on Quality and Quantity	Change in the Continuous Spectrum	Change in the Discrete Spectrum
Generator phase (voltage waveform)	Increase in quality and quantity	Amplitude increases	Shift to right
kVp	Increase in quality and quantity	Amplitude increases	Shift to right
mA	Increase in quantity; no change in quality	Amplitude increases	No shift
mAs	Increase in quantity; no change in quality	Amplitude increases	No shift
Added filtration	Increase in quality; decrease in quantity	Amplitude increases	No shift
Target material	Increase in quantity and quality	Amplitude increases slightly	Shift to right
SID	No change	No change	No change

equipment may be purchased as a single device, which has the capability of performing multiple tests, or as individual devices that perform one type of test. One such multitest instrument is the Non-invasive Evaluator of Radiation Outputs (NERO mAx) Model 8000 (see Fig. 4-14). This particular instrument has the capability of measuring kilovoltage, mAs, mA, exposure time, HVL, radiation exposure, and radiation rate. The data obtained from the various tests can is placed directly in a spreadsheet for easy access and report generation.

The QC tests discussed in this section include phantom images, kVp accuracy and reproducibility, radiation output rate, average glandular dose, breast exposure, AEC reproducibility, AEC performance, AEC density control, and beam quality assessment (HVL).

Phantom Images

Rationale

This test is designed to confirm that film density, differences in contrast, uniformity, and image quality are maintained at optimum levels.

Testing Frequency

This test should be performed weekly, when the mammographic unit is serviced, when the automatic processor has been worked on, or when changes in image quality are suspected or noticed.

Equipment

- Mammographic phantom (see Fig. 6-14)
- Mammographic image receptor and film
- Original phantom image and previous phantom image
- Magnifying glass
- Densitometer

Procedure

A. Place the image receptor in the image receptor holder of the mammographic unit.
B. Place the phantom on top of the image receptor holder.
C. Position the phantom so that the edge is aligned with the chest wall side of the image receptor.
D. Lower the compression device so that it is in contact with the phantom.
E. Confirm that the AEC sensor is in the same position as previous phantom test films.
F. Select a technique that would be most commonly used for 4.5-centimeter compressed breast.
G. Record the exposure factors in the phantom image log.
H. Expose and process the film (Fig. 6-26).
 I. Measure the density of the film in the area of the disk and in the background adjacent to the disk.
J. Record the densities in phantom log (Fig. 6-27).

K. From the image determine the number of fibers, specks, and masses visible in the image. Record the number in the log (Fig. 6-28).

Acceptance Parameters

- The phantom image background density should be never less than 1.2 ± 0.20.
- The overall level for phantom image background optical density should be at least 1.40.
- For the 4-millimeter-thick disk the density difference should be 0.40 ± 0.05 for films exposed at 28 kVp.
- ACR Mammography Accreditation requires a minimum of the four largest fibers, the three largest speck groups, and the three largest mass groups to pass.

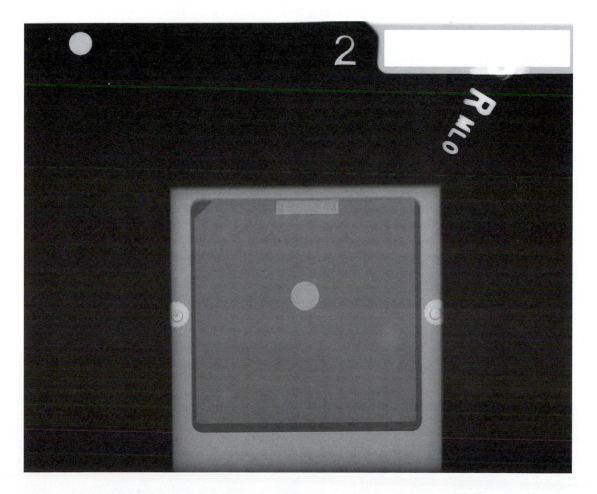

Figure 6-26 Phantom image.

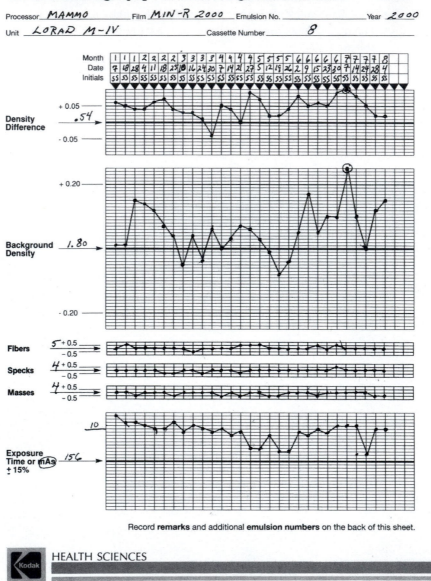

Record **remarks** and additional **emulsion numbers** on the back of this sheet.

Figure 6-27 Mammography phantom control chart.

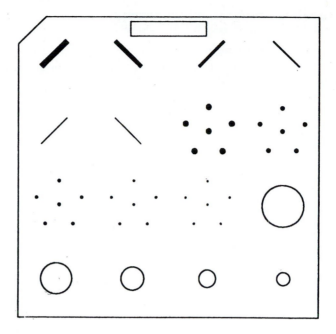

Figure 6-28 Diagram of wax insert from mammography phantom showing the location of the fibers, specks, and masses. *(Courtesy of Nuclear Associates, used with permission.)*

- The object sizes are listed below.

Nuclear Associates ACR Approved Phantom

Fibers	Specks	Masses (Thickness)
(1) 1.56 mm	(7) 0.54 mm	(12) 2.00 mm
(2) 1.12 mm	(8) 0.40 mm	(13) 1.00 mm
(3) 0.89 mm	(9) 0.32 mm	(14) 0.75 mm
(4) 0.75 mm	(10) 0.24 mm	(15) 0.50 mm
(5) 0.54 mm	(11) 0.16 mm	
(6) 0.40 mm		

Record Keeping

A record should be kept that documents the date of the test, who performed the test, the results of the test, and the corrective action taken.

Potential Problems

Failure to follow test protocol may cause an error in results.

kVp Accuracy and Reproducibility

Rationale

This test is designed to confirm that the generator is accurately producing the kVp as indicated on the control panel and that it is reproducible.

Testing Frequency

The kilovoltage should be checked annually.

Equipment

- Mammography digital kVp meter (Fig. 6-29)
- kVp record form

Procedure

A. Before performing the test, it is important to follow the appropriate tube warm-up procedure.
B. Turn the kVp meter on and allow it to warm up as recommended by the manufacturer.
C. Place the kVp meter on top of image receptor holder.
D. Perform the following tasks.
- Collimate the beam to a size just slightly larger than the test device.
- Select the manual timing mode.
- Select the most commonly used clinical kVp.
E. Make four exposures and record the readings.
- After each exposure reset the kVp meter.
- Average the four readings and compare them to the preset kVp.
F. For reproducibility repeat this procedure for other important clinical kVps, but make only one exposure for each selected kVp and record this data on the record form.
G. Reproducibility is checked at the lowest and highest kVp used to produce clinical images.

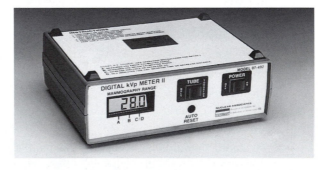

Figure 6-29 Mammography digital kVp meter. *(Courtesy of Nuclear Associates, used with permission.)*

H. Reproducibility is determined by (see example)
- averaging the kVp
- calculating the SD and CV.
I. Record the coefficient of variation on the record form.

Acceptance Parameters

- MQSA requires that the kilovoltage be within ±5% of the selected kVp.
- MQSA requires that the COV of reproducibility of the kVp shall be equal to or less than 0.02 (≤ 0.02)

Record Keeping

A record should be kept that documents the date of the test, who performed the test, the results of the test, and the corrective action taken.

Potential Problems

- Inaccurate readings may be obtained during times of high electrical power demand.
- Inaccurate readings may be obtained if the incoming power supply is constantly fluctuating.

kVp Accuracy and Reproducibility Example

Nominal kVp setting	23	24	25	26	27	28	29	30	35
Nominal focal spot size	0.3	0.3	0.3	0.3	0.3	0.3	0.3	0.3	0.3
mA/mAs setting									
Measured kVp values									
kVp_1	23.3	24.4	25.2	26.2	27.2	27.9	29	29.9	34.7
kVp_2				26.3					
kVp_3				26.3					
kVp_4				25.2					
Mean kVp SD	23.3	24.4	25.2	26.25	27.2	27.9	29	29.9	34.7
				0.058					
Mean − nominal kVp	0.3	0.4	0.2	0.25	0.2	−0.1	0.0	−0.1	−0.3
0.05 × nominal kVp	1.15	1.20	1.25	1.30	1.35	1.40	1.45	1.50	1.75
CV = mean ÷ SD				0.002					

Radiation Output

Rationale

This test is designed to measure the radiation output of the mammography unit.

Testing Frequency

This test should be performed annually.

Equipment

Mammography digital R-meter with ionization chamber (Fig. 6-30)

Procedure

A. Initially, perform the following tasks.
- Prepare the mammography unit for operation in the manual mode.
- Place the 18- × 24-centimeter mammography image receptor in the Bucky tray.
- Use 28 kVp and the Mo/Mo target/filter combination.
- The exposure time should be set for an exposure of at least 3 seconds.

B. Place the ionization chamber 4.5 centimeters above the breast support plate and 4 centimeters in from the chest wall. The ionization chamber should be completely exposed.

C. Collimate the beam to just slightly larger than the ionization chamber.

D. The compression paddle is positioned to just above the ionization chamber or in contact with it.

E. Secure the ionization chamber and do not change its position for subsequent exposures.

F. Make an exposure and record the readings on the record form.

G. For all clinically used SIDs repeat Steps A through F.

Acceptance Parameters

- Currently the ACR and MQSA require that a mammography unit shall be capable of producing a minimum output of 4.5 mGy air kerma per second (513 mR/sec) when operating at 28 kVp in the standard mammography (Mo/Mo) mode.

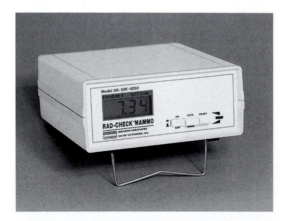
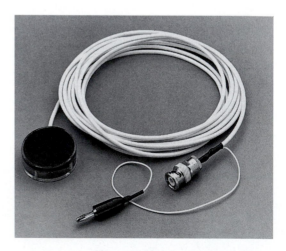

Figure 6-30 Mammography digital R-meter and ionization chamber. *(Courtesy of Nuclear Associates, used with permission.)*

- After October 28, 2002, the ACR and MQSA will require that a mammography unit shall be capable of producing a minimum output of 7.0 mGy air kerma per second (800 mR/sec) when operating at 28 kVp in the standard mammography (Mo/Mo) mode.

Record Keeping
A record should be kept that documents the date of the test, who performed the test, the results of the test, and the corrective action taken.

Potential Problem
Failure to properly secure the ionization chamber for all exposures will lead to erroneous results.

Average Glandular Dose and Breast Entrance Exposure

Rationale
This test is designed to determine the **average glandular dose** and breast entrance exposure of the mammography unit.

Testing Frequency
This test should be performed annually or when the AEC has been serviced.

Equipment
- Mammography digital R-meter with ionization chamber (Fig. 6-30)
- Mammographic phantom
- 18- × 24-centimeter mammography image receptor

Procedure
A. Initially, perform the following tasks.
  - Set the mammography unit for operation in the most commonly used mode.
  - Place the 18- × 24-centimeter mammography image receptor in the image receptor holder.
  - Collimate the beam to the film size being used.
  - For units that have a variable SID, use the most commonly used SID for mammography.
  - Select the AEC density control setting that is normally used for the clinically average patient.
  - Select the kVp, target material, and filtration that are most commonly used for mammography.
B. Positioning of the test equipment:
  - Align the chest wall side of the phantom with the chest wall side of the image receptor.
    Center the phantom left to right.
  - Place the ionization chamber of the R-meter in the x-ray field next to the phantom.

The ionization chamber needs to be centered 4 centimeters from the chest wall side of the image receptor.

The center of the ionization chamber should be level with the phantom.

Secure the ionization so that it will not move during the measurements.

C. The compression paddle is positioned to just above the ionization chamber or in contact with it.

D. Make an exposure and record the readings on the appropriate record form.

E. Repeat Step D until four exposures have been made.

F. Calculate the mean exposure.

G. Using each mean exposure value, calculate the average glandular dose.
- Refer to pages 280 to 283 of the ACR QC manual for a complete description calculation process.
- The average glandular dose is an approximation of the breast entrance exposure.

H. Calculate the exposure rate for each clinically used SID.
- Divide measured exposure by the measured or indicated exposure time.
- Air kerma (mGy/s) = exposure rate (mR/s) × 0.00873 mGy/mR

I. Using the mean exposure values, calculate the standard deviation and the coefficient of variation for breast exposure.

Acceptance Parameters

- The ACR and MQSA state that the average glandular dose shall not exceed 3.0 mGy per exposure (0.3 rad per exposure).
- The coefficient of variation for breast entrance air kerma and mAs shall not exceed 0.05.

Record Keeping

A record should be kept that documents the date of the test, who performed the test, the results of the test, and the corrective action taken.

Potential Problem

Failure to follow the test protocol may lead to erroneous results.

Automatic Exposure Control

The mammography AEC device works on the same principal as the AEC device used in general radiography. The **automatic exposure control (AEC)** device for mammography consists of a solid state detector, which is also called a sensor. The detector senses the amount of radiation passing through the patient and terminates the exposure when a predetermined exposure has been reached. Depending on the type of mammography unit, the sensor will be either one large detector (~10 cm^2) or three small detectors (~1 cm^2), which are between the Bucky assembly and breast support plate of the unit. The detector assembly can be adjusted either forward or backward to be positioned under the glandular region of the breast.

The mammography QC tests that are performed on an AEC device require a minimum of equipment. The required equipment includes the mammographic phantom (see Fig. 6-14), mammography digital R-meter (see Fig. 6-30), and the mammography AEC consistency test tool (Fig. 6-31). There are two types of commercially available mammography AEC consistency test tools. One is made from acrylic and the other from tissue equivalent BR-12 material. Both tools have four slabs that measure 10 × 12.5 × 2 centimeters thick. The BR-12 test tool is more expensive because of the technology involved to make it.

The tests performed on the AEC include reproducibility, performance capability, and density control function.

Automatic Exposure Control Reproducibility

Rationale
To assess AEC reproducibility.

Testing Frequency
This test should be performed annually.

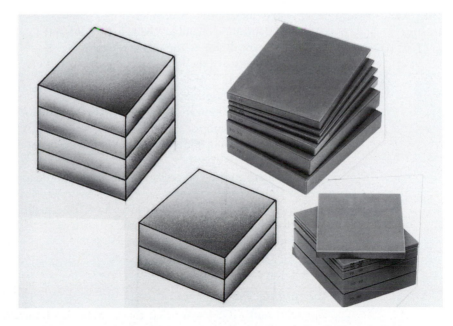

Figure 6-31 Mammography AEC consistency test tool. *(Courtesy of Nuclear Associates, used with permission.)*

Equipment
- Mammography digital R-meter with ionization chamber (see Fig. 6-30)
- Mammographic phantom
- 18- × 24-centimeter mammography image receptor

Procedure
A. Initially, perform the following tasks.
- Set the mammography unit for operation in the most commonly used mode.
- Place the 18- × 24-centimeter mammography image receptor in the image receptor holder.
- Collimate the beam to the film size being used.
- For units that have a variable SID, use the most commonly used SID for mammography.
- Select the AEC density control setting that is normally used for the clinically average patient.
- Select the kVp, target material, and filtration is most commonly used for mammography.

B. Positioning of the test equipment:
- Align the chest wall side of the phantom with the chest wall side of the image receptor.
  Center the phantom left to right.
- Place the ionization chamber of the R-meter in the x-ray field next to the phantom.
  The ionization chamber needs to be centered 4 centimeters from the chest wall side of the image receptor.
  The center of the ionization chamber should be level with the phantom.
  The entire ionization should be exposed.
  Secure the ionization chamber so that it will not move during the measurements.

C. The compression paddle is positioned to just above the ionization chamber or in contact with it.

D. Make an exposure and record the readings on the appropriate record form.

E. Repeat Step D until four exposures have been made.

F. Perform the following calculations:
- mean of the exposure and mAs.
- SD of exposure and mAs.
- CV for the exposure and mAs.

Acceptance Parameters
The ACR and MQSA state that the coefficient of variation for AEC reproducibility should not exceed 0.05.

Record Keeping

A record should be kept that documents the date of the test, who performed the test, the results of the test, and the corrective action taken.

Potential Problem

Failure to follow the test protocol may lead to erroneous results.

Automatic Exposure Control Performance

Rationale

This test is designed to assure that the AEC system maintains consistent optical density with changes in imaging modes and breast thickness.

Testing Frequency

This test should be performed annually or when the AEC has been serviced.

Equipment

- Mammographic AEC consistency test tool (see Fig. 6-31)
- Most commonly used mammography image receptor (i.e., 18 × 24 centimeters)
- Lead numbers
- Densitometer
- Box of mammography film

Procedure

A. Initially, perform the following tasks.
- Select the density control setting that is clinically used.
- Select the focal spot, mA, AEC mode, target material, filtration, and kVp that are routinely used for mammography.

B. Load a single mammography image receptor.

C. Place the mammography image receptor in the image receptor holder.

D. To indicate image sequence, place a lead number in the upper right quadrant of the image receptor holder.

E. Place a 2-centimeter-thick slab on the image receptor holder.
- The slab is placed in the position that is normally occupied by the breast.
- Confirm that the slab covers the entire active area of the AEC sensor.

F. The compression paddle is positioned in contact with the slab.

G. Make an exposure and record the readings on the record form.

H. Process the film in the processor normally used for mammographic images.

I. For a range of breast thicknesses (2 to 8 centimeters), repeat Steps A through H.

J. For a 4-centimeter slab, repeat Steps A through H for various imaging modes that are used to produce clinical images.

K. Measure and record the optical density at the center of each image.

L. Over all performance capability tests calculate the mean optical density.

Acceptance Parameters

- The ACR and MQSA state that the AEC should maintain a constant film density to within ±0.30 of the average over the 2- to 8-centimeter images.
- For a narrower range of conditions (2 to 6 centimeters), the optical density must be maintained to within ±0.15.
- After October 28, 2002, the ACR and MQSW will require that the AEC be capable of maintaining film optical density within ±0.15 of the mean optical density when the thickness of a homogeneous material is varied over a range of 2 to 6 centimeters and kVp is varied for such thicknesses over the clinical kVp.

Record Keeping

A record should be kept that documents the date of the test, who performed the test, the results of the test, and the corrective action taken.

Potential Problem

Failure to follow the test protocol may lead to erroneous results.

Automatic Exposure Control Density Control

Rationale

This test is designed to ensure that the AEC system maintains consistent optical density is maintained when density control selection is changed.

Testing Frequency

This test should be performed annually or when the AEC has been serviced.

Equipment

- Mammographic AEC consistency test tool (see Fig. 6-31)
- Most commonly used mammography image receptor (i.e., 18 × 24 centimeters)
- Lead numbers
- Densitometer
- Box of mammography film

Procedure

A. Initially, perform the following tasks.
   - Select the density control setting that is clinically used.
   - Select the most commonly used clinical kVp.
   - Select the focal spot, mA, AEC mode, target material, and filtration that are used routinely used for mammography.
B. Load a single mammography image receptor.
C. Place the mammography image receptor in the image receptor holder.
D. To indicate image sequence, place a lead number in the upper right quadrant of the image receptor holder.
E. Place a 4-centimeter-thick slab on the image receptor holder.

- The slab is placed in the position that is normally occupied by the breast.
- Confirm that the slab covers the entire active area of the AEC sensor.
F. The compression paddle is positioned in contact with the slab.
G. Make an exposure and record the readings on the record form.
H. Process the film in the processor normally used for mammographic images.
I. Repeat Steps A through H for all clinical settings of the AEC's density control selector.
J. Calculate the relative mAs and relative image optical density from the recorded data for measured mAs and image optical density.
  - Relative mAs is the mAs ratio at each density control setting to that at the "normal" setting.
  - Relative image optical density is the difference between the optical density at each density control setting to that at the "normal" setting.

Acceptance Parameters

- The ACR and MQSA state that the optical density of the film in the center of the images shall not be less than 1.20.
- The ACR and MQSA recommend that there be two plus and two minus density settings.
  - Each step should result in a 12% to 15% change in mAs, or approximately a 0.15 change in film density.

Record Keeping

A record should be kept that documents the date of the test, who performed the test, the results of the test, and the corrective action taken.

Potential Problem

Failure to follow the test protocol may lead to erroneous results.

Half Value Layer

When x-rays are produced, they exit the tube as a polyenergetic beam. The beam consists of different wavelengths and frequencies. The x-ray beam is often described as having "soft" and "hard" rays. The "soft" rays of the beam have low energy and are absorbed in the soft tissues, which result in increased exposure to the patient. These low energy x-rays can be eliminated or reduced by placing an absorbing material in the path of the x-ray beam which attenuates the beam and makes it more homogenous.

The amount of material (usually aluminum) needed to reduce the intensity of an x-ray beam by 50% is called the **half value layer (HVL).** The HVL provides information about the penetrating ability (quality) of the x-ray beam. It is also used to determine that the filtration placed in the path of the x-ray beam is sufficient. Information regarding the minimum HVLs required are found in Table 6-32.

Table 6-32
Minimum Half-Value Layers (mm Al)
for Mammography Units

Tube Potential (kVp)	Minimum HVL (mm Al)
20	0.20
25	0.25
30	0.30

Beam Quality Assessment (HVL)

Rationale

This procedure is designed to confirm that the filtration installed at the x-ray tube is kept at a suitable level to help minimize exposure to the patient.

Testing Frequency

This test should be performed annually or when the x-ray tube has been replaced.

Equipment

- Digital R-meter with ionization chamber attachment
- 6 pieces of 0.1-millimeter-thick aluminum

Procedure

A. Initially, perform the following tasks.
- Set a manual exposure time that is sufficiently long enough to produce an exposure of approximately 500 mR.
- Select the most commonly used kVp.
- Place the compression as close to the x-ray tube as possible.

B. Place the ionization chamber about 4.5 centimeters above the image receptor holder.
- The ionization chamber should be centered left to right and 4 centimeters in from the chest wall side of the image receptor.
- The ionization chamber should be completely in the x-ray field.
- Turn the R-meter on and allow it to warm up for approximately 2 minutes.

C. Collimate the beam to an area just slightly larger than the ionization chamber.

D. Perform the following tasks.
- Make an exposure with no aluminum in the beam and record the results.
- Place 0.2 mm Al on the compression paddle; make an exposure and record the results.
- Add 0.1 mm Al to the x-ray beam; make an exposure and record the results.

Continue to make exposures and add 0.1 mm Al until the reading is half of the original exposure reading.

Record the results of each additional exposure.

E. Remove all of the Al sheets from the compression paddle and make a final exposure.
- If the final reading differs from the initial reading by 2%, the entire exposure sequence must be repeated.

F. Repeat Steps A through E for other kVp/target/filter settings ranging from the lowest to the highest.

G. Calculate the HVL.

Acceptance Parameters

- The ACR and MQSA state that at a given setting in the mammographic kV range (below 50 kV), the measured HVL with the compression paddle in place must be equal to or greater than the value:

$$HVL > \frac{kVp}{100} + 0.03 \text{ mm Al}$$

- The ACR and MQSA recommend, that for units using Mo/Mo, Mo/Rh, Rh/Rh, or W/Rh target/filtration combinations, the HVL be within a constant value (C) of the minimum acceptable HVL:

$$HVL < \frac{kVp}{100} + C \text{ mm Al}$$

For Mo/Mo C = 0.12 mm Al
For Mo/Rh C = 0.19 mm Al
For Rh/Rh C = 0.22 mm Al
For W/Rh C = 0.30 mm Al

Record Keeping

A record should be kept that documents the date of the test, who performed the test, the results of the test, and the corrective action taken.

Potential Problem

Failure to follow the test protocol will lead to erroneous results.

COMPRESSION

In mammography, compression is used to improve image quality by compressing the breast tissue over a uniform area that reduces the amount of scatter produced and therefore improves contrast of the image. The compression device is independent of the tube assembly. It is important that the compression device work properly at all times. Therefore, the functionality of the compression device should be checked on a regular basis for **compression force** and **compression deflection.**

Compression Force Test

Rationale

This test is designed to confirm that the mammographic compression device can provide adequate compression with both the automatic and manual modes and that the unit does not allow too much compression to be used.

Testing Frequency

This test should be performed semiannually or when decreased compression is suspected.

Equipment

- Mammographic unit
- Bathroom scales
- Three or four towels

Procedure

A. Place a towel on top of the image receptor holder.
B. Place the bathroom scales on top of the towel. The central part of the scales should be directly under the compression device.
C. Place two or three towels on top of the bathroom scales.
D. Use the power drive to lower the compression device until it stops automatically.
E. Read the amount of compression on the scales and record the amount.
F. Release the compression device.
G. Use the manual drive to lower the compression device until it stops and then repeat Steps E and F.

Acceptance Parameters

- MQSA requires that in the power and manual modes a compression force of at least 25 pounds (111 newtons) shall be provided.
- Effective October 28, 2002, MQSA will require that the maximum compression force initial power drive must be between 25 pounds (111 newtons) and 45 pounds (200 newtons).

Record Keeping

The compression force readings for both the power and manual drives must be documented.

Potential Problems

- Failure to follow the test protocol can damage the compression device.
- Failure to follow the test protocol can result in reading errors.

Compression Paddle Deflection Test

Rationale

This test is designed to confirm that the compression paddle deflection mechanism is functioning properly.

Testing Frequency

This test should be performed on installation of new equipment and annually thereafter.

Equipment

- 18 × 24 and 24 × 30 centimeter compression paddles
- 30 × 30 centimeter support plate (lucan or masonite)
- Ruler with centimeter markings
- Test objects
  - Two compressible foam sponges: one 18 × 24 and one 24 × 30 *or*
  - Nine tennis balls: three for the 18 × 24 paddle and six for the 24 × 30 paddle
    - The tennis balls should be taped together in the shape of a triangle (Figs. 6-32A and B)
- Towel

Procedure

A. Cover the Bucky with a towel and place the support plate on the Bucky.
B. Place the widest edge of the test object along the chest wall edge of the Bucky.
C. Attach the compression paddle to the unit.
D. Apply a compression force of 25 pounds (111 newtons).
E. Measure each corner of the paddle from its bottom to the support plate.
F. The amount of deflection is calculated by subtracting the smallest distance from the largest distance.
G. Repeat Steps D through F for the remaining compression paddle.

Acceptance Parameters

MQSA requires that the deflection of the paddles must be less than 1 centimeter.

Record Keeping

The amount of deflection for each compression paddle must be documented.

Potential Problems

- Failure to follow the test protocol can damage the compression device.
- Failure to follow the test protocol can result in reading errors.

IMPORTANT REMINDER

- If the mammography unit does not have a compression force readout, bathroom scales may be be substituted for the test objects.

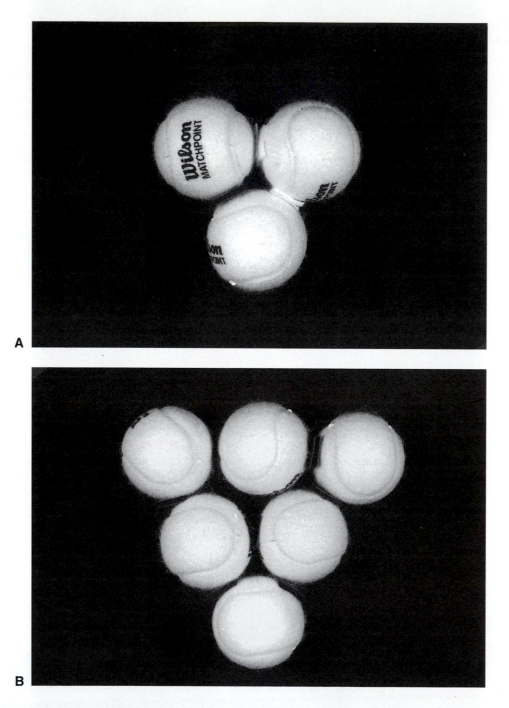

Figure 6-32 *A.* Three ball configuration that is used for the compression deflection test. *B.* Six ball configuration that is used for the compression deflection test.

CHAPTER REVIEW

- MQM is governed by the institution's mission statement, the need to personalize services, and MQSA.
- The goals of MQM are to provide quality images, accurate image interpretation, and the speedy delivery of results.
- The MQM program focuses on the responsibilities of the personnel, reporting, record keeping, the medical outcomes audit, consumer complaint mechanism, infection control, radiologist QA, suboptimal film tracking, mammography QA, and mammography QC.
- The responsibilities of the radiologist, technologist, and medical physicist are clearly defined by MQSA.
- The mammography report must contain specific information regarding the facility, the patient, the examination, and the final assessment.
- Record keeping involves not only the patient's films, but also the records that pertain to the radiologist, the technologist, and the medical physicist. The records that are maintained on the radiologist, technologist, and medical physicist include documentation of formal training, license, certification, and evidence of continuing education, and continuing experience.
- The primary goal of the medical outcomes audit is to ensure the reliability, clarity, and accuracy of interpretation. The outcomes audit consists of a data collection phase and a data analysis phase.
- The data obtained for the audit are categorized as true positive, true negative, false positive, and false negative.
- The collected data should be analyzed with respect sensitivity, specificity, positive predictive value, positive biopsy rate, and cancer detection rate.
- The BI-RADS system is an assessment mechanism that makes the interpretation process easier for the radiologist. It consists of six categories ranging from 0 to 5.
- All mammography facilities must have a mechanism for addressing consumer complaints.
- All mammography facilities must have an infection control policy for cleaning and disinfecting mammography equipment that has come into contact with blood or other potentially infectious materials.
- Radiologist QA may be achieved through correlation of mammography reports and ultrasound reports, correlation of mammography reports and pathology reports, and double reading of films.
- The tracking of suboptimal mammographic images is a mechanism that can be used to provide both positive and negative feedback to the technologist.
- Mammography QA focuses on the improvement of image quality through a systematic program of record keeping, equipment selection, and acceptance testing.
- Mammography QC focuses on the testing and monitoring of equipment in all areas of the mammography facility.

- The computer is the most powerful tool that can be used in MQM because of its ability to store and manipulate tremendous amounts of data. The ability of the computer to perform the necessary tasks is directly related to its processing speed and storage capabilities.
- Measures of central tendency include the mean, median, and mode. The most commonly used measure of central tendency is the mean. The mean is the average of a group of numbers, and is very stable. The median and mode are not used as frequently because they are unstable measures.
- Measures of spread (dispersion) are the range, percentile, standard deviation, and coefficient of variation. The range is the highest and lowest number in a group of numbers. The most commonly used percentiles are the 25th, 50th, and 75th. Standard deviation is the range of variation around the mean. Coefficient of variation is a relative measure of dispersion and is used to compare two or more measures of dispersion.
- Frequency distributions are used to describe data by how often an event or a situation occurs.
- Sample size is dictated by what is being studied. The ideal sample size should be no less than 30 and no greater than 100.
- X-ray film should be stored in an area that is environmentally controlled area where the relative humidity is between 30% and 50% and the temperature is between 50° and 70°F.
- Boxes of x-ray film should be stored vertically either on end or on the side.
- Artifacts that appear on a finished radiograph are caused either by the processor or inappropriate handling of the film before or after exposure and prior to processing. Processor artifacts can be eliminated through processor maintenance. Film handling artifacts can be reduced through proper education of the darkroom personnel and department staff. Artifacts will never be completely eliminated.
- Repeat analysis is used to identify areas where there are problems or potential problems. Repeat rates should be between 2% and 5%.
- Causal repeat analysis is used to determine what portion of the overall repeat rate is the result of a specific cause.
- The UV light is used to determine how clean the darkroom is. The ACR and MQSA require that the darkroom and loading bench be totally free of dirt and dust.
- The safelight test is used determine if fog on the film is being caused by a crack in the filter or the wrong wattage of bulb in the safelight. The density readings from the fogged area should not exceed 0.05.
- The tools that are required for processor monitoring are the thermometer, sensitometer, densitometer, a box of QC film, and processor control chart.
- The ACR requires that both the sensitometer and densitometer be recalibrated every 18 months.
- Monitoring of the automatic processor is done daily, and it is important for the person responsible to analyze the processor control charts for any trends that develop. Failure to do this will have an impact on image quality.

- Sensitometric films are run through each processor at the same time every day.
- Processor control charts reflect the b + f density, speed index, contrast index, and developer temperature. The midrange density of the control strip reflects the speed index. The density difference between the high and low densities reflects the contrast index.
- Checking films for fixer retention should be done quarterly and should not exceed 5 micrograms per square centimeter.
- The TIS test is a critical test that should be done annually to ensure that the film is in the developer for the proper amount of time. The manufacturer of the specific processor being tested sets the acceptance parameters for this test.
- The crossover procedure has been developed to ensure that established processing parameters are maintained from one film lot to another.
- The loss of image receptor film-screen contact will result in a loss of detail and resolution within the image. The loss of image detail results in increased exposure to the patient and increased departmental costs. Image receptors that cause a loss of detail should be removed from circulation. Image receptors that have areas greater than 1 centimeter of poor contact should be removed from circulation. Image receptors that have multiple areas of poor screen contact less than 1 centimeter should also be removed from circulation.
- All image receptors should be checked with UV light after they have been cleaned. The UV light will demonstrate visible and invisible defects in the screens of the image receptor. The use of the UV light will confirm that the image receptor is free of dirt, dust, and particulate matter.
- Illuminators used for mammography should have an illumination level of 3000 cd/m^2.
- The ambient lighting for the mammography reading room should be no higher than 50 lux.
- Illuminance is the amount of light that falls on a surface. The unit for illuminance is the lux; 1 lux is equal to 1 lumen/m^2.
- Luminance is the brightness of the illuminator. The unit for luminance is the candela per square meter; 1 cd/m^2 is equal to 1 nit.
- Lead protective devices must be checked annually by either radiographic or fluoroscopic means. When a defect is demonstrated, the particular protective device must be removed from use. A defect allows radiation through, exposing the person wearing the device.
- Mammography grids must be checked annually. Grid test films should be uniform with an optical density of ±0.10.
- NEMA establishes the acceptance parameters for focal spot size.
- Collimation acceptance parameters for mammography are ± 2% of the SID.
- Light field illuminance should be no less than 160 lux.
- ACR mammography accreditation requires a minimum of the four largest fibers, the three largest speck groups, and the three largest mass groups be visualized to pass the phantom image test.

- The mammographic kilovoltage must be accurate to within 5% of the set kVp. kVp reproducibility must have a CV ≤0.02.
- Mammography units shall be capable of producing a minimum radiation output of 7 mGy/sec (800mR/sec) when operating at 28 kVp in the standard mammography mode.
- The average glandular dose shall not exceed 3 mGy/exposure (0.3 rad/exposure). The average glandular dose is an approximation of the breast entrance exposure.
- The CV for AEC reproducibility should not exceed 0.05.
- AEC performance should maintain a constant film density to within ±0.30 of the average.
- The minimum HVL for a mammography unit operating at 30 kVp should be 0.3 mm Al.
- The compression force test should be at least 25 pounds (111 newtons) in the power and manual modes.
- Effective October 28, 2002, the maximum compression for initial power drive must be between 25 pounds (111 newtons) and 45 pounds (200 Newtons).
- The compression deflection test results must be less than 1 centimeter.

DISCUSSION QUESTIONS

1. Why is darkroom cleanliness important?
2. Why is the crossover procedure important?
3. What viewing conditions are necessary for viewing finished radiographs?
4. How is image quality affected by poor film-screen contact?
5. What is the rationale for performing a repeat/reject analysis?
6. What are acceptance parameters for the QC tests described in this chapter?
7. Why are the darkroom UV test and the image receptor test necessary?

REVIEW QUESTIONS

1. Mammography viewboxes should have a minimum luminance of
   a. 1500 cd/m²
   b. 2000 cd/m²
   c. 2500 cd/m²
   d. 3000 cd/m²
2. When performing processor quality control, what is the acceptable b × f parameter?
   a. ±0.01 of the total b + f
   b. ±0.03 of the total b + f
   c. ±0.05 of the total b + f
   d. ±0.1 of the total b + f

3. When performing processor quality control, what is the acceptable temperature parameter?
   a. ±3°F
   b. ±2°F
   c. ±1°F
   d. ±0.5°F

4. When performing processor quality control, what is the acceptable contrast index parameter?
   a. ±0.01
   b. ±0.03
   c. ±0.05
   d. ±0.15

5. When performing processor quality control, what is the acceptable speed index parameter?
   a. ±0.05
   b. ±0.10
   c. ±0.15
   d. ±0.20

6. The ideal repeat rate for a breast imaging facility should be approximately
   a. 2%
   b. 5%
   c. 10%
   d. 20%

7. Which of the following statements is correct regarding optimum viewing conditions for mammographic images?
   a. Background or ambient lighting should be as bright as possible.
   b. The color of light produced by illuminators is not important.
   c. Individual light bulbs should be replaced as they burn out.
   d. All illuminators used mammography should produce the same light level.

8. The ambient lighting for a mammography reading room should not exceed
   a. 45 lux
   b. 50 lux
   c. 55 lux
   d. 60 lux

9. Which of the following statements is correct?
   a. The contrast index is determined by the density difference between the high density and midrange density of the processor control strip.
   b. The contrast index is determined by the density difference between the high density and low density of the processor control strip.
   c. The contrast index is determined by the density difference between the midrange density and low density of the processor control strip.
   d. The contrast index is determined by the density difference between the high density and b + f density of the processor control strip.

10. Which of the following statements is correct?
    a. The b + f density of the processor control strip determines the speed index.
    b. The high density step of the processor control strip determines the speed index.
    c. The low fog density step of the processor control strip determines the speed index.
    d. The midrange density step of the processor control strip determines the speed index.

11. At a 40 inches (100 centimeters) SID the light field illumination of a mammography unit should not be less than
    a. 50 lux
    b. 75 lux
    c. 100 lux
    d. 160 lux

12. When the power drive is in operation, the compression device should provide a compression force of
    a. 5 to 10 pounds
    b. 10 to 15 pounds
    c. 15 to 25 pounds
    d. 25 to 40 pounds

13. Fixer retention should not exceed
    a. 5 micrograms per square centimeter
    b. 10 micrograms per square centimeter
    c. 15 micrograms per square centimeter
    d. 20 micrograms per square centimeter

14. What material is most commonly used for the target of a mammography x-ray tube?
    a. Yttrium
    b. Tungsten
    c. Rhodium
    d. Molybdenum

15. The basic unit of illuminance is the
    a. cd/m^2
    b. footlambert
    c. lux
    d. nit

16. Characteristic radiation is associated with the
    a. continuous x-ray emission spectrum
    b. discrete x-ray emission spectrum
    c. both a and b
    d. neither a nor b

17. Which of the following statements is correct?
    a. Repeat analysis needs a patient volume of at least 50 patients for it to be meaningful.

b. Repeat analysis needs a patient volume of at least 150 patients for it to be meaningful.

c. Repeat analysis needs a patient volume of at least 100 patients for it to be meaningful.

d. Repeat analysis needs a patient volume of at least 250 patients for it to be meaningful.

18. Which of the following statements is correct?

a. Film should stored in an environmentally controlled area with the relative humidity between 20% and 30%.

b. Film should stored in an environmentally controlled area with the relative humidity between 30% and 50%.

c. Film should stored in an environmentally controlled area with the relative humidity between 50% and 60%.

d. Film should stored in an environmentally controlled area with the relative humidity between 70% and 80%.

19. In mammography at 30 kVp the HVL should be

a. 0.2 mm Al

b. 0.25 mm Al

c. 0.3 mm Al

d. 0.5 mm Al

20. Which of the following statements is correct?

a. Characteristic radiation is produced when incident electrons interact with an inner shell electron.

b. Characteristic radiation is produced when incident electrons interact with the nucleus.

c. Characteristic radiation is produced when incident electrons interact with an outer shell electron.

d. Characteristic radiation is produced when incident electrons interact with an inner shell electron and the nucleus.

21. The phantom image background optical density should never be less than

a. 1.0

b. 1.2

c. 1.4

d. 1.6

22. The basic unit of luminance is the

a. cd/m^2

b. footlambert

c. lambert

d. lux

23. Which of the following statements is correct?

a. The amount of light either scattered or emitted by a surface is called illuminance.

b. The amount of light falling on a surface is called illuminance.

    c. The amount of light being reflected is called illuminance.

    d. The amount of light falling, being scattered, or emitted by a surface is called illuminance.

24. The optical density attributable to darkroom fog shall not exceed

    a. 0.01

    b. 0.03

    c. 0.05

    d. 0.06

25. Which of the following statements is correct?

    a. The amount of light either scattered or emitted by a surface is called luminance.

    b. The amount of light falling on a surface is called luminance.

    c. The amount of light being reflected is called luminance.

    d. The amount of light falling, being scattered, or emitted by a surface is called luminance.

26. In mammography at 20 kVp the HVL should be

    a. 0.2 mm Al

    b. 0.25 mm Al

    c. 0.3 mm Al

    d. 0.5 mm Al

27. Densitometers and sensitometers should be recalibrated every

    a. 6 to 8 months.

    b. 12 to 18 months

    c. 20 to 24 months

    d. 30 to 36 months

28. Bremsstrahlung radiation is associated with the

    a. continuous x-ray emission spectrum

    b. discrete x-ray emission spectrum

    c. both a and b

    d. neither a nor b

29. Repeat analysis is done

    a. daily

    b. weekly

    c. monthly

    d. quarterly

30. Phantom images are done

    a. daily

    b. weekly

    c. monthly

    d. quarterly

Bibliography

Adams HG, Arora S. *Total Quality in Radiology: A Guide to Implementation*. Delray Beach, Fla: St. Lucie Press; 1994.

American College of Radiology Committee on Quality Assurance in Mammography. *Mammography Quality Control Manual*. Reston, Va: American College of Radiology; 1999.

Andolina VF, Lille SL, Willison KM. *Mammographic Imaging: A Practical Guide*. Philadelphia: Lippincott; 1992.

Ballinger PW, Frank ED. *Merrill's Atlas of Radiographic Positions and Radiologic Procedures*. 9th ed. St. Louis: Mosby; 1999.

Bassett LW, et al. *Breast Imaging Reporting and Data System (BI-RADS™)*. 3rd ed. Reston, Va: American College of Radiology; 1998.

Bassett LW, et al. *Quality Determinants of Mammography*. Rockville, Md: U.S. Department of Health and Human Services; October 1994. AHCPR publication 95-0632.

Berwick DM, Godfrey AB, Roessner J. *Curing Health Care: New Strategies for Quality Improvement*. San Francisco: Jossey-Bass; 1990.

Blanchard K, Bowles S. *Raving Fans: A Revolutionary Approach to Customer Service*. New York: William Morrow and Company; 1993.

Bothe DR. *Measuring Process Capability*. New York: McGraw-Hill; 1997.

Bouchard E. *Radiology Management: An Introduction*. Denver: Multi-Media Publishing; 1983.

Bowles J, Hammond J. *Beyond Quality*. New York: Putnam; 1991.

Brassard M, Ritter D. *The Memory Jogger II: A Pocket Guide of Tools for Continuous Improvement & Effective Planning*. Methuen, Mass: GOAL/QPC; 1994.

Burkhart RL. *Checklist for Establishing a Diagnostic Radiology Quality Assurance Program*. Rockville, Md: U.S. Department of Health, Education, and Welfare; 1983.

Burns C. Achieving darkroom and processing quality control in mammography: A step beyond minimum recommendations. *Seminars in Radiologic Technology*. 1995;3:68–85.

Burns EF. *Radiographic Imaging: A Guide for Producing Quality Radiographs*. Philadelphia: Saunders; 1992.

Bushberg JT, Seibert JA, Leidholt EM, Boone JM. *The Essential Physics of Medical Imaging*. Baltimore: Williams & Wilkins; 1994.

Bushong SC. *Radiologic Science for Technologists: Physics, Biology, and Protection*. 6th ed. St. Louis: Mosby; 1997.

Carlton R, Adler A. *Introduction to Radiography and Patient Care*. Philadelphia: Saunders; 1994.

Carlton R, Adler A. *Principles of Radiographic Imaging*. 2nd ed. Albany, NY: Delmar; 1996.

Carlton R. Establishing a total quality assurance program in diagnostic radiology. *Radiol Technol.* 1980;52(1): 23–38.

Carroll QB. *Fuch's Principles of Radiographic Exposure, Processing, and Quality Control.* 5th ed. Springfield, Il: Charles C. Thomas; 1993.

Carter PH. *Chesneys' Equipment for Student Radiographers.* 4th ed. Oxford: Blackwell Scientific Publications; 1994.

Chu RY, et al. *Standardized Methods for Measuring Diagnostic X-ray Exposures.* AAPM Report No. 31, 1990.

Code of Federal Regulations, Title 21, Vol 8, Part 900, Section 12; U.S. Government Printing Office.

Code of Federal Regulations, Title 21, Vol 8, Part 1020, Section 30-33; U.S. Government Printing Office.

Cotton L, Sparrow M. Creating a successful relationship with customers. *Radiology Management.* 1998;20(3): 40–45.

Corr B. Quality control in radiology: An administrative overview. *The Canadian Journal of Radiography, Radiotherapy, and Nuclear Medicine.* 1985;16(1):4–16.

Cullinan AM, Cullinan, JE. *Producing Quality Radiographs.* 2nd ed. Philadelphia: Lippincott; 1994.

Dawson-Saunders B, Trapp RG. *Basic & Clinical Biostatistics.* 2nd ed. Norwalk, Conn: Appleton & Lange; 1994.

Deming WE. *Out of the Crisis.* Cambridge, Mass: MIT Press; 1986.

Dodd BC. Repeat analysis in radiology: A method of quality control. *The Canadian Journal of Radiography, Radiotherapy, and Nuclear Medicine.* 1983;14(2):37–40.

Dowd SB, Wilson BG. *Encyclopedia of Radiographic Positioning.* Philadelphia: Saunders; 1995.

Duffey RM. Quality assurance/departmental audits—New buzzwords in health care. *The Canadian Journal of Radiography, Radiotherapy, and Nuclear Medicine.* 1989;15(4):134–139.

Eastman TR. Reject audits. *Radiol Technol.* 1996;68:166.

Eisenberg RL. *Radiology: An Illustrated History.* St. Louis: Mosby-Year Book; 1992.

Fellers G. *The Deming Vision.* Milwaukee: ASQC Press; 1992.

Freedman D, Pisani R, Purves R, Adhikari A. *Statistics.* 2nd ed. New York: W.W. Norton; 1991.

Gaucher E, Coffey R. *Total Quality in Health Care.* San Francisco: Jossey-Bass; 1993.

Goldfield N, Pine M, Pine J. *The Health Care Manager's Guide to Continuous Quality Improvement.* Gaithersburg, Md: Aspen; 1991.

Graham N. *Quality in Health Care.* Gaithersburg, Md: Aspen; 1995.

Grant EL, Leavenworth RS. *Statistical Quality Control.* New York: McGraw-Hill; 1988.

Gray JE, Winkler NT, Stears J, et al. *Quality Control in Diagnostic Imaging.* Rockville, Md: Aspen; 1983.

Gurley LT, Callaway, WJ. *Introduction to Radiologic Technology.* 4th ed. St. Louis: Mosby, 1996.

Handbook for Improvement: A Reference Guide for Tools & Concepts. 2nd ed. Brentwood, Tenn: Executive Learning, Inc.; 1997.

Haus AG, Jaskulski SM. *The Basics of Film Processing in Medical Imaging.* Madison, Wis: Medical Physics Publishing; 1997.

Hendrick RE, et al. Quality control in mammography. *Radiol Clin North Am.* 1998;207:663–668.

Hill C. Introducing a radiographic quality control system at crawley district general hospital. *Radiography Today.* 1991;57(649):16–21.

Hiss SS. *Introduction to Health Care Delivery and Radiology Administration.* Philadelphia: Saunders; 1997.

How Safe Is Your Safelight?: A Guide To Darkroom Illumination. Rochester, NY: Eastman Kodak Company; 1994. Kodak Publication no. K-4.

Joint Commission on Accreditation of Healthcare Organizations. *Forms, Charts, and Other Tools for Performance Improvement.* Oak Brook Terrace, Il: Author; 1994.

Juran JM. *Juran on Planning for Quality.* New York: The Free Press—Macmillan; 1998.

Kelsey CA. *Essentials of Radiology Physics.* St. Louis: Warren H. Green, Inc.; 1985.

Kodak X-omat Processing 101—Fundamentals of Radiographic Film Processing. Rochester, NY: Eastman Kodak Company; 1995. Publication no. TM3058-1.

Lam R, Golden L. Continuous Quality Improvement for Hospital Radiology Services Part 1: Understanding the JCAHO Process. *ASRT Homestudy Series.* 1996;1(2): 1–21

Lam R, Golden L. Continuous Quality Improvement for Hospital Radiology Services Part 2: Implementing a Successful CQI Program. *ASRT Homestudy Series.* 1996;1(3): 1–21.

Leland K, Bailey K. *Customer Service for Dummies.* Foster City, Calif: IDG Books Worldwide; 1995.

Lin P, et al. *Protocols for the Radiation Safety Surveys of Diagnostic Radiological Equipment.* AAPM Report No. 25, 1988. New York: American Institute of Physics.

Linver M, Newman J. MQSA: The Final Rule. *Radiologic Technology.* 1999;70(4):338–353.

Mason RD, Lind DA, Marchal WG. *Statistics: An Introduction.* 3rd ed. New York: Harcourt Brace Jovanovich; 1983.

McCloskey LA, Collett DN. *TQM A Basic Text: A Primer Guide to Total Quality Management.* Methuen, Mass: GOAL/QPC Publishing; 1993.

McKinney WEJ. *Radiographic Processing and Quality Control.* Philadelphia: Lippincott, 1988.

McKinney WEJ. Sensitometric processing quality. *Seminars in Radiologic Technology.* 1998:6(4):140–149.

McLemore J. *Quality Assurance in Diagnostic Radiology.* Chicago: Year Book Medical Publishers, Inc; 1981.

Meisenheimer C. *Improving Quality.* 2nd ed. Gaithersburg, Md: Aspen; 1997.

Myers CP. *Mammography Quality Control: The Why and How Book.* Madison, Wi: Medical Physics Publishing; 1997.

National Council on Radiation Protection and Measurements. *Mammography—User's Guide.* Bethesda, Md: Author; 1986. NCRP Report No. 85.

National Council on Radiation Protection and Measurements. *Maintaining Radiation Protection Records.* Bethesda, Md: Author; 1992. NCRP Report No. 114.

National Council on Radiation Protection and Measurements. *Medical X-ray, Electron Beam and Gamma-Ray Protection For Energies Up to 50 MeV.* Bethesda, Md: Author; 1989. NCRP Report No. 102.

National Council on Radiation Protection and Measurements. *Quality Assurance for Diagnostic Imaging Equipment.* Bethesda, Md: Author; 1988. NCRP Report No. 99.

National Electrical Manufacturers Association. *Measurement of Dimensions and Properties of Focal Spots of Diagnostic Tubes.* Washington, DC: Author; 1992.

Newman J. Quality control and artifacts in mammography. *Radiol. Technol.* 1998;70(1):61–76.

Paleen R, Skundberg PA, Schwartz H. How much is quality assurance costing your department? *Radiology Management.* 1989;11(1):24–26.

Papp J. *Quality Management in the Imaging Sciences.* St. Louis: Mosby; 1998.

Papp J. Quality management in radiology. *Seminars in Radiologic Technology.* 1998:6(4):129–139.

Plesk P. *Methods and Tools of Quality Improvement: Theory into Action.* Brookline, Mass: Institute for Healthcare Improvement; 1992.

Process Control Procedure for Mammographic Processors. Technical Chart Kodak Health Sciences. Rochester, NY: Eastman Kodak Company.

Process Control Procedure for Radiographic Processors. Technical Chart Kodak Health Sciences. Rochester, NY: Eastman Kodak Company.

Quality Assurance in Mammography. Ridgefield Park, NJ: AGFA Corporation; 1990.

Radiation Protection for Medical and Allied Health Personnel. Bethesda, Md. National Committee on Radiation Protection and Measurements (NCRP) Publications; 1989. Report No. 105.

Rush B. *MQSA Made Easy: Understanding and Implementing the Facility-Based Final Regulations.* San Diego, Calif: Breast Imaging Specialists; 1999.

Saia DA. *PREP: Radiography.* 2nd ed. Stamford, Conn: Appleton & Lange; 1999.

Schroeder P. *Improving Quality and Performance: Concepts, Programs, and Techniques.* St. Louis: Mosby; 1994.

Seeram E. *X-ray Imaging Equipment: An Introduction.* Springfield, Il: Charles C. Thomas; 1985.

Sickles EA. Quality assurance: How to audit your own mammography practice. *Radiol Clin North Am.* 1992;30(1):265–275.

Siedband M, et al. *Basic Quality Control in Diagnostic Radiology.* 1978. AAPM Report No. 4. New York: American Institute of Physics.

Slater R. *Integrated Process Management: A Quality Model.* New York: McGraw-Hill; 1991.

Spatz C, Johnston JO. *Basic Statistics: Tales of Distribution.* 4th ed. Pacific Grove, Calif: Brooks/Cole; 1989.

Spence JT, Cotton JW, Underwood BJ, Duncan CP. *Elementary Statistics.* 4th ed. Englewood Cliffs, NJ: Prentice-Hall; 1983.

Sprawls P. *Physical Principles of Medical Imaging.* Rockville, Md: Aspen; 1987.

Stockley SM. *A Manual of Radiographic Equipment.* Edinburgh: Churchill Livingstone; 1986.

Tague NR. *The Quality Toolbox.* Milwaukee, Wi: ASQC Press; 1995.

Taylor JK. *Statistical Techniques for Data Analysis.* Boca Raton, Fla: Lewis-CRC Press; 1990.

Thompson MA, Hattaway MP, Hall JD, Dowd SB. *Principles of Imaging Science and Protection.* Philadelphia: Saunders; 1993.

Thompson TT. *A Practical Guide to Modern Imaging Equipment.* 2nd ed. Boston: Little, Brown, and Company; 1985.

Thornhill PJ. Quality assurance in diagnostic radiography: Are we using it correctly and what is its future? *Radiography.* 1987;53(609):161–163.

Tomlinson D, Stapleman K. A new concept in radiology qa in a large setting. *Radiology Management.* 1998;20(2):30–37.

Tortorici MR, Apfel PJ. *Advanced Radiographic and Angiographic Procedures.* Philadelphia: FA Davis; 1995.

Tortorici MR. *Concepts in Medical Radiographic Imaging.* Philadelphia: Saunders; 1992.

Using Control Charts to Improve Performance. Brentwood, Tenn: Executive Learning, Inc; 1997.

Walton M. *Deming Management at Work.* New York: Putnam; 1990.

Watkinson SA. Economic aspects of quality assurance. *Radiography.* 1985; 51(597)133–140.

Wentz G. *Mammography for Technologists.* 2nd ed. New York: McGraw-Hill; 1997.

Wheeler DJ, Lyday RW. *Evaluating the Measurement Process.* 2nd ed. Knoxville, Tenn: SPC Press; 1989.

Winters R. The origins and applications of quality initiatives in diagnostic imaging settings. *Seminars in Radiologic Technology.* 1998;6(4):150–159.

Wolbarst AB. *Physics of Radiology.* Norwalk, Conn: Appleton & Lange; 1993.

Wright M. Employee satisfaction: Creating a positive work force. *Radiology Management.* 1998;20(3):34–38.

Yaffe M, et al. *Equipment Requirements and Quality Control for Mammography.* 1990. AAPM Report No. 29. New York: American Institute of Physics.

Review Question and Brain Teaser Answers

REVIEW QUESTION ANSWERS

Chapter 1		*Chapter 2*		*Chapter 3*	
1.	d	1.	b	1.	d
2.	c	2.	c	2.	d
3.	b	3.	b	3.	b
4.	d	4.	a	4.	b
5.	c	5.	d	5.	b
6.	d	6.	b	6.	a
7.	d	7.	d	7.	b
8.	b	8.	a	8.	c
9.	c	9.	c	9.	d
10.	b	10.	a	10.	d
11.	a	11.	d	11.	a
12.	b	12.	a	12.	c
13.	d	13.	a	13.	a
14.	d	14.	c	14.	b
15.	d	15.	d	15.	c
16.	c	16.	a	16.	a
17.	a	17.	b	17.	c
18.	b	18.	b	18.	a
19.	a	19.	c	19.	b
20.	c	20.	c	20.	d
21.	c	21.	c	21.	a
22.	a	22.	c	22.	b
23.	c	23.	b	23.	b
24.	a	24.	b	24.	c
25.	b	25.	d	25.	b

Chapter 4		*Chapter 5*		*Chapter 6*	
1.	c	1.	c	1.	d
2.	c	2.	a	2.	b
3.	b	3.	c	3.	d
4.	a	4.	d	4.	d
5.	b	5.	c	5.	c
6.	a	6.	c	6.	a
7.	d	7.	b	7.	d
8.	b	8.	b	8.	b
9.	d	9.	a	9.	b
10.	a	10.	d	10.	d
11.	b	11.	c	11.	d
12.	a	12.	b	12.	d
13.	c	13.	d	13.	a
14.	a	14.	a	14.	d
15.	c	15.	d	15.	c
16.	a	16.	b	16.	b
17.	a	17.	d	17.	d
18.	a	18.	a	18.	b
19.	b	19.	c	19.	c
20.	a	20.	b	20.	a
21.	a	21.	d	21.	b
22.	b	22.	b	22.	a
23.	d	23.	d	23.	b
24.	b	24.	a	24.	c
25.	a	25.	c	25.	a
26.	c			26.	a
				27.	b
				28.	a
				29.	d
				30.	b

BRAIN TEASER ANSWERS

Brain Teaser 1

The stated focal spot sizes for a conventional tomography tube are 0.4 and 0.8 millimeter. After performing the focal spot test using the star test pattern you have determined that the small focal spot is actually 0.9 millimeter and the large focal spot is actually 1.8 millimeter. Are the focal spots within acceptance parameters? What would be your recommendations?

ANSWER

An x-ray tube with stated focal spot sizes of 0.4 and 0.8 millimeter when measured can have a maximum size of 0.6 and 1.2 millimeters. Because the measured sizes of this tube are 0.9 and 1.8 millimeters, it would not be acceptable for use in such areas as special procedures and body section radiography where imaging fine detail structures is critical. However, this tube would be satisfactory in a general radiography room.

Brain Teaser 2

The light field/beam alignment indicates that the light field is greater on the longitudinal axis and half as much on the vertical axis of the film. Can you identify the possible cause or causes for this finding?

ANSWER

According to field service engineers the most frequently occurring cause of this problem is that the collimator is used at the same SID and the same film sizes therefore the feedback potentiometers used in the sizing stop on the same area of the potentiometer. This causes them to wear out and causes one or both blades to size incorrectly. Another potential cause is the collimator mirror was knocked out of alignment when the collimator light bulb was replaced.

Brain Teaser 3

The light field/beam alignment indicates that the light field is greater on both the longitudinal axis and vertical axis of the film. Can you identify the possible cause or causes for this finding?

ANSWER

There are several possible causes for this problem and all of them need to be checked out before the field service engineer is called. The collimator mirror may be out of alignment. The wrong SID was used. Finally, the SID indicator may need adjustment. According to field service engineers the most common cause of this problem is that the collimator blades do not respond when the Bucky tray is pushed in.

Brain Teaser 4

The radiograph from the beam perpendicularity test demonstrates that the upper bead is outside the second ring. Can you identify the possible cause or causes for this finding?

ANSWER

There are three possible causes for this problem. When the test was performed, the tube, the table, or both may not have been level. It is important to repeat the test to ensure that the tube and table are level (parallel) with each other. Once the test has been repeated and the problem still exists, the most logical cause is the tube has moved out of alignment and the field service engineer will need to be called.

Brain Teaser 5

You have just completed a manual spin top test in a single-phase radiographic room. All four of your images demonstrate the appropriate number of dots, but in each image you observe that every other dot is light. Can you identify the cause of this anomaly?

ANSWER

The solution to this is very simple—a rectifier has gone bad and instead of having full wave rectification you are getting half wave rectification.

Brain Teaser 6

You have just completed a manual spin top test in a single-phase radiographic room. All of the images demonstrate half the expected number of dots. Can you identify the probable cause for this?

ANSWER

A rectifier has gone bad and the test results obtained reflect half wave rectification.

Brain Teaser 7

You have just completed a mechanized test tool in a three-phase radiographic room. The image for the 1/5-second timer station indicates an angle of 80°. Is the time station accurate? If the timer is not accurate, is the exposure time too short or too long?

ANSWER

The acceptance parameters for this particular time station are between 69° and 75°; therefore the 1/5-second time station is not accurate. Based on the information provided the exposure time is too long and a field service engineer should be called in to recalibrate the timer.

Brain Teaser 8

You have just completed testing the 60 to 100 kV ranges in 10-kV increments with the digital kVp meter. You determined that you were obtaining 62 kVp, 68 kVp, 81 kVp, 90 kVp, and 100 kVp at the designated kVp selections. Are the kVp selections within accepted parameters?

ANSWER

Yes, all of the kilovoltages tested are within ±4 kV of the selected kV.

Brain Teaser 9

You have just completed testing the 60 to 100 kV ranges in 10-kVp increments. The results you obtained were as follows: 57 kVp, 74 kVp, 85 kVp, 95 kVp, and 95 kVp. Are the kVp selections within accepted parameters? If they are not what are the possible causes for this?

ANSWER

The 60 kV and 70 kV selections are within the ±4 kVp acceptance parameters. However, the selected 80 kV, 90 kV, and 100 kV are not within the acceptance parameters and they would need to be recalibrated by the field service engineer.

Brain Teaser 10

It was found that the mAs reciprocity variation was 12%. What would be the probable cause for this?

ANSWER

It is impossible to make a determination of cause without further diagnostic tests of the timer and mA settings.

Brain Teaser 11

It was found that the exposure in mR from the 100 mA station to the 200 mA station tripled. Is this acceptable? What would cause this?

ANSWER

It is important to remember that mA is directly proportional to mR output. If mA doubles, mR output doubles. Answering the first part of this problem is simple; it is not acceptable. To answer the second, a field service engineer would need to be called. The

most logical cause would be that the 200 mA station is in need of calibration. It is remotely possible that there may be a problem with the x-ray tube or exposure timer. Also, on some generators the kVp is calibrated separately for each mA station and this problem could be caused if the kVp was off for one station. Both of these would need to be checked at the time the mA calibration is checked.

Brain Teaser 12

It was found that the exposure reproducibility for a single phase generator was 6%. What would cause this?

ANSWER

The exposure reproducibility of this generator is not within the ±5% acceptance standard. The cause for this could be related to either the exposure timer or mA. The field service engineer would need to be called to run further diagnostic tests in order to determine the exact cause of the problem.

Survey Forms
and Record Forms

Radiology Survey

<u>Your Opinion Counts</u>

Will you take a few moments to share your thoughts with us?

Test(s) performed during your visit:

_____ **X-ray** _____ **Mammogram** _____ **Nuclear medicine**

_____ **CAT scan** _____ **Other**

What other departments did you visit today? _____

How long did you wait to be registered at Outpatient Registration? (Circle one of the following):

| No wait | Less than 15 mins. | Less than 30 mins. | Longer than 30 mins. | Don't know |

Approximate waiting time for procedure (Circle one of the following):

| No wait | Less than 15 mins. | Less than 30 mins. | Longer than 30 mins. | Don't know |

	YES	NO
1. Was the receptionist courteous?	_____	_____
2. Did the receptionist answer your questions?	_____	_____
3. Was the receptionist neat in appearance?	_____	_____
4. Was the waiting room clean?	_____	_____
5. Was the technologist courteous?	_____	_____
6. Did the technologist answer your questions?	_____	_____
7. Was the technologist organized?	_____	_____
8. Did the technologist make you feel comfortable?	_____	_____
9. Was your procedure(s) clearly explained?	_____	_____
10. Was your procedure(s) performed in a timely fashion?	_____	_____
11. When your procedure(s) were completed, were you promptly released?	_____	_____
12. Was the technologist neat in appearance?	_____	_____
13. Was the x-ray room clean?	_____	_____
14. Were the restrooms clean?	_____	_____

Please grade us on our services (check one): ☐ **Outstanding** ☐ **Good** ☐ **Fair** ☐ **Poor**

Thank you for completing this survey.
Any suggestions may be placed on the back of the survey.

Department of Radiology

The Radiology Department strives to provide quality services to you and our mutual patients. As a frequent referrer to the Radiology Department, your opinions regarding our level of service are very important to us.

Please take a moment to answer the following questions to help us serve you better. Any suggestions you wish to offer outside the questions asked would be appreciated. Please fax your completed survey to the Quality Assurance Coordinator for Radiology or mail it in the enclosed envelope.

1. How long did you wait at the customer service counter in the Radiology Department to receive your films?

   a. 1 – 10 minutes   b. 11 – 20 minutes   c. 21 – 30 minutes   d. > 30 minutes

2. How long did you wait to receive your radiology reports?

   a. < 24 hours   b. 24 hours   c. 24 – 36 hours   d. 36 – 48 hours   e. > 48 hours

	Poor	Fair	Good	Very Good	Excellent	NA
3. How would you rate the following qualities of the file room staff?						
a. Caring	___	___	___	___	___	___
b. Courtesy	___	___	___	___	___	___
c. Professional appearance	___	___	___	___	___	___
4. How would you rate the following qualities of the technical staff?						
a. Caring	___	___	___	___	___	___
b. Courtesy	___	___	___	___	___	___
c. Professional	___	___	___	___	___	___
5. How would you rate the following features of radiology department?						
a. Report turnaround time	___	___	___	___	___	___
b. Availability of appointment times	___	___	___	___	___	___
c. Customer service desk	___	___	___	___	___	___
d. Film quality	___	___	___	___	___	___
e. Availability of the radiologists	___	___	___	___	___	___
6. How would you rate the following features of the radiology department?						
a. Cleanliness of the waiting room	___	___	___	___	___	___
b. Comfort of the waiting room	___	___	___	___	___	___
c. Cleanliness of the x-ray room	___	___	___	___	___	___
d. Cleanliness of the restrooms	___	___	___	___	___	___
e. Privacy of the dressing room	___	___	___	___	___	___
7. How would you rate us on the services that we provide?	___	___	___	___	___	___

8. What do you perceive is the greatest opportunity for improvement regarding Radiology Services at the hospital?

Thank you for completing this survey.
Any comments may be placed on the back of the survey.

Radiology Survey

Directions: We are constantly striving to improve the service that we offer our customers. Please take the time to complete the following survey.

1. How long did you wait in the Radiology Department for the start of your examination? (Circle one of the following):

   a. 1 – 10 minutes   b. 11 – 20 minutes   c. 21 – 30 minutes   d. > 30 minutes

	Poor	Fair	Good	Very Good	Excellent	NA
2. How would you rate the following qualities of the reception staff?						
a. Caring	___	___	___	___	___	___
b. Courtesy	___	___	___	___	___	___
c. Professional appearance	___	___	___	___	___	___
3. How would you rate the following qualities of the technical staff?						
a. Caring	___	___	___	___	___	___
b. Courtesy	___	___	___	___	___	___
c. Professional	___	___	___	___	___	___
4. How would you rate the following aspects of your exam?						
a. Instructions given to you by the technologist	___	___	___	___	___	___
b. Time in room until your exam began	___	___	___	___	___	___
c. Organization of the technologist	___	___	___	___	___	___
d. Procedure performed promptly	___	___	___	___	___	___
e. Prompt release following procedure	___	___	___	___	___	___
f. Courtesy of the radiologist	___	___	___	___	___	___
g. The ability of the radiologist to answer your questions	___	___	___	___	___	___
5. How would you rate the following features of the radiology department?						
a. Cleanliness of the waiting room	___	___	___	___	___	___
b. Comfort of the waiting room	___	___	___	___	___	___
c. Cleanliness of the x-ray room	___	___	___	___	___	___
d. Cleanliness of the restrooms	___	___	___	___	___	___
e. Privacy of the dressing room	___	___	___	___	___	___
6. How would you rate your visit today?	___	___	___	___	___	___
7. How would you rate us on the service provided today?	___	___	___	___	___	___
8. How would you compare today's exam with previous exams?	___	___	___	___	___	___

Thank you for completing this survey.
Any comments may be placed on the back of the survey.

Department of Radiology

Dear Doctor,

The Radiology Department strives to provide quality services to you and our mutual patients. As a frequent referrer to the Radiology Department, your opinions regarding our level of service are very important to us.

Please take a moment to answer the following questions to help us serve you better. Any suggestions you wish to offer outside the questions asked would be appreciated. Please fax your completed survey to the Technical Director for Radiology or mail it in the enclosed envelope.

1. Are you able to schedule procedures in a timely manner?   Yes   No

   Comments:

2. Do you feel you always get the earliest appointment available?   Yes   No

   Comments:

3. Are certain procedures harder to schedule than others?   Yes   No

   Please name specific procedures.

4. Are receptionists in Radiology helpful and friendly?   Yes   No

   Comments:

5. If you view your films, do they meet your quality expectations? Yes   No

   Comments:

6. Does report turnaround time meet your expectations?   Yes   No

   If not, what is acceptable to you?

7. Do the hours the radiologist are available meet your needs?   Yes   No

   Comments:

8. What do you perceive is the greatest opportunity for improvement regarding Radiology Services at the hospital?

Radiologist QA

QA REF # _____

Radiology/Physician QA

Aspect of Care: Performance improvement/Peer review

Indicator: Cross-readings

Threshold: 100% agreement with original dictation

Radiologist: _____   Date of review: _____

Note to transcriptionist: Please send this QA form/request and typed report to the QA office.

Patient name: _____   DOB _____

Patient MR# _____

Exam/exams: _____

Pertinent HX: _____

Comparison films pulled: Yes _____   No _____

Review by QA radiologist

Were readings in agreement?   Yes   No

Peer review determination:

_____ 1. Not a variance   _____ 4. Marginal deviation from S.O.C.

_____ 2. Predictable/acceptable, within S.O.C.   _____ 5. Significant deviation from S.O.C.

_____ 3. Unpredictable, within S.O.C.

Comments: _____

_____

Signature of QA radiologist: _____   Date: _____

Original radiologist: _____

Diagnostic Radiology

Image Quality Action

Please return to the QA Coordinator at Box #155 within seven days of receipt.

Technologist: _____ Number: _____

Student: _____ Number: _____

Complaint lodged by: _____

Facility: _____

Patient: _____

MR#: _____

Exam: _____

Date of procedure: _____

1. Film identification

    a. Wrong ID stamp on film _____

    b. No ID stamp on film _____

    c. Not clear or legible _____

2. Film quality

    a. Overexposed _____

    b. Underexposed _____

    c. Poor positioning _____

    d. Motion _____

    e. Artifacts _____

    f. Double exposed _____

    g. Part excluded _____

    h. Part obscured _____

    i. Grid cut-off _____

    j. Other _____

3. Film marking

    a. No right or left marker _____

    b. Improper marking of film _____

    c. No technologist number _____

    d. No date and/or time on films _____

    e. Wrong date and/or time _____

4. Wrong exam done _____

5. Wrong patient done _____

6. All views not done _____

7. No evidence of collimation _____

8. No evidence of gonadal shielding _____

9. No pertinent patient history _____

10. Film size (too large/small) _____

11. Processor _____

12. Other _____

QA comments:

_____

_____

_____

_____

_____

_____

_____

_____

_____

Date _____ _____
                                 Signature

Technologist comments:

_____

_____

_____

_____

_____

_____

_____

_____

_____

Date _____ _____
                                 Signature

Supervisor comments:

_____

_____

_____

_____

_____

Date _____ _____
                                 Signature

CROSSOVER PROCEDURE RECORD FORM

Processor: _____   Date: _____

Old emulsion # _____

Strip #	B + F	MD (Step 11)	HD (Step 13)	LD (Step 9)	DD (13–9)
1					
2					
3					
4					
5					
Average					

New emulsion # _____

Strip #	B + F	MD (Step 11)	HD (Step 13)	LD (Step 9)	DD (13–9)
1					
2					
3					
4					
5					
Average					

Calculate the change in film by subtracting the old average from the new average for each aim value.

	B + F	MD	DD
New average			
(–) Old average			
Change			

New aim values: Add the change in film by subtracting the old average from the new average for each film.

	B + F	MD	DD
Present aim			
Change			
New aim			

To obtain the new aim add the change to the present aim.

If the new b + f aim is greater than 0.02 of the present aim, investigate the cause or contact the service engineer and/or the film manufacturer.

Repeat Analysis Record Form

Department Area: _____ **Quarter:** _____ **Month:** _____ **Year:** _____

	Cause	Chest	Abd	Extremity	Cranium	C. Spine	T. Spine	L. Spine	Sacrum Coccyx	Pelvic Girdle	Bony Thorax	UGI	BE	GU	Total
1	Positioning														
2	Motion														
3	Overexposed														
4	Underexposed														
5	Artifact														
6	Fogged														
7	Processor														
8	Misc (?)														
9	Total														
10	Black														
11	Green														
12	Clear														
13	Sensitometry														
14	Copy Film														
15	Laser Film														
	Total														

FILM ILLUMINATOR RECORD FORM

Date: Location:				Units of measurement (check the appropriate box) Illuminance: EV ☐ footcandles ☐ Luminance: nits ☐ cd/m² ☐		
Lower Panel *(Left to Right)*	*LUQ*	*LLQ*	*Middle*	*RUQ*	*RLQ*	*Average*
Panel #1						
Panel #2						
Panel #3						
Panel #4						
Panel #5						
Panel #6						
Panel #7						
Panel #8						
Upper Panel *(Left to Right)*						
Panel #1						
Panel #2						
Panel #3						
Panel #4						
Panel #5						
Panel #6						
Panel #7						
Panel #8						

Comments:

_____

Signature

Lead Protective Devices Survey

Area: _____

Date of survey: _____ Date of survey: _____

Date of survey: _____ Date of survey: _____

Date of survey: _____ Date of survey: _____

Inventory Number	Assigned To	Color	Inspection Results											Inspector					Comments
			1999	2000	2001	2002	2003	99	00	01	02	03							

1 = No defects 2 = Small pinholes; left in service 3 = Small holes\small multiple defects; left in service 4 = Large holes\multiple defects; remove from service

mAs Reciprocity Record Form (Stepwedge Method)

Room _____   Unit _____   Single phase ☐   Three phase ☐

Exposure time _____   kVp _____

Acceptance parameters

Step	Densitometer Readings at 100 mA	200 mA	300 mA	400 mA
1				
2				
3				
4				
5				
6				
7				
8				
9				
10				
11				
12				
13				
14				
15				
16				
17				
18				
19				
20				
21				

Comments:

_____   _____
        Signature   Date

Light Field Illumination Record Form

Room _____   Unit _____   Single phase ☐   Three phase ☐

Quadrant	Reading
1	
2	
3	
4	
Average	

Comments:

_____   _____

Signature   **Date**

EXPOSURE TIME RECORD FORM

Room _____   Unit _____   Single phase ☐   Three phase ☐

Timer Accuracy (Spin Top)	
Exposure Time	*Number of Dots*
1/5 sec	
1/10 sec	
1/20 sec	
1/30 sec	

Comments:

Room _____   Unit _____   Single phase ☐   Three phase ☐

Timer Accuracy (Mechanized Spin Top)	
Exposure Time	*Number of Degrees*
1/5 sec	
1/10 sec	
1/20 sec	
1/30 sec	

Comments:

Room _____   Unit _____   Single phase ☐   Three phase ☐

Timer Accuracy (Digital Device)			
Selected		*Measured*	

Comments:

_____
Signature

kVp Record Form

Room _____   **Unit** _____

Single phase ☐   **Three phase** ☐

Acceptance parameters

Exposure	50 kVp	60 kVp	70 kVp	80 kVp	90 kVp	100 kVp
#1						
#2						
#3						
#4						
#5						
#6						
Average						

Comments:

_____   _____

Signature   **Date**

mA/mAs LINEARITY RECORD FORM

Room _____ Unit _____ Single phase ☐ Three phase ☐

mA/mAs Linearity					
80 kVp ____.____ Factor adjacent ____.____ Factor any					
mA	Measured Seconds	mAs	kVp	mR	mR/mAs

Comments:

_____ _____
Signature   Date

GRID UNIFORMITY RECORD FORM

Type of grid: _____   Grid ratio: _____

_____ mA   _____ Exposure time   _____ kVp   _____ SID

Grid Uniformity	
Area	Density Reading
Upper right quadrant	
Upper left quadrant	
Lower right quadrant	
Lower left quadrant	
Center	

Comments:

_____   _____
Signature   Date

HALF VALUE LAYER RECORD FORM

Room _____   Unit _____   Single phase ☐   Three phase ☐

Half Value Layer	
Half Value Layer at 80 kVp	
mR	*mm Added Al*

mm Al added filtration	
mm Al measured HVL	

Comments:

_____   _____
Signature   Date

AEC EXPOSURE REPRODUCIBILITY RECORD FORM (R-METER)

Room _____   Unit _____   Single phase ☐   Three phase ☐

Exposure	Sensor Location	mR	mR/mAs
#1			
#2			
#3			
		Percent Variation	

Comments:

Signature   Date

AUTOMATIC EXPOSURE CONTROL RECORD FORM

Room _____   Unit _____   Single phase ☐   Three phase ☐

mA Exposure Consistency		
Acceptance: ±0.2 OD		
mA	*kVp*	*OD*
100	70	
200	70	
300	70	
400	70	

kVp Exposure Consistency		
Acceptance: ±0.3 OD		
mA	*kVp*	*OD*
200	60	
200	70	
200	80	
200	90	

Sensor Chamber Consistency		
Acceptance: ±0.2 OD		
Exposure	*Cm of Attenuation*	*OD*
One		
Two		
Three		

Exposure Reproducibility		
Acceptance: ±0.1 OD		
mA	*kVp*	*OD*
200	80	
200	80	
200	80	

Consistency of Exposure with Varying Field Size	
Acceptance: ±0.1 OD	
Field Size	*OD*
6 × 6	
10 × 10	
14 × 14	

Consistency of Exposure with Varying Patient Thicknesses	
Acceptance: ±0.1 OD	
Phantom Size	*OD*
10 cm	
20 cm	
30 cm	

Backup Exposure Time	
mAs	
Sec	
Pass	
Fail	

Comments:

_____   _____
Signature   Date

mR/mAs Output Record Form

Room _____ Unit _____ Single phase ☐ Three phase ☐

Radiation Output			
Selected kVp	**Measured kVp**	**Free-in-air mR/mAs**	

kVp	Single phase (mR/mAs)	Three phase (mR/mAs)
60	5.12	7.68
80	8.96	13.44
100	14.08	20.48
125	22.40	30.72

Technique: _____ mA

_____ mAs

@ _____ " SCD

Comments:

_____ _____

Signature   Date

COEFFICIENT OF VARIATION FORM

Room _____   Unit _____   Single phase ☐   Three phase ☐

Coefficient of Variation			
Selected— _____kVp	_____mA	_____sec	_____mAs
Measured—	mR	kVp	seconds
Mean			
SD			
COV			

Comments:

_____   _____
Signature   Date

EXPOSURE REPRODUCIBILITY RECORD FORM

Room _____   Unit _____   Single phase ☐   Three phase ☐

mA _____   Time _____   SID _____

Exposure	mAs	kVp	mR
#1			
#2			
#3			
#4			
#5			
#6			
		Percent Variation	

Comments:

_____   _____
Signature   Date

Timer Linearity Record Form

Room number: _____   Generator phase: _____   Date: _____

mA	Exp Time	mAs	kVp	mR	mR/mAs
200					
200					
200					
200					
			Percent Variation		

Comments:

_____   _____
Signature   Date

Fluoroscopy Record Form

Room: _____   Unit: _____

Half Value Layer

Half Value Layer At _____ kVp

R/min		mm Added Al	

_____ mm Al HVL

Image Recording Mode

kVp	mR	mAs	Attenuator	
				Digital Spot film
				100 mm 105 mm
				Imaging mode:
				Density setting:

Reproducibility factor: Pass   Fail   N/A

kVp Compensation and mA Linearity

Selected kVp	Measured kVp	mA	mAs	mR	Optical Density	Attenuator

Image Quality

Low Contrast Resolution

	kVp	Mode	Focal Spot	Resolution				
Fluoro mode:					%	P	F	N/A
Image recording mode:					%	P	F	N/A

High Contrast Resolution

	kVp	Mode	Focal Spot	Resolution				
Fluoro mode:					mesh	P	F	N/A
Image recording mode:					mesh	P	F	N/A

Image Intensifier Exposure Rates

Sid: _____   Grid: _____   Detail/Gain: _____   Minimum kVp: _____

R/min	kVp	mA	Attenuation	Image Mode	Fluoro Mode

_____   _____
Signature   **Date**

Mammography Image Quality Action

Technologist: _____   Date: _____

Facility: _____   Radiologist: _____

Comments: _____

_____

_____

Patient name: _____   Medical Record #: _____

<u>Repeat/suboptimal reason:</u>   (Circle Breast)   (Circle Projection)

Positioning	R	L	MLO	CC	Other _____
Patient motion	R	L	MLO	CC	Other _____
Blur	R	L	MLO	CC	Other _____
Light films	R	L	MLO	CC	Other _____
Dark films	R	L	MLO	CC	Other _____
Static	R	L	MLO	CC	Other _____
Artifact	R	L	MLO	CC	Other _____
Processor marks	R	L	MLO	CC	Other _____
Fog	R	L	MLO	CC	Other _____
Incorrect patient identification	R	L	MLO	CC	Other _____
Double exposure	R	L	MLO	CC	Other _____
Date of film missing	R	L	MLO	CC	Other _____
Missing films	R	L	MLO	CC	Other _____
Improper marking of lesions	R	L	MLO	CC	Other _____

<u>Place an "X" in the box:</u>

Mammo folder not written up   [ ]   **Missing paperwork**   [ ]

Incomplete history form   [ ]   **Old/previous films not included**   [ ]

Other: _____

Please place technologist and supervisor response on back.

Technologist's Response: _____

_____

_____

_____

_____

Technologist's Signature: _____   **Date:** _____

Supervisor's Response: _____

_____

_____

_____

_____

_____

Supervisor's Signature: _____   **Date:** _____

Plan of Action: _____

_____

_____

_____

_____

_____

_____

MAMMOGRAPHY IMAGING SERVICES

Dear Patient,

As stated in our hospitals mission statement, we are committed to proving compassionate patient care of the highest quality. To accomplish this, we need your help. By sharing your opinions, both positive and negative, with us through this survey, you can allow us to see what we are doing right and where we need to improve. Your comments about your experience will be kept confidential. Thank you for taking the time to help us improve.

PLEASE CHECK THE BEST ANSWER FOR EACH QUESTION.

	Excellent	Very Good	Good	Fair	Poor	Does Not Apply
1. The technologist listened closely to my needs.						
2. The technologist took prompt action to meet my needs.						
3. The technologist was friendly and respectful.						
4. The technologist demonstrated caring and concern.						
5. The technologist asked questions about my breast history.						
6. The technologist explained my test to me.						
7. The technologist answered my questions in a way that I could understand.						
8. The technologist demonstrated skill and knowledge.						
9. The exam room was clean and comfortable.						
10. The exam room was quiet and private.						
11. The registration process was simple and wait time was kept to a minimum.						
12. How well were you able to find your way around the Medical Center?						
13. How do you rate the overall quality of the care you received?						

	<20	20-29	30-39	40-49	50-59	60+
14. How old are you?						

					Male	Female
15. What is your gender?						

					Yes	No
16. Have you been a patient at any Medical Center health care facility?						
17. Will you return to the Medical Center the next time you need health care?						
18. Will you recommend the Medical Center to your friends?						
19. Would you like to talk with a manager about a concern or issue?						

Is there anything else you would like to tell us? Please use back of form.

Optional Information

Name _____

Phone number _____

Thank You from the Staff

KODAK Mammography Processing Control Chart

Processor _____ Film _____ Emulsion No. _____ Year _____

Date Crossover Performed _____ Crossover Emulsion No. _____

Month
Date
Initials

+ 0.15
+ 0.10

**Medium
Density MD**
(Speed Index)

Step # _____

− 0.10
− 0.15

+ 0.15
+ 0.10

**Density
Difference DD**
(Contrast Index)

Step # _____
Step # _____ − 0.10
− 0.15

+ .03

Base plus Fog
(B+F)

**Developer
Temperature**

Replenishment Rates per
      # of films _____
      film size _____
length of film travel _____

Date	Developer	Fixer

Record **remarks** on the back of this sheet.

 HEALTH SCIENCES

Remarks

Date	Action

Remarks

Date	Action

More than quality imaging

M7-173   Printed in U.S.A.   © Eastman Kodak Company, 1995   Kodak is a trademark.

KODAK Mammography Phantom Image Worksheet

Unit _____ Processor _____ Initials_____ Date _____

Exposure Factors

☐ MANUAL   ☐ AUTOMATIC EXPOSURE CONTROL

kVp_____   mA_____   kVp_____   mAs _____

Exposure time (seconds) _____   Photocell position_____

Density Information

Optical density of background   _____

Optical density of disc   _____

Density difference   _____
(Optical density of background minus optical density of disc)

Technique

☐ GRID   ☐ NON-GRID

Mammographic Phantom *(Score objects seen)*

Fibers

_____ 1) 1.56 mm nylon fiber
_____ 2) 1.12 mm nylon fiber
_____ 3) 0.89 mm nylon fiber
_____ 4) 0.75 mm nylon fiber
_____ 5) 0.54 mm nylon fiber
_____ 6) 0.40 mm nylon fiber

_____ **Total score of fibers**

Specks

_____ 7) 0.54 mm Al_2O_3 specks
_____ 8) 0.40 mm Al_2O_3 specks
_____ 9) 0.32 mm Al_2O_3 specks
_____ 10) 0.24 mm Al_2O_3 specks
_____ 11) 0.16 mm Al_2O_3 specks

_____ **Total score of specks**

Masses

_____ 12) 2.00 mm mass
_____ 13) 1.00 mm mass
_____ 14) 0.75 mm mass
_____ 15) 0.50 mm mass
_____ 16) 0.25 mm mass

_____ **Total score of masses**

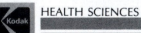

HEALTH SCIENCES

Practice Examination and Answers

PRACTICE EXAMINATION

1. Which of the following are considered forms of peer review?
   1. Suboptimal film tracking
   2. Radiologist QA
   3. Medical imaging audits
   a. 1 and 2 only
   b. 1 and 3 only
   c. 2 and 3 only
   d. 1, 2, and 3
2. Which of the following statements is correct?
   a. The primary purpose of radiographic QA is to maintain a standard of image quality that benefits the patient, physician, Medical Imaging Department, and the institution.
   b. The primary purpose of image quality improvement is to maintain a standard of image quality that benefits the patient, physician, Medical Imaging Department, and the institution.
   c. The primary purpose of radiographic QC is to maintain a standard of image quality that benefits the patient, physician, Medical Imaging Department, and the institution.
   d. None of the above
3. An increase in the amount of time it takes to do an examination will result in
   a. a decrease in patient satisfaction and customer service.
   b. an increase in patient satisfaction and customer service.
   c. increased patient satisfaction and decreased customer service.
   d. decreased patient satisfaction and increased customer service.

4. What level of customer service would a patient get if they were to receive the correct examination and the physician were to receive a report within 7 days?
   a. An average level
   b. A high level
   c. A minimal level
   d. None of the above
5. Noninvasive equipment testing is considered
   a. complex.
   b. simple.
   c. both a and b
   d. neither a nor b
6. Which of the following is not considered a form of peer review?
   a. Examination tracking
   b. Medical imaging audits
   c. Radiologist QA
   d. Suboptimal film tracking
7. The majority of problems are the result of the minority of causes is best described by the
   a. 70/15 rule.
   b. 70/20 rule.
   c. 80/15 rule.
   d. 80/20 rule.
8. Which of the following statements is correct?
   a. Patients that are referred by their personal physician are considered internal customers.
   b. Patients that are referred by their personal physician are considered external customers.
   c. Personnel from another department are considered external customers.
   d. Housestaff are considered external customers.
9. Which of the following is a form of peer review?
   a. Cost analysis
   b. Examination tracking
   c. Medical imaging audits
   d. Turnaround times
10. What level of customer service would a patient get if they were to receive the correct examination and the physician were to receive a report within 2 days?
    a. An average level
    b. A high level
    c. A minimal level
    d. None of the above
11. Processes, not people, are the root of quality problems is best described by the

  a. 70/15 rule.

  b. 70/20 rule.

  c. 85/15 rule.

  d. 80/20 rule.

12. QM deals with

  1. Image quality improvement

  2. QA

  3. Performance improvement

  4. QC

  a. 1 only

  b. 3 only

  c. 1 and 3 only

  d. 2 and 4 only

13. Drs. Deming and Juran introduced

  a. QA as a management tool in post-war Japan.

  b. QC as a management tool in post-war Japan.

  c. quality concepts as a management tool in post-war Japan.

  d. performance improvement as a management tool in post-war Japan.

14. Which of the following did the 1981 Consumer Patient Radiation Health and Safety Act do?

  1. Reduce repeat exposure

  2. Reduce unnecessary exposure to patients

  3. Provide minimum training standards for radiography programs

  4. Require certification of operators

  a. 1 and 3 only

  b. 1, 2, and 3 only

  c. 1, 2, and 4 only

  d. 1, 2, 3, and 4

15. The 14 points for management were developed by

  a. W. Edwards Deming.

  b. J.M. Juran.

  c. W.A. Shewhart.

  d. Fredrick Winslow Taylor.

16. Focusing on those aspects of departmental operations that directly pertain to improving the standard of patient care and outcomes is the goal of

  a. QM.

  b. image quality improvement.

  c. performance improvement.

  d. QC.

17. Maintaining standards of image quality that benefit the patient, physician, Medical Imaging Department, and the institution is the primary purpose of

  a. radiographic QC.

  b. image quality improvement.

  c. radiographic QA.

  d. performance improvement.

18. The testing and monitoring of equipment in all areas of the Medical Imaging Department is the focus of
    a. radiographic QA.
    b. radiographic QC.
    c. image quality improvement.
    d. none of the above.

19. Which of the following is a method used to pinpoint waste in the Medical Imaging Department?
    a. Cost analysis
    b. Examination tracking
    c. Medical imaging audits
    d. Timeliness of service

20. A medical imaging audit is a mechanism for looking at the
    a. financial health of the Medical Imaging Department.
    b. internal operations of the Medical Imaging Department.
    c. overall operations of the Medical Imaging Department.
    d. timeliness of service.

21. Suboptimal image tracking is a mechanism for looking at the
    a. financial operations of the Medical Imaging Department.
    b. internal operations of the Medical Imaging Department.
    c. overall operations of the Medical Imaging Department.
    d. technical operations of the Medical Imaging Department.

22. Turnaround times are a reflection of
    a. financial operations of the Medical Imaging Department.
    b. internal operations of the Medical Imaging Department.
    c. overall operations of the Medical Imaging Department.
    d. timeliness of service of the Medical Imaging Department.

23. Examination tracking is a mechanism for looking at the
    a. financial health of the Medical Imaging Department.
    b. internal operations of the Medical Imaging Department.
    c. overall operations of the Medical Imaging Department.
    d. timeliness of service.

24. A systematic program of record keeping, equipment selection, imaging criteria, and continuing education is the goal of
    a. radiographic QC.
    b. image quality improvement.
    c. radiographic QA.
    d. none of the above.

25. What statistical tool would be used to describe how often an event or situation occurs?
    a. Check sheet
    b. Frequency distribution
    c. Mode
    d. Range

26. What does a circle with an A inside represent in the detailed flowchart?
    a. Decision point
    b. Starting and ending point
    c. Step in the process
    d. Continuation of the flowchart onto the next page
27. What is the coefficient of variation when the mean is 8 and the standard deviation is 4.6?
    a. 0.505
    b. 0.555
    c. 0.575
    d. 0.605
28. What does a rectangle represent in the detailed flowchart?
    a. Decision point
    b. Starting and ending point
    c. Step in the process
    d. Continuation of the flowchart onto the next page
29. What does a diamond represent in the detailed flowchart?
    a. Decision point
    b. Starting and ending point
    c. Step in the process
    d. Continuation of the flowchart onto the next page
30. Which of the following detailed flowcharts would be the least complex?
    a. Intermediate level
    b. Macro level
    c. Micro level
    d. None of the above
31. Which of the following statements is correct?
    a. An intermediate-level flowchart will show minute items within the process.
    b. A macro-level flowchart will show minute items within the process.
    c. A micro-level flowchart will show minute items within the process.
    d. None of the above

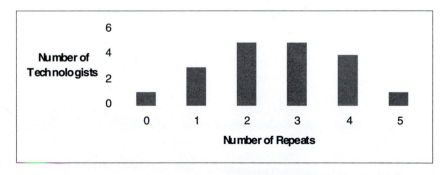

32. The diagram above is representative of a

    a. control chart.
    b. histogram.
    c. Pareto chart.
    d. scatter plot.

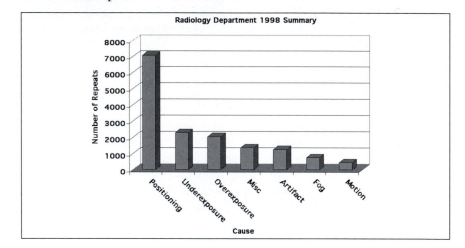

33. The diagram above is representative of a
    a. control chart.
    b. histogram.
    c. Pareto chart.
    d. scatter plot.
34. What is the standard deviation of 3, 4, 5, and 6?
    a. 1.1
    b. 1.6
    c. 1.9
    d. 2.2
35. Free thought is best seen in which of the following?
    a. Brainstorming
    b. Data collection
    c. Team work
    d. None of the above
36. What does the "C" stand for in PDCA?
    a. Check
    b. Clarify
    c. Correct
    d. Contact
37. Which of the following statistics is used to compare two institutions?
    a. Coefficient of variation
    b. Standard deviation
    c. Mean
    d. Percentile

38. What does the "C" stand for in FOCUS?
    a. Check
    b. Clarify
    c. Correct
    d. Contact
39. What type of chart would be used to analyze the cause and effect of different variables on a process?
    a. Detailed flowchart
    b. Histogram
    c. Fishbone diagram
    d. Top-down flowchart
40. Range is best described by the
    a. lowest and middle numbers.
    b. middle and highest numbers.
    c. lowest and highest numbers.
    d. highest number only.
41. Which of the following tools is used to compare two or more variables?
    a. Check sheets
    b. Control charts
    c. Flowcharts
    d. Matrices

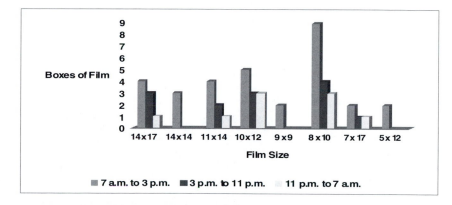

42. The diagram above is representative of a
    a. bar graph.
    b. histogram.
    c. Pareto chart.
    d. pie chart.

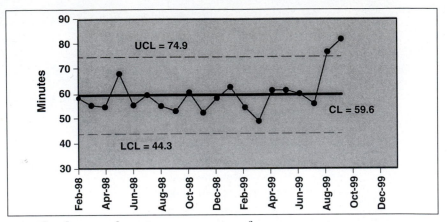

43. The diagram above is representative of a
    a. control chart.
    b. line chart.
    c. scatter plot.
    d. run chart.
44. What does an oval represent in the detailed flowchart?
    a. Decision point
    b. Starting and ending point
    c. Step in the process
    d. Continuation of the flowchart onto the next page

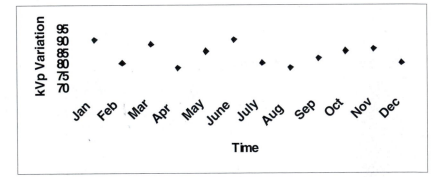

45. The diagram above is representative of a
    a. control chart.
    b. line chart.
    c. scatter plot.
    d. run chart.
46. How many levels of detailed flowcharts are there?
    a. 1
    b. 2
    c. 3
    d. 4

47. What is the range of 33, 25, 55, 44, 21, 18, and 22?
    a. 18 and 55
    b. 25 and 44
    c. 33 and 55
    d. 21 and 44
48. What is the mode of the following data 5%, 15%, 20%, 10%, 15%, 8%, 9%, 25%, 15%, and 10%?
    a. 25%
    b. 15%
    c. 10%
    d. 5%
49. What is the mean of 3, 4, 5, and 6?
    a. 4.5
    b. 6.4
    c. 9.2
    d. 18
50. The basic unit of luminance is the
    a. footcandle.
    b. footlambert.
    c. lux.
    d. cd/m^2.
51. If the total processing time from dry film to dry film exceeds 2% of the manufacturer's recommended processing time, what will the finished radiograph look like?
    a. The finished film will not be affected.
    b. The finished film will be light.
    c. The finished film will be dark.
    d. There is not enough information given.
52. The basic unit of illuminance is the
    a. cd/m^2.
    b. footlambert.
    c. lux.
    d. nit.
53. As developer temperature and immersion time increases
    a. density and contrast increase.
    b. density and contrast decrease.
    c. density increases and contrast decreases.
    d. density decreases and contrast increases.
54. Which of the following statements is correct?
    a. The sensitometer is used to imprint 11-step stepwedge on a film.
    b. The sensitometer is used to imprint 15-step stepwedge on a film.
    c. The sensitometer is used to imprint 21-step stepwedge on a film.
    d. The sensitometer is used to imprint 31-step stepwedge on a film.
55. An unexposed and processed x-ray film has a small but measurable density called

   a. fog.

   b. polyester tint.

   c. background fog.

   d. base plus fog.

56. The luminance level of a group of viewboxes used in general radiography was tested and found to have a luminance of 2500 nit. What conclusion could be made regarding these particular viewboxes?

   a. The luminance level of the viewboxes is within the acceptance parameters.

   b. The luminance level of the viewboxes is not within the acceptance parameters.

   c. The luminance level of the viewboxes exceeded the acceptance parameters.

57. What causes a film to turn brown?

   a. Inadequate developing or fixing of the film

   b. Inadequate washing or fixing of the film

   c. Inadequate washing or drying of the film

   d. Inadequate developing of the film

58. Which of the following statements is correct?

   a. A trend is a series of five consecutive points that has a downward pattern on the processor control chart.

   b. A trend is a series of five consecutive points that has an upward pattern on the processor control chart.

   c. A trend is a series of five consecutive points that has a downward or upward pattern on the processor control chart.

   d. None of the above

Questions 59 to 62 pertain to the information below.

Parameter	Aim
Speed index	1.35
Contrast index	2.15
Base plus fog	0.18
Temperature	94°F

59. The contrast index reading for the 24th of the month was 1.96. What conclusion could be made?

   a. The contrast index was within normal limits.

   b. The contrast index was below the minimum acceptable limits.

   c. The contrast index exceeded the maximum acceptable limits.

60. The speed index for the 15th of the month was 1.49. What conclusion could be made?

   a. The speed index was within normal limits.

   b. The speed index was below the minimum acceptable limits.

   c. The speed index exceeded the maximum acceptable limits.

61. The temperature reading for the 12th of the month was 94.6°F. What conclusion could be made?
  a. The temperature was within normal limits.
  b. The temperature was below the minimum acceptable limits.
  c. The temperature exceeded the maximum acceptable limits.

62. The speed index reading for the 30th of the month was 1.19. What conclusion could be made?
  a. The speed index was within normal limits.
  b. The speed index was below the minimum acceptable limits.
  c. The speed index exceeded the maximum acceptable limits.

63. Which of the following statements is correct?
  a. A run is a series of two points that fall either above or below the target aim.
  b. A run is a series of three points that fall either above or below the target aim.
  c. A run is a series of five points that fall either above or below the target aim.
  d. A run is a series of seven points that fall either above or below the target aim.

64. Which of the following statements is correct?
  a. Cycling is a series of two points that alternate above and below the mean.
  b. Cycling is a series of three points that alternate above and below the mean.
  c. Cycling is a series of five points that alternate above and below the mean.
  d. Cycling is a series of seven points that alternate above and below the mean.

65. Which of the following statements is correct?
  a. A radiograph of an intensifying screen with poor screen contact would show areas of decreased density.
  b. A radiograph of an intensifying screen with poor screen contact would show areas of increased density.
  c. A radiograph of an intensifying screen with poor screen contact would show areas of decreased and increased density.
  d. A radiograph of an intensifying screen with poor screen contact would not show areas of decreased or increased density.

Questions 66 to 70 pertain to the information below.

Total number of repeats	630
Total number of waste films	525
Initial film inventory	12,500
Final film inventory	11,600
New film shipments	16,500
Total number of films repeated for positioning	235

66. What is the total film used for the month?
    a. 16,900
    b. 17,200
    c. 17,400
    d. 17,900
67. What is the waste rate?
    a. 3%
    b. 4%
    c. 5%
    d. 6%
68. What is the reject rate?
    a. 3.2%
    b. 3.6%
    c. 6.6%
    d. 7.6%
69. How many films were rejected?
    a. 235
    b. 525
    c. 630
    d. 1155
70. What was the causal repeat rate for positioning for the month?
    a. 37.3%
    b. 43.6%
    c. 53.1%
    d. 69.0%
71. The density difference between the exposed and unexposed portion a safelight test film should not exceed a density of
    a. 0.01.
    b. 0.03.
    c. 0.05.
    d. 0.06.
72. Processor monitoring is done
    a. daily.
    b. weekly.
    c. monthly.
    d. quarterly.
73. The density difference between the high density reading and low density reading of the processor control strip determines the
    a. base plus fog.
    b. contrast index.
    c. contrast index and speed index.
    d. speed index.
74. The midrange density of the processor control strip determines the
    a. base plus fog.
    b. contrast index.

    c. contrast index and speed index.

    d. speed index.

75. Individual illuminator variations within the department should not exceed

    a. 5%.

    b. 10%.

    c. 15%.

    d. 20%.

76. A three phase timer can be tested for accuracy using a synchronous spinning top. The resulting image looks like a

    a. series of dots or dashes, each representative of a radiation pulse.

    b. solid arc; the angle (in degrees) representative of the exposure time.

    c. series of gray tones, from white to black.

    d. multitude of small, mesh like squares of uniform sharpness.

77. It was determined that the x-ray field size was off by 1 centimeter on three of four sides at 100 centimeters. Is the collimator within acceptable parameters?

    a. Yes

    b. No

    c. Not enough information has been given

78. A comprehensive quality control program includes the testing and/or monitoring of the

    1. kVp.

    2. focal spot size.

    3. exposure time accuracy.

    a. 1 only

    b. 1 and 2 only

    c. 1 and 3 only

    d. 1, 2, and 3

Questions 79 to 82 deal with the chart below.

mA	Exp. Time	mAs	mR	mR/mAs
100	1/10	10	.044	
200	1/20	10	.045	
300	1/30	10	.041	
400	1/40	10	.050	
				Percent Variation =

79. What is the mR/mAs ratio for the 300 mA station?

    a. 0.0041

    b. 0.0044

    c. 0.0045

    d. 0.0050

80. What is the average mR/mAs?
    a. 0.0041
    b. 0.0044
    c. 0.0045
    d. 0.0050
81. What is the percent of mAs reciprocity?
    a. 6%
    b. 10%
    c. 16%
    d. 21%
82. Based on the answer from question 81, is mAs reciprocity within acceptable parameters?
    a. Yes
    b. No
    c. Not enough information has been given
83. You have been assigned to check the 50 kVp on a particular generator. You found the average kVp for this unit is 55 kVp. What conclusions can you make about this generator at 50 kVp?
    a. The 50 kVp setting is accurate.
    b. The 50 kVp setting is inaccurate.
    c. The information provided is not adequate.
84. The focal spot on an x-ray tube has been determined to have an actual focal spot of 1.0 millimeter, is this within accepted limits?
    a. Yes
    b. No
    c. Not enough information has been given

Questions 85 to 88 pertain to the information presented below.

General Information	Exposure Time	Test Results
Single-phase generator	1/5 second	23 dots
Test tool used: Spinning top	1/10 second	15 dots
Last calibration: 6-25-97	1/20 second	6 dots
Last service call: 5-30-99	1/30 second	2 dots

85. What conclusion can be made about the 1/5 second time station?
    a. the exposure time is too long
    b. the exposure time is too short
    c. the exposure time is accurate
86. What conclusion can be made about the 1/30 second time station?
    a. the exposure time is too long
    b. the exposure time is too short
    c. the exposure time is accurate

87. What conclusion can be made about the 1/10 second time station?
    a. The exposure time is too long.
    b. The exposure time is too short.
    c. The exposure time is accurate.
88. What conclusion can be made about the 1/20 second time station?
    a. The exposure time is too long.
    b. The exposure time is too short.
    c. The exposure time is accurate.

Questions 89 to 95 pertain to the information presented below.

General Information	Exposure Time	Test Results
Three-phase generator	1/5 second	75° arc
Test tool used: Mechanized spin top	1/10 second	39° arc
Last calibration: 6-25-97	1/20 second	22° arc
Last service call: 5-30-99	1/30 second	9° arc

89. What conclusion can be made about the 1/20 second time station?
    a. The exposure time is too long.
    b. The exposure time is too short.
    c. The exposure time is accurate.
90. What conclusion can be made about the 1/30 second time station?
    a. The exposure time is too long.
    b. The exposure time is too short.
    c. The exposure time is accurate.
91. What conclusion can be made about the 1/5 second time station?
    a. The exposure time is too long.
    b. The exposure time is too short.
    c. The exposure time is accurate.
92. What conclusion can be made about 1/10 second time station?
    a. The exposure time is too long.
    b. The exposure time is too short.
    c. The exposure time is accurate.
93. Based on the information in question 92, which of the following statements is correct?
    a. The film would be correctly exposed.
    b. The film would be overexposed.
    c. The film would be underexposed.
94. Based on the information in question 89, which of the following statements is correct?
    a. The film would be correctly exposed.
    b. The film would be overexposed.
    c. The film would be underexposed.

95. Based on the information in question 91, which of the following statements is correct?
  a. The film would be correctly exposed.
  b. The film would be overexposed.
  c. The film would be underexposed.
96. An x-ray tube has stated focal spot sizes of 0.8 and 1.2 millimeters. Focal spot test determined that the actual focal spots were 1.0 and 2.0 millimeters. Are both focal spots within acceptable parameters?
  a. Yes
  b. No
  c. Not enough information has been given
97. Which of the statements is correct?
  a. Digital timers may be used only with single-phase x-ray equipment.
  b. Digital timers may be used only with three-phase x-ray equipment.
  c. Digital timers may be used only with high frequency x-ray equipment.
  d. Digital timers may be used with all types of x-ray equipment.
98. Which of the following statements would be correct about positive beam limitation?
  a. At a 36-inch SID, the light field should be within ± 1.0 inches.
  b. At a 36-inch SID, the light field should be within ± 1.2 inches.
  c. At a 40-inch SID, the light field should be within ± 1.0 inches.
  d. At a 40-inch SID, the light field should be within ± 1.2 inches.

Questions 99 to 100 pertain to the mR/mAs output data below.

mA	Time	mAs	kVp	1st Exposure	2nd Exposure	3rd Exposure	4th Exposure	Average	mR/mAs
50	.80	40	80	222	222	223	223	222.5	
100	.40	40	80	226	225	225	225	225.25	
200	.20	40	80	232	231	231	232	231.5	
400	.10	40	80	238	238	239	240	238.75	
500	.080	40	80	232	232	231	230	231.25	

99. What is the mR/mAs ratio for the 50 mA station?
  a. 5.56
  b. 5.63
  c. 5.66
  d. 5.78
100. What is the mR/mAs ratio for the 500 mA station?
  a. 5.56
  b. 5.63
  c. 5.66
  d. 5.78

101. What are the acceptance parameters for fluoroscopic kVp?
    a. ±2%
    b. ±3%
    c. ±4%
    d. ±5%

102. It was determined that the maximum fluoroscopic rate for a particular fluoroscopic unit was 6 R/min. What conclusions can you make about the fluoroscopic rate?
    a. The fluoroscopic rate was within acceptable limits.
    b. The fluoroscopic rate was outside of acceptable limits.
    c. There is not enough information given to make an assessment.

103. Fluoroscopic mA linearity should be within _____ of the set mA.
    a. 0.05
    b. 0.1
    c. 0.15
    d. 0.2

104. In general standard fluoroscopic exposure rates should be between
    a. 0.5 to 1 R/min.
    b. 1 to 3 R/min.
    c. 4 to 6 R/min.
    d. 7 to 10 R/min.

105. Fluoroscopic beam limitation should be no greater than
    a. 2%.
    b. 3%.
    c. 4%.
    d. 5%.

106. The standard fluoroscopic exposure level for an image intensifier in the 6-inch mode without a grid was found to be 0.7 mC/kg/min. Is this acceptable?
    a. Yes
    b. No
    c. There is not enough information given

107. Which of the following statements is correct?
    a. The typical mA used for fluoroscopic procedures is 200 to 500.
    b. The typical mA used for fluoroscopic procedures is 5 to 10.
    c. The typical mA used for fluoroscopic procedures is 1 to 3.
    d. The typical mA used for fluoroscopic procedures is 0.5 to 1.

108. When the image intensifier is in the automatic mode, what are the acceptance parameters for maximum fluoroscopic exposure rate?
    a. <2.6 mC/kg/min
    b. 2.7 to 3.0 mC/kg/min
    c. 3.0 to 3.4 mC/kg/min
    d. >3.4 mC/kg/min

109. The standard fluoroscopic exposure level for an image intensifier in the 9-inch mode without a grid was found to be 0.5 mC/kg/min. Is this acceptable?

    a. Yes

    b. No

    c. There is not enough information given

110. The maximum fluoroscopic rate in the automatic mode for an image intensifier was found to be 2.8 mC/kg/min. What conclusions can you make about the fluoroscopic rate?

    a. The fluoroscopic rate was within acceptable limits.

    b. The fluoroscopic rate was outside of acceptable limits.

    c. There is not enough information given to make an assessment.

111. Fluoroscopic QC tests are performed

    a. annually.

    b. monthly.

    c. quarterly.

    d. semiannually.

112. The maximum fluoroscopic rate in the manual mode for an image intensifier was found to be 5 R/min. What conclusions can you make about the fluoroscopic rate?

    a. The fluoroscopic rate was within acceptable limits.

    b. The fluoroscopic rate was outside of acceptable limits.

    c. There is not enough information given to make an assessment.

113. When the image intensifier is in the manual mode, what are the acceptance parameters for maximum fluoroscopic exposure rate?

    a. <1.4 mC/kg/min

    b. 1.5 to 2.0 mC/kg/min

    c. 2.0 to 2.2 mC/kg/min

    d. >2.2 mC/kg/min

114. Fluoroscopic resolution should be checked on which of the following?

    a. Spot film device

    b. TV

    c. Both a and b

    d. Neither a nor b

115. The standard fluoroscopic exposure level for an image intensifier in the 9-inch mode without a grid was found to be 1 mC/kg/min. Is this acceptable?

    a. Yes

    b. No

    c. There is not enough information given

116. The operating level for phantom image background optical density should be at least

    a. 1.0.

    b. 1.2.

    c. 1.4.

    d. 1.6.

117. The CV of variation for breast exposure and AEC reproducibility should be

    a. <0.02.

    b. <0.03.

    c. <0.04.

    d. <0.05.

118. Which of the following factors affects the x-ray emission spectrum?

    1. Added filtration

    2. Anode angle

    3. Voltage waveform

    4. Source-to-image distance

    a. 1 and 3 only

    b. 2 and 4 only

    c. 1, 2, and 3 only

    d. 1, 2, 3, and 4

119. Mammographic kVp should be accurate to within _____ of the set kVp.

    a. ±1%

    b. ±3%

    c. ±5%

    d. ±7%

120. Base-plus-fog is measured on

    a. any blank area of the film.

    b. a high density step.

    c. a medium density step.

    d. a low density step.

121. Which of the following statements is correct?

    a. The room temperature for film should be maintained between 50° and 70°F.

    b. The room temperature for film should be maintained between 40° and 60°F.

    c. The room temperature for film should be maintained between 30° and 50°F.

    d. The room temperature for film is not a critical issue in mammography.

122. In mammography which of the following determines focal spot size?

    1. Anode angle

    2. Filament size

    3. Filament shape

    4. Distance between the anode and cathode

    a. 1 and 3 only

    b. 2 and 4 only

    c. 1, 2, and 3 only

    d. 1, 2, 3, and 4

123. Which of the following statements is correct?

    a. Film should be stored in an area free of temperature extremes.

    b. Film should be stored in an area free of any potential exposure to x-radiation.

   c. Film should be stored in an area free of temperature and humidity extremes.
   d. Film should be stored in an area free of temperature and humidity extremes and any potential exposure to x-radiation.
124. A processed image that has a milky appearance is the result of improper
   1. developing.
   2. fixing.
   3. washing.
   a. 1 and 2 only
   b. 1 and 3 only
   c. 2 and 3 only
   d. 1, 2, and 3
125. In mammography at 25 kVp the HVL should be
   a. 0.2 mm Al.
   b. 0.25 mm Al.
   c. 0.3 mm Al.
   d. 0.5 mm Al.
126. The repeat rate for breast imaging should not exceed
   a. 2%.
   b. 3%.
   c. 4%.
   d. 5%.
127. The interaction of an incident electron and an inner shell orbital electron results in the production of
   a. Bremsstrahlung radiation.
   b. characteristic radiation.
   c. Compton scatter.
   d. Rayliegh radiation.
128. As atomic number of the target material decreases there is a shift in the
   a. continuous portion of the x-ray emission spectrum to the left.
   b. continuous portion of the x-ray emission spectrum to the right.
   c. discrete portion of the x-ray emission spectrum to the left.
   d. discrete portion of the x-ray emission spectrum to the right.
129. Which of the following determines when a repeat analysis for breast imaging is done?
   a. Number of examinations
   b. Number of exposures
   c. Number of films
   d. Number of patients
130. The interaction of an incident electron with the nucleus of the atom results in the production of
   a. Bremsstrahlung radiation.
   b. characteristic radiation.
   c. Compton scatter.
   d. Rayliegh radiation.

131. As SID increases there is
    a. a decrease in quantity.
    b. an increase in quantity.
    c. no change in quantity.
    d. none of the above.

132. Which of the following statements is true?
    a. As filtration is added there is an increase in quality and quantity.
    b. As filtration is added there is a decrease in quality and quantity.
    c. As filtration is removed there is a decrease in quality and quantity.
    d. As filtration is removed there is an increase in quality and a decrease in quantity.

133. The use of low kVp in mammography results in
    a. a decrease in quality and quantity.
    b. an increase in quality and quantity.
    c. a decrease in quality and an increase in quantity.
    d. an increase in quantity and a decrease in quality.

134. The probability of detecting a new cancer when a cancer exists is called
    a. positive biopsy rate.
    b. positive predictive value.
    c. sensitivity.
    d. specificity.

135. The CV for kVp reproducibility should be
    a. ≤0.02.
    b. ≤0.03.
    c. ≤0.04.
    d. ≤0.05.

136. The percentage of all known biopsies as a result of positive screening is called the
    a. positive biopsy rate.
    b. positive predictive value.
    c. sensitivity.
    d. specificity.

137. The cancer detection rate is based on how patients examined by mammography?
    a. 250
    b. 500
    c. 1000
    d. 1500

138. MQSA requires that the x-ray field size does not extend beyond any edge of the image receptor more than
    a. 1% of the SID.
    b. 2% of the SID.
    c. 3% of the SID.
    d. 4% of the SID.

139. The probability of a normal mammogram report when no cancer exists is called the
    a. positive biopsy rate.
    b. positive predictive value.
    c. sensitivity.
    d. specificity.

140. How does SID affect beam quality and quantity?
    a. There is a decrease.
    b. There is an increase.
    c. There is no change.

ANSWERS TO THE PRACTICE EXAMINATION

1.	d	31.	c	61.	c
2.	b	32.	b	62.	b
3.	a	33.	c	63.	d
4.	c	34.	a	64.	d
5.	c	35.	a	65.	b
6.	a	36.	a	66.	c
7.	d	37.	d	67.	a
8.	b	38.	b	68.	c
9.	c	39.	c	69.	d
10.	b	40.	c	70.	a
11.	c	41.	d	71.	b
12.	c	42.	a	72.	a
13.	b	43.	a	73.	b
14.	d	44.	b	74.	d
15.	a	45.	d	75.	b
16.	c	46.	c	76.	b
17.	b	47.	a	77.	b
18.	b	48.	b	78.	d
19.	a	49.	a	79.	a
20.	c	50.	d	80.	c
21.	d	51.	c	81.	b
22.	d	52.	c	82.	a
23.	b	53.	c	83.	b
24.	c	54.	c	84.	c
25.	b	55.	d	85.	c
26.	d	56.	a	86.	b
27.	c	57.	b	87.	a
28.	c	58.	c	88.	c
29.	a	59.	b	89.	a
30.	b	60.	a	90.	b

91.	c	108.	a	125.	b
92.	a	109.	a	126.	d
93.	b	110.	b	127.	b
94.	b	111.	d	128.	c
95.	a	112.	a	129.	d
96.	a	113.	a	130.	a
97.	d	114.	c	131.	c
98.	d	115.	b	132.	d
99.	a	116.	b	133.	a
100.	d	117.	d	134.	c
101.	d	118.	a	135.	a
102.	c	119.	c	136.	a
103.	b	120.	a	137.	c
104.	b	121.	a	138.	b
105.	b	122.	d	139.	d
106.	a	123.	d	140.	c
107.	c	124.	c		

Index

Note: Page numbers followed by *f* refer to figures. Page numbers followed by *t* refer to tables.

V

Viewbox. *See* Illuminator

X

X-rays
Bremsstrahlung, 152
characteristic, 152

ISBN 0-8385-8249-4

9 780838 582497